UNDERSTANDING THE BEHAVIORAL HEALTHCARE CRISIS

UNDERSTANDING THE BEHAVIORAL HEALTHCARE CRISIS

The Promise of Integrated Care and Diagnostic Reform

Edited by
Nicholas A. Cummings
and William T. O'Donohue

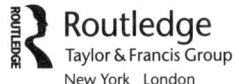
Routledge
Taylor & Francis Group
New York London

Routledge
Taylor & Francis Group
270 Madison Avenue
New York, NY 10016

Routledge
Taylor & Francis Group
27 Church Road
Hove, East Sussex BN3 2FA

© 2011 by Taylor and Francis Group, LLC
Routledge is an imprint of Taylor & Francis Group, an Informa business

Printed in the United States of America on acid-free paper
10 9 8 7 6 5 4 3 2 1

International Standard Book Number: 978-0-415-87643-8 (Hardback)

For permission to photocopy or use material electronically from this work, please access www.copyright.com (http://www.copyright.com/) or contact the Copyright Clearance Center, Inc. (CCC), 222 Rosewood Drive, Danvers, MA 01923, 978-750-8400. CCC is a not-for-profit organization that provides licenses and registration for a variety of users. For organizations that have been granted a photocopy license by the CCC, a separate system of payment has been arranged.

Trademark Notice: Product or corporate names may be trademarks or registered trademarks, and are used only for identification and explanation without intent to infringe.

Library of Congress Cataloging-in-Publication Data

Understanding the behavioral healthcare crisis : the promise of integrated care and
   diagnostic reform / edited by Nicholas Cummings, William T. O'Donohue.
       p. cm.
    Summary: "The Promise of Integrated Healthcare is a necessary book, edited and contributed to by a great variety of authors from academia, government, and industry. The book takes a bold look at what reforms are needed in healthcare and provides reforms and specific recommendations. Some of the serious concerns about the healthcare system that Cummings, O'Donohue, and contributors address include access problems, safety problems, costs problems, the uninsured, and problems with efficacy. When students, practitioners, researchers, and policy makers finish reading this book they will have not just a greater idea of what problems still exist in healthcare, but, more importantly, a clearer idea of how to tackle them and provide much-needed reform"-- Provided by publisher.
    Includes bibliographical references and index.
    ISBN 978-0-415-87643-8 (hardback : acid-free paper)
   1. Mental health services--United States. 2. Health care reform--United States. 3. Integrated delivery of health care--United States. I. Cummings, Nicholas A. II. O'Donohue, William T. III. Title.

RA790.6.U53 2011
362.196'89--dc22   2010043255

Visit the Taylor & Francis Web site at
http://www.taylorandfrancis.com

and the Routledge Web site at
http://www.routledgementalhealth.com

Contents

Acknowledgment ix
Editors xi
Contributors xiii

Chapter 1 Where We Are, How We Got There, and Where We Need to Go: The Promise of Integrated Care 1

Nicholas A. Cummings and William T. O'Donohue

Chapter 2 Our 50-Minute Hour in the Nanosecond Era. The Need for a Third "E" in Behavioral Healthcare: Efficiency 19

Nicholas A. Cummings

Chapter 3 The Financial Dimension of Integrated Behavioral/Primary Care 33

Nicholas A. Cummings, William T. O'Donohue, and Janet L. Cummings

Chapter 4 Mental Health Informatics 59

Bruce Lubotsky Levin and Ardis Hanson

Chapter 5 E-health and Telehealth 83

Anthony Papa and Crissa Draper

Chapter 6 Can Prescribing Psychologists Assist in Providing More Cost-Effective, Quality Mental Healthcare? 129

Morgan T. Sammons

Chapter 7 Diagnostic System Innovations 149

Thomas A. Widiger

Chapter 8	Evidence-Based Treatment 171
	E. David Klonsky
Chapter 9	The Quality Improvement Agenda in Behavioral Healthcare Reform: Using Science to Reduce Error 203
	William O'Donohue, Rachel Ammirati, and Scott O. Lilienfeld
Chapter 10	The Behavioral Health Medical Home 227
	Dennis Freeman
Chapter 11	Reforms in Professional Education 257
	Ronald R. O'Donnell
Chapter 12	Pay for Performance and Other Innovations in Reimbursement for Behavioral Care Services 279
	Nicholas A. Cummings and Janet L. Cummings
Chapter 13	Trends in Behavioral Healthcare for an Aging America 299
	Christina Garrison-Diehn, Clair Rummel, Casey Catlin, and Jane E. Fisher
Chapter 14	Failure to Serve: The Use of Medications as a First-Line Treatment and Misuse in Behavioral Interventions 327
	John L. Caccavale With the collaboration of Joseph Casciani, Nicholas A. Cummings, Jerry Morris, Dave Reinhardt, Howard Rubin, Elle Walker, and Jack G. Wiggins
Chapter 15	Reforms in Treating Children and Families 343
	James H. Bray

Chapter 16 Reforms for Ethnic Minorities and Women ... 367

Lorraine Benuto and Brian D. Leany

Chapter 17 Wellness and Prevention: Key Elements in the Next Generation of Behavioral Health Service Delivery Systems 395

Monica E. Oss

Chapter 18 Reforms in Veteran and Military Behavioral Health................................. 417

R. Blake Chaffee

Chapter 19 Biofeedback 441

James Lawrence Thomas

Index 469

Acknowledgment

The editors express their deep appreciation to Linda Goddard, executive assistant, Cummings Foundation for Behavioral Health, for her extensive administrative skills, which rendered possible the timely completion of this book.

Editors

Nicholas A. Cummings, PhD, ScD, is distinguished professor at the University of Nevada, Reno, and the Arizona State University, Tempe, Arizona, as well as president of the Cummings Foundation for Behavioral Health and the board chair of the Nicholas & Dorothy Cummings Foundation. He is a past president of the American Psychological Association as well as the American Psychological Foundation. He founded the first professional school with the four campuses of the California School of Professional Psychology, now Alliant University, as well as over two dozen other organizations, including the National Association of Schools and Programs in Professional Psychology (NASPP), the National Academies of Practice in Washington, DC, and American Biodyne, the only national healthcare delivery system (25 million enrollees in 50 states) that was psychology driven. He is an innovator who has anticipated by decades the future morphology of psychology and has formed successful organizations to demonstrate to the disbelieving profession what was to come. He conducted his first project in colocated integrated behavioral/primary care in 1963, fully 46 years before it became APA policy.

William T. O'Donohue, PhD, is a full professor of psychology at the University of Nevada, Reno, and held the Cummings Chair in Mental Healthcare Delivery in that university for several years. He holds a master's degree in philosophy and is honorary associate professor in the Department of Philosophy at UNR. He served for 10 years as the CEO of CareIntegra and also as the executive director of the Cummings Foundation for Behavioral Health; he continues as a senior fellow of the latter. On a part-time basis, he conducts a successful forensic practice as well as a unique consulting practice in integrated behavioral/primary care. Working with CareIntegra, he has conducted pioneering integrated behavioral care projects in the military, TriCare, the Veterans Administration, and a number of national healthcare companies.

Contributors

Rachel Ammirati
Emory University
Atlanta, Georgia

Lorraine Benuto
University of Nevada
Reno, Nevada

James H. Bray
Department of Family &
 Community Medicine
Baylor College of Medicine
Houston, Texas

John L. Caccavale
National Alliance of
 Professional Psychology
 Providers

Casey Catlin
University of Nevada
Reno, Nevada

R. Blake Chaffee
TriWest Healthcare Alliance
Phoenix, Arizona

Janet L. Cummings
Doctor of Behavioral Health
 Program
Arizona State University
Tempe, Arizona
University of Nevada
Reno, Nevada

Crissa Draper
University of Nevada
Reno, Nevada

Jane E. Fisher
University of Nevada
Reno, Nevada

Dennis Freeman
Cherokee Health Systems
Knoxville, Tennessee

Christina Garrison-Diehn
University of Nevada
Reno, Nevada

Ardis Hanson
Louis de la Parte Florida
 Mental Health Institute
University of South Florida
Tampa, Florida

E. David Klonsky
Department of Psychology
University of British
 Columbia
Vancouver, British Columbia

Brian D. Leany
University of Nevada
Reno, Nevada

Scott O. Lilienfeld
Emory University
Atlanta, Georgia

Bruce Lubotsky Levin
University of South Florida
Tampa, Florida

Ronald R. O'Donnell
Arizona State University
Tempe, Arizona

Monica E. Oss
OPEN MINDS
Gettysburg, Pennsylvania

Anthony Papa
University of Nevada
Reno, Nevada

Clair Rummel
University of Nevada
Reno, Nevada

Morgan T. Sammons
California School of
   Professional Psychology
San Francisco, California

James Lawrence Thomas
The Brain Clinic
Penthouse, New York

Thomas A. Widiger
Department of Psychology
University of Kentucky
Lexington, Kentucky

One

Where We Are, How We Got There, and Where We Need to Go
The Promise of Integrated Care

NICHOLAS A. CUMMINGS AND WILLIAM T. O'DONOHUE

INTRODUCTION

This is the era of health reform, stemming from a growing consensus that our broken system cannot be sustained. The percent of the overall budget for mental health has steadily declined in the past decade, and when one deducts the expenditures for psychotropic medications, all behavior care services comprise but 1.5% of the total national health budget (see Chapter 3 in this volume). The American Psychological Association, which is usually reticent about the dismal statistic on psychotherapy, was unusually candid in a recent article by its president. In the past decade, when healthcare went from 7% to almost 16% of the gross domestic product, mental healthcare remained static at 1% even though the number of people receiving services has increased dramatically, according to Goodheart (2010). She goes on to state that, in 2006, 51% of mental health spending was for prescription drugs, 16% went to hospitalization, and the 33% remaining had to cover all other mental health services.

The recent health reform legislation (Patient Protection and Affordable Care Act, the PPACA, signed by President Obama in 2010) has recognized the importance of behavioral health as an integral part of primary care; to accomplish this, the legislation places the primary care physician in charge of behavioral health delivery (Dentzer, 2010). This reflects the urgency and the need, but while legislation can enable, it cannot deliver. It is the responsibility of behavioral health to transcend its current moribund status and thus to deliver effective, quality services.

This volume addresses the advances needed in the various areas of behavioral practice and will demonstrate how the profession can meet the challenge of twenty-first century health reform through the development of effective, evidence-based interventions. This would restore the rightful place of behavioral health, which is to be integrated into the mainstream healthcare system. In the broadest sense, this is what is proffered as integration, with the specific term "integrated behavioral/primary care" regarded as a prime specific, as delineated in Chapter 3.

AN HISTORICAL PERSPECTIVE OF WHERE WE ARE AND HOW WE GOT THERE

In the early 1980s, the profession of psychiatry began to "remedicalize"—its own word for a process in which it was to transition from a psychotherapeutic treatment profession to one it considered akin to medicine. It abandoned psychotherapy, which it disdainfully began to call "talk therapy," in favor of becoming what it named "biological psychiatry." The concept intended that, by prescribing medication instead of dispensing talk therapy, it would be treating actual diseases, as did fellow physicians and that psychiatry would be more aligned with medicine than with psychologists, who had matured as a profession and were rapidly becoming the nation's premier psychotherapists. By becoming "biological," psychiatrists would eliminate competition from psychologists, who could not prescribe medications. The psychiatric residencies quickly fell in line and the transition was made in a remarkably short time.

As of this writing, five outcomes of this transition, affecting all mental health, have evolved:

1. It is very rare to find a psychiatrist under age 50 who performs psychotherapy.
2. Psychiatry has become an "every fifteen minute per patient pill-pushing" profession (Shorter, 2010) that has proven unattractive to medical school graduates,

who shun it as a career. Consequently, there is now a severe shortage of psychiatrists.
3. As a result, 85% of all psychotropic drugs are prescribed by nonpsychiatric physicians, an inevitable outcome predicted by psychiatrist Stan Lesse 30 years ago (Lesse, 1982).
4. The vast majority of mental health simply involves the dispensing of psychotropic medications, with the portion attributable to behavioral care services continuing to shrink.
5. Masters-level psychotherapists have proliferated to where they far outnumber doctoral psychologists. They are now licensed to practice and, because their fees are somewhat less than doctoral-level providers, they now perform the vast majority of psychotherapy in America. Because psychiatrists by virtue of being physicians are in control of most mental health delivery systems, they supervise these masters-level providers in the "talk therapy" they long ago gave up and in which they are no longer experts. This is tantamount to a kiwi (a nonflier) telling pilots how to fly.

And where has psychology been all this time? In its fervent antagonism to psychiatry and in rejecting what it calls the "medical model," it isolated itself from mainstream healthcare by creating its own separate silo. The result has been lack of access, the stigmatization of the referral for psychotherapy, and a decline in funding.

The consequences to mental health and its failure to deliver appropriate behavioral care parallel and are largely reflected in the challenges of the peculiar diagnostic system in which mental health operates.

THE ADVENT OF THE DSMS

The *Diagnostic and Statistical Manual of Mental Disorders,* known as the DSM for short, has undergone a series of iterations in the past half century since the inception of DSM-I by the American Psychiatric Association. Known colloquially as the "psychiatric bible," the DSM is the basis for reimbursement for services, as well as the nomenclature by which government and other agencies collect statistical data on aspects of mental and emotional illness. In spite of its seemingly universal utility, however, it has been fraught with controversy.

As the DSM proceeds through it iterations, the controversy has increased steadily, now reaching a crescendo as DSM-5 is being constructed.

Few if any mental health professionals practicing today are aware of the void—perhaps better described as incredulity—that existed in diagnosis prior to the inception of the first DSM. The senior author entered independent practice in California in 1948, and, thumbing through some early diagnostic reports, he has gleaned a host of archaically colorful diagnoses that were once accepted parlance. Consider, for example, "anal retentive personality culminating in rectal cancer." Or you can look at the one that would be resented by every woman living today: "Exaggerated female masochism, conveniently married to a sadistic husband who emotionally rewards her by becoming contrite after each occasion in which he beats her." Often these atavistic diagnoses sought to embody causation, such as "severe Oedipus complex inevitably resulting in homosexuality and effeminate personality." And, of course, there is the all-time favorite: "idiot, imbecile grade."

But the now apparent absurdity of these diagnoses reflects the fact that each school of psychiatry (and even of then budding clinical psychology) used its own esoteric nomenclature. In other words, diagnoses were parochial, with each "system" disdaining all others. That this was hampering interchangeability among various practitioners soon became subordinate to the greater problems that emerged in the 1950s as government and private insurance began to reimburse for psychiatric services. (Note that reimbursement of psychiatric services preceded that for services of psychologists by a number of years, with that for social workers and counselors occurring much later.) Diagnoses were so diverse that third-party payers struggled to discern which claims were proper and deserving of reimbursement. Hence, the real impetus for DSM-I was unmistakably economic, which in time propelled the DSMs to the status of the "psychiatric bible." As will be seen in this chapter, the economic purpose remains the dominant impetus inasmuch as the so-called diagnostic categories are collections of symptoms rather than reflective of actual disease processes such as those seen in medical diagnoses.

DSM-I: The Age of Anxiety

Published in 1952, the first *Diagnostic and Statistical Manual* was a relatively succinct and simple document compared to its most recent successors. In the 1950s and 1960s, when psychiatry was still under the influence of the European scientific tradition, there was a striving for reasonably accurate diagnoses, as is reflected in the DSM-I (Shorter, 2010). Furthermore, it must be remembered—although this has grown more difficult to believe in the last two decades—that psychiatry was still psychotherapeutically oriented. "Psychoneurosis" was the principal diagnosis of the day; simply put, if a patient complained of being "blue, uneasy or generally jumpy, 'nerves' was the common diagnosis. To the psychotherapeutically oriented psychiatrists of the day, 'psychoneurosis' was the equivalent of nerves" (Shorter, 2010, p. 1). There was no reason to delineate this further as both doctor and patient understood "a case of nerves."

The DSM-I was not widely used in the 1950s, which is in stark contrast with the must-use dictum since the 1980s. It did serve as a centrifugal force, bringing order to the jumble of nomenclatures proffered by what Cummings long ago named the "psychoreligions"; its simplicity seemed to satisfy widely divergent practitioners. The notion that anxiety was central to all psychological conditions was the subject of two widely read and generally highly regarded books: Rollo May's *The Meaning of Anxiety* (1950, 1977) and Hans Selye's *The Stressors of Life* (1956). In coining the term "stressor," Selye added a word universally invoked by the psychiatrists (and psychologists) of the era (Menand, 2010).

The then universal nature of anxiety fostered the fiasco of the earliest psychotropic medications. In 1955 meprobamate (brand name: Miltown) was introduced as an anxiolytic, and soon it became the largest selling drug in American history up to that time (Tone, 2009). In fact, it accounted for one third of *all* prescriptions written by American physicians. It is startling to recall that Miltown was soon eclipsed by two other anxiolytics, Librium and Valium, introduced in 1960 and 1963, respectively. By 1968, Valium had become the most prescribed drug in the Western world, and the stock of its manufacturer, Hoffman-La Roche, increased in 1972 to $73,000 a share (Tone, 2009).

Although these anxiolytics were marketed with FDA approval as nonaddictive, the senior author became alarmed as a legion of patients heavily addicted to them filled his practice. His early attempts to sound an alarm were dismissed by both the manufacturer and the FDA, but by 1980 the research findings were incontrovertible and the FDA issued a warning label that stated the stressors of everyday life did not warrant the use of such addictive drugs (Tone, 2009). The crash of Librium and Valium sales marked the end of the age of anxiety, but there was an overlap with the introduction of DSM-II.

DSM-II: A Freudian Document, While Personality Disorders Become Mental Illnesses

The second DSM was more complicated and it was based on the concepts put forth by Sigmund Freud and Adolph Meyer, who came to the United States from Switzerland (Menand, 2010). Thus, it was based on psychoanalytic theory and reflected Meyer's emphasis on the importance of the patients, which led to the inclusion of a vast population that had not been regarded as patients.

Introduced in 1968 as Axis II disorders, the second DSM gave character disorders the new name of personality disorders and made them the province of psychiatric treatment. Heretofore, they had been termed "characterological" because they were regarded as enduring aspects of one's character and impervious to treatment. Changing the designation added millions of new potential paying patients to psychiatry. This forever cluttered the field with intractable but demanding patients to the detriment of non-Axis II patients and the severely mentally ill, both of whom do not bombard the besieged system with vociferous demands for immediate attention. But this was only the beginning of the now self-serving expansion of psychiatric diagnoses into aspects of daily life's vicissitudes.

DSM-III: The End of Psychopathology

The publication of the third iteration in 1980 brought about a sea change and destined mental health to the eventual crisis in which it now finds itself. With energetic and engaging psychiatrist Robert Spitzer at the helm, it was determined to solve the problem of reliability so that every practitioner given a set of symptoms would come out with the same diagnosis. In so doing, however, the manual did not address an even greater problem—namely, validity, which is defined as the correspondence of symptoms to organic conditions (Greenberg, 2010; Menand, 2010). In other words, rather than diseases, the end result was a set of "conditions" or "syndromes" characterized by common signs and symptoms, often loosely woven, whose existence and validity could not be proven.

Spitzer did accomplish one positive reform: He purged the DSM of the Freudian jargon that had plagued the previous editions. In so doing, however, he threw out the baby with the bathwater. Psychoanalysis at least struggled to base itself on psychopathology, but Spitzer inadvertently omitted psychopathology altogether. Consider where medicine would be without pathophysiology: exactly where it was over a century ago, dealing with conditions and syndromes instead of diseases. This is perhaps why psychiatry has paradoxically gone overboard in espousing psychopharmacology before there are any known diseases to medicate (Kirsch, 2010).

DSM-III also began the process of "diagnoses by ballot," which would be perfected in the next iteration.

DSM-IV-TR: Our Beleaguered Present

The current manual comprises a series of controversial and arbitrary positions that have not abated but rather have increased the questionable aspects of its predecessors. It has led to a groundswell of dissatisfaction both inside and outside the profession.

The series of signs and symptoms that comprise our syndromes do not lead to behavioral interventions, but rather facilitate the prescribing of medication. For every symptom there is ostensibly a medication. Although a large inventory of psychotropic drugs exists, there are a limited number of different classes, and often the same medication is prescribed for a variety of different conditions. For example, antidepressants may be prescribed not only for depression, but also for obsessive-compulsive disorder, smoking cessation, job dissatisfaction, low libido, premature ejaculation, eating disorders, or whatever else the diverse but questionable literature might suggest. Furthermore, depression and anxiety are not diagnoses any more than a headache or fever is, as these are symptoms manifest a disease. Because the current DSM constitutes a reshuffling of the same old symptoms to describe conditions with new names, this has led critics like Menand (2010) to ask whether we may not be dealing with one yet unnamed disease (mental illness) with a variety of stages and symptoms.

The current DSM has resulted in an "age of depression" similar to the "age of anxiety" with its Miltown, Librium, and Valium in the 1960s; predictions are that we may be heading for the same train wreck with antidepressants (Greenberg, 2010; Herzberg, 2008; Kirsch, 2010). In addressing the propensity to prescribe antidepressants for the problems of daily living, Wakefield and Horwitz (2007) deplore the elimination of sadness as a normal and informative emotion in daily living. These same authors have summarized the growing body of literature revealing the relative ineffectiveness of antidepressants, especially in milder cases, along with the startling array of harmful side effects, many of them quite serious.

Psychiatrist Carlat (2010) concludes flatly that psychotherapy might be more effective and less physically destructive than antidepressants, a position espoused by an ever increasing number of critics both inside and outside the profession.

DIAGNOSIS BY CONSENSUS: POLITICAL CORRECTNESS TRUMPS SCIENCE

In the absence of validity and with the emphasis on reliability alone, determination of diagnoses by consensus is perhaps as good as it can get. Yet this is far from scientific validity, bringing with it flaws that expose the consensus to well-meaning biases that reflect the social and political pressures and beliefs of the time more than actual diseases that require specific medicating. To be sure, the consensus may be the result of extensive clinical experience, but the ability to diagnose a fever gives only limited knowledge. For a skilled clinician the symptoms throwing out the baby with the Freudian bathwater in DSM-II we also deemphasized both the taking of an extensive history and the administration of psychological tests. The brief paper-and-pencil tests of depression currently in use are so obvious that many Axis II patients manipulate them to obtain the desired diagnosis.

Let us look at some of the more flagrantly unscientific nomenclature decisions that have been the result of beliefs or biases:

- In formulating the DSM-III, there was considerable horse-trading. The younger biology-oriented psychiatrists were able to dump some of the previous designations that sounded like psychoanalytic mumbo-jumbo with the new term "major depression," but as a concession to their older colleagues, they coined the addition of "dysthymia." To the psychoanalysts, this sounded like their beloved neurotic depression, and the compromise was effected. With the further addition to bipolar of a separate unipolar, there were now enough categories for nearly everyone to qualify as a depressive, even though all these "depressions" may be the same condition with slightly varying symptom formations (Shorter, 2010). Anxiety was finished, and the stage was set for almost everyone to be eligible for treatment with antidepressants. Greenberg (2010) goes

so far as to accuse the profession of a conspiracy to render sadness a chemical disease of the brain.
- With consensus and compromise determining diagnoses, it was inevitable that political correctness would insert itself in the process. In 1973 the American Psychiatric Association removed homosexuality as a treatable aberrant condition. The question here is not the right or wrong of that decision, but rather the way it was done. A political firestorm had been created by gay activist groups within psychiatry; intense opposition to normalizing homosexuality came from a few outspoken psychiatrists who were demonized and even threatened, rather than scientifically refuted. Psychiatry's house of delegates sidestepped the conflict by putting the matter to a vote of the membership, marking the first time in the history of healthcare that a diagnosis or lack of a diagnosis was decided by popular vote rather than by scientific evidence. Similarly, a number of issues sensitive to feminist and other activists were determined politically (see Wright & Cummings, 2005, for a comprehensive delineation), underscoring the arbitrary nature of psychiatric diagnoses. Could this occur with the diagnosis of pancreatic cancer or any other such diagnosis based on scientific validity? Yet this trend continues, one example being the disturbing effort to normalize pedophilia in the forthcoming DSM-5.
- The preliminary history of the proposed DSM-5 emphasizes the arbitrariness of psychiatric diagnoses. After the task force deliberated secretly for almost 3 years, enough disturbing information as to what was being contemplated was leaked, creating a storm of controversy. As a result, the completion was delayed for 2 years while widespread comment is being solicited. At best, the outcome can only be consensus, not validity.
- Since new diagnoses are based on votes of committees rather than neurobiological testing, the field is vulnerable to "disease mongering" (Carlat, 2010), which is defined as the expansion of "disease" definitions in order to pump up the market for medication treatment. We have already seen how the inclusion of personality disorders more than doubled our potential patients. The redefinition in 2001 of ADHD quadrupled the number of children eligible to be so diagnosed (Cummings

& Wiggins, 2001), while the increase in the number of categories of depression eliminated sadness and rendered almost anyone eligible to be prescribed antidepressants. At times the expansion became colorful, with seasonal affective disorder (SAD) to be followed by reverse seasonal affective disorder (reverse SAD) for people who are depressed in the summer rather than in winter. When the existence of multiple personality disorder was questioned (Lilienfeld & Lynn, 2003), the category was deftly changed to dissociative identity disorder, and in so doing it was quietly expanded. These are just a few examples of why some critics have referred to this process as *psychosprawl* (Carlat, 2010).

PSYCHOLOGY VERSUS PSYCHIATRY

Although a very limited number of psychologists have participated in the formulations of the DSMs, psychology has had no meaningful role in the treatment/reimbursement "bible" that has shaped behavioral services and brought the field to its current beleaguered pseudobiological status. In contrast to the arbitrary nature of psychiatric diagnoses, psychology has been remarkably active and successful in transitioning psychotherapy into evidence-based treatments (Chambless et al., 1996, 1998; see also Fisher & O'Donohue, 2006) and the development of effective cognitive behavioral therapy (O'Donohue, Fisher, & Hayes, 2003). Unfortunately, referrals for psychotherapy have declined; at the present time, up to 80% of patients are prescribed psychotropic medication, principally antidepressants, by their physicians in lieu of even a referral to psychotherapy. In response, psychology has advanced two initiatives:

- A legislative campaign by the American Psychological Association would permit specially trained psychologists to prescribe psychotropic medication. To date, psychiatric opposition, along with some internal dissension among psychologists, has stalled the effort. As of this writing, only two states (Louisiana and New Mexico) and the U.S. military have enacted prescribing psychologists (see Chapter 6, this volume).
- The first integrated primary/behavioral care project was launched by the senior author at Kaiser Permanente in 1963, and there have been a number of such projects, particularly in the military, with the

emerging research being unequivocally positive (for an historical perspective, see Cummings, Cummings, & Johnson, 1997). After half a century of insisting on a separate silo for mental health, in 2009 the American Psychological Association espoused the integration of behavioral health into mainstream healthcare. Undoubtedly, the impetus was the fact that mainstream healthcare was moving in that direction, and the enactment of the PPACA catapulted the heretofore most resistant sectors of mental health in that direction. Seemingly, at this juncture everyone has become an expert in integrated behavioral health, among them even some of its recently most vocal opponents.

Among many psychologists there is dissatisfaction with the American Psychological Association's tepid address of two important issues. The first is the scientists who see the accreditation process in clinical psychology as too lacking in scientific training. They broke away almost 20 years ago, forming what is now known as the Association for Psychological Science (APS) that is challenging the APA's accreditation process (Richard McFall, personal communication, 2009). The second is at the opposite end of the spectrum. Composed of practitioners who believe the APA is neglecting practice issues, the National Alliance of Professional Psychology Providers (NAPPP) is undertaking the tasks that it believes the APA is neglecting. A recently adopted white paper (NAPPP, 2010) challenges the common medical practice of prescribing medication as the first treatment, and the organization will launch a national education campaign on the merits of medication versus psychotherapy.

WHITHER THE DSM-5?

Although the committee formulating the forthcoming edition of the DSM is still seeking feedback, there are some changes that seem destined for approval. For one thing, the roman numerals of the previous DSMs have been officially abandoned in favor of the title "DSM-5." More substantive likely changes are not expected to fix the problems of the previous DSM series and may even create some new ones. Certainly, it will accelerate the previous drive to make more of the spectrum of everyday behaviors into disorders. For example, schizophrenia is extended to a larger population with the new "psychosis risk syndrome."

To be certain, one of the deficiencies of the recent DSMs has been the lack of pathophysiology, such as the thought disorder that is present in various forms and is discernible and even measurable in persons who one day *might* become overtly psychotic. This knowledge was useful in times of stress for the appropriate choice of brief, nonpsychologically invasive behavioral interventions that brought rapid stabilization and avoided any pending psychosis and did not need medication. The new disorder, however, would bypass behavioral intervention and render a large, essentially benign population eligible for psychotropic medication.

Perhaps one positive proposal will turn the jumble of children's developmental syndromes into one: autism spectrum disorders, with the elimination of the confusing Asperger's syndrome, stuck amid autism and childhood schizophrenia. However, the decades-long trend will doubtlessly be accelerated, turning everyday behavior into diseases, apprehension into anxiety, sadness into depression, sexual promiscuity into addiction, and boyishness into hyperactivity.

WHERE WE NEED TO GO

Behavioral healthcare often is unjustifiably ignored in discussions of or plans for healthcare reform because of the naïve view that, because substance abuse and mental health expenditures are only 5% or less of the current budget, they deserve an amount of attention commensurate with this. This is naïve because it ignores all the behavioral health pathways to medical utilization. It has been documented that lifestyle problems like obesity, lack of exercise, poor nutrition, poor social support, and stress can be experienced as somatic complaints (Cummings, O'Donohue, & Naylor, 2005). In addition, often undiagnosed DSM disorders are motivating medical presentations; these can range from major depression, to substance abuse, to anxiety disorders, to personality disorders, to bereavement, and so on (Cucciarre & O'Donohue, 2005).

Many physicians are either not interested in or not skilled at appropriately diagnosing these; when they are missed in the medical setting, these can involve patients with expensive courses of physical diagnosis (e.g., CAT scans) or treatment (medications, hospitalizations). In addition, it is well known now that behavioral health pathways, such as poor treatment compliance with chronic medical conditions such as diabetes, asthma, coronary heart disease, emphysema, and arthritis, result in large expenditures in healthcare (Cummings et al., 2005). There is no "treatment compliance" pill or surgery. Thus, it is our contention that, in order to be effective, health reform must consider the explicit current cost as well as the somewhat hidden costs of behavioral health problems.

There has been recognition of the role of behavioral health pathways in medical expenditures, but the recognition has been partial and has not resulted in a systematic approach to addressing these problems. The disease management industry has arisen in the past few decades and has grown to a multibillion dollar enterprise. These interventions have certainly done some good, but sometimes they are often ill conceived (i.e., the patient requires only information needed to remedy the problem or there is no comorbidity such as substance abuse or depression) and thus the results of this industry are ultimately disappointing. It is not enough to parachute single chronic disease interventions into a medical setting (e.g., a depression program) while ignoring anxiety, obesity, substance abuse, and so on.

Moreover, in many individual cases, psychoeducational information or e-mails or a few phone calls from a case manager are not sufficient. These may be sufficient in a population management approach to handle the "low hanging fruit" inexpensively, but sometimes a more intensive clinical approach is needed due to the severity or the complexity of the case. The disease management industry has been slow to recognize this due to their business and clinical model.

In addition, there have been some initial efforts at integrated care, but these have been sporadic, although increasing in recent years. The American Psychological Association has begun to recognize the importance of integrated care as can be seen in the recent presidential addresses of Ron Levant and James Bray. Recently, much faith has been placed on a cousin of integrated care—the medical home (see Chapter 10, this volume). However, the interest in this greatly outstrips the data of its effectiveness. This needs to be seen more as a promise as opposed to a demonstrated improvement.

There is a very limited movement toward electronic health records as compared to what is happening on the medical side. The evidence-based practice movement is gaining momentum in some corners although there is less effect on actual practice than many would like (see Chapter 8, this volume). There is little systematic acceptance of a quality improvement prospective in behavioral health, although again this movement is much stronger inside physical medicine (see Chapter 9, this volume). It is noteworthy that President Obama recently appointed Dr. Daniel Berwick as head of the CMS (Centers for Medicare & Medicaid Services)—we applaud this appointment and expect that a new paradigm may emerge because Dr. Berwick has been one of the most important voices in the quality improvement movement in medicine.

New payment schemes such as pay for performance are also not widely practiced (see Chapter 12, this volume), but these are necessary in order to address the incentives to overtreat in fee-for-service or undertreat in capitation contracts. There is certainly a lot of unexplored territory regarding behavioral healthcare reform, and very little territory has been systematically evaluated so that a reasonable understanding of possible reform effectiveness can be reached.

The responses to the behavioral healthcare crisis have been overly piecemeal and uncoordinated: Some reforms only concentrate on electronic health records while ignoring reforms in practice such as integrated care, evidence-based care, and telehealth or while ignoring possible improvements in payment mechanisms. We propose that one of the first things needed is a comprehensive coordinated strategic plan for behavioral health reform. The healthcare system needs to be seen as a system, and systematic reforms are needed. This plan should look at all facets—not just a favored one—and should be based on the best research evidence as well as a reasonable vision of what might work in reforming the system as a whole.

It is a regrettable state of affairs that our professional organizations such as the American Psychological Association have not already put together such a blueprint for an effective, safe, affordable, accessible, consumer-centric healthcare delivery system. But one has to recognize that some of the guild issues protect existing turf, even if it is eroding away, rather than take the risk of innovating into a brighter future. We hope this book may educate professionals so that they can serve as visionaries for reform. But, again, we think reform should not continue in the unorganized, unsystematic, incomplete, and myopic way it has to date. We think such a blueprint with appropriate input from all stakeholders ought to be the immediate goal.

This book can outline the broad parameters of this reform, though. The reform needs to embrace a quality improvement perspective and technology: The goal should not be "good enough" but rather "exceeding stakeholders expectations," constantly improving the value proposition, and in general embracing constant innovations to produce improvements always. No doubt there is plenty of room for improvement. Integrated care that breaks the silos of healthcare also certainly needs to be a part of any reformed system. It simply does not make sense to treat the "body" and "mind" as separate entities.

Electronic health records (EHRs) need to replace the inefficient, incomplete, illegible, and difficult to access paper records. David Merritt (2007) has appropriately edited and entitled a book, *Paper Kills;* the unfortunate state of affairs is that paper will keep killing for many years to come in behavioral health. These EHRs need to have tools that can help both the clinician and the patient, such as hot buttons to literature reviews of treatment effectiveness and hot buttons to basic information and questions about the diagnosis. This is doable *now:* The VA system and the military both have first-rate EHRs, but innovation in the civilian sector is limping along.

The evidence-based treatment movement also needs more traction: We cannot afford to spend money on ineffective treatments that strike the fancy of some therapist following what Cummings has appropriately called a "psychoreligion." Spending money this way is what the Japanese call *muda*—waste. The field needs reforms in professional training, but the tenure system in academia and the lack of contact of many academics with real-world healthcare problems makes this process too slow also. Our field and healthcare consumers need to be able to train professionals to better handle chronic diseases such as diabetes. We also need to train professionals to better meet the needs of the elderly (see Chapter 13, this volume). Too few properly trained professionals and too few training programs recognize the demographic shift that has occurred and will continue to occur. It is still much more likely for a professional to be trained in child psychology than gerontology.

We hope that professionals can recognize these problems without being risk averse. Change involves risk and the unknown. It is psychologically tempting to be nostalgic: to wish that we could make the future more like the past. But this is not possible in healthcare. Technological changes in medicine, demographic shifts—particularly an increase in life span—and the rise of behavioral patterns that result in large medical expenses (obesity, sedentary lifestyle, smoking, stressful lives) simply make this impossible.

In an important book, Cutler (2004) states the problem simply: The reason why 1950s medicine was relatively inexpensive was because it was also relatively ineffective. Since the 1950s, we have had significant improvements in a wide variety of treatments (from antibiotics to oncological treatments, from cognitive behavior therapy for anxiety disorders to antipsychotics) and a wide variety of diagnoses (from CAT scans to MRIs), but these improved effectiveness comes at a cost. Future technological improvements will also have a price tag.

Thus, we hope the future will first recognize that the future will require a consistent commitment to innovation in the entire healthcare system and that this innovation needs to be deep and thoroughgoing as well as systematic and coordinated. This requires an education into the problems and a comprehensive response to these problems. We hope this book will at least be a beginning to this all-important venture.

REFERENCES

Carlat, D. J. (2010). *Unhinged: The trouble with psychiatry—A doctor's revelations about a profession in crisis.* New York, NY: Free Press.

Chambless, D. L., Baker, M. J., Baucom, D. H., Beutler, L., Calhoun, K. S., Crits-Christoph, P.,...Woody, S. A. (1998). Update on empirically validated therapies, II. *Clinical Psychologist, 51,* 3–16.

Chambless, D. L., Sanderson, W. C., Shoham, V., Bennett Johnson, S., Pope, K. S., Crits-Christoph, P.,...McCurry, S. (1996). An update on empirically validated therapies. *Clinical Psychologist, 49,* 5–18.

Cucciare, M., & O'Donohue, W. (2005). Pathways to medical utilization. *Journal of Clinical Psychology in Medical Settings 12*(2), 185–197.

Cummings, N. A., Cummings, J. L., & Johnson, J. N. (Eds.). (1997). *Behavioral health in primary care: A guide for clinical integration.* Madison, CT: Psychosocial Press.

Cummings, N. A., O'Donohue, W. T., & Naylor, E. (2005). *Psychological approaches to chronic disease management.* Reno, NV: Context Press.

Cummings, N. A., & Wiggins, J. G. (2001). A collaborative primary care/behavioral health model for the use of psychotropic medication with children and adolescents. *Issues in Interdisciplinary Care, 3*(2), 121–128.

Cutler, P. (2004). Problem solving in clinical medicine. New York, NY: Basic Books.

Dentzer, S. (2010). Reinventing primary care: A task that is far "too important to fail." *Health Affairs, 29*(5), 757–759.

Fisher, J. E., & O'Donohue, W. T. (2006). *Practitioner's guide to evidence-based psychotherapy.* New York, NY: Springer.

Goodheart, C. D. (2010). The economic realities of health care. *Monitor on Psychology, 45*(6), 5.

Greenberg, G. (2010). *Manufacturing depression.* New York, NY: Simon & Schuster.

Herzberg, D. (2008). *Happy pills in America.* Baltimore, MD: John Hopkins University Press.

Kirsch, I. (2010). *The emperor's new drugs.* New York, NY: Basic Books.

Lesse, S. (1982). The uncertain future of clinical psychiatry. *American Journal of Psychotherapy, 37*(2), 306–312.

Lilienfeld, S. O., & Lynn, S. J. (2003). Dissociation identity disorder: Multiple personalities, multiple controversies. In S. O. Lilienfield, S. J. Lynn (Eds.), *Science and pseudoscience in clinical psychology.* New York, NY: Guilford (109–142).

May, R. (1950). *The meaning of anxiety.* New York, NY: Norton.

May, R. (1977). *The meaning of anxiety* (Rev. Ed.). New York, NY: Norton.

Menand, L. (2010). Can psychiatry be a science? *New Yorker,* March 10: http://www.newyorker.com/arts/critics/2010/03/01/100301crat_atlargw_menand?curr

Merrit, D. (2007). Paper kills. Washington, DC: Center for Health Transformation.

NAPPP (National Alliance of Professional Psychology Providers). (2010). Failure to serve: A white paper on the use of medications as a first line treatment and misuse in behavioral interventions. www.NAPPP.org

O'Donohue, W. T., Fisher, J. E., & Hayes, S. C. (2003). *Cognitive behavior therapy.* Hoboken, NJ: Wiley.

Selye, H. (1956). *The stressors of life.* New York, NY: McGraw–Hill.

Shorter, E. (2010). Why psychiatry needs therapy. *Wall Street Journal (WSJ.com).* http://online.wsj.com/article_email/SB10001424052748704188104570081370022760116

Tone, A. (2009). *The age of anxiety: A history of America's turbulent affair with tranquilizers.* New York, NY: Basic Books.

Wakefield, J., & Horwitz, A. (2007). *The loss of sadness.* New Brunswick, NJ: Rutgers University Press.

Wright, R. H., & Cummings, N. A. (Eds.). (2005). *Destructive trends in mental health: The well-intentioned path to harm.* New York, NY: Routledge.

Two

Our 50-Minute Hour in the Nanosecond Era. The Need for a Third "E" in Behavioral Healthcare *Efficiency**

NICHOLAS A. CUMMINGS

INTRODUCTION

A nanosecond is not just a minuscule fraction of a second, but a seemingly incomprehensible one billionth of a second. Similarly, a nanometer is one billionth of a meter. These are not abstract oddities, but rather measures that science employs daily. In medicine, for example, some intricate parts of the inner ear are so small as to be invisible in a traditional laboratory microscope, and they are measured in nanometers that require a whole new technology. This does not mean that medicine has abandoned the traditional measures that remain useful, but it has moved on to address the advances of modern technology and biological discoveries. In the meantime, our 50-minute hour remains five sixths of an hour, and constitutes an antiquated limitation on the practice of psychotherapy.

This is not to demean in any way the continued usefulness of the 50-minute hour, but rather is meant to address the failure of the profession to move beyond it. Just because medicine now possesses handheld imaging technology has not led to the

---

* Portions of this chapter were presented by the author as part of the 32nd Annual Grimes Lecture (2010), La Salle University, Philadelphia, PA.

abandonment of the stethoscope, which still is useful in the physical examination of the patient. The 50-minute hour will always have its place.

EFFICACY, EFFECTIVENESS, AND NOW EFFICIENCY

After over 60 years of contentious debate (see Reisman, 1976, and Chapter 8 in this volume), there is now a decided emphasis on evidence-based care (APA, 2006), while the integration of science and practice continues to be a bumpy road (Norcross, Klonsky, & Tropiano, 2008). Working closely with the American Psychological Association, Chambless and Honlon (1998) defined empirically supported therapies as *efficacy,* the first of our three *E*s. Psychology is still far behind medicine in the role of evidence-based therapies (EBTs) and, while the debate continues, David Barlow (2004) has introduced *effectiveness,* the second of our three *E*s. Many therapies that seem to work well in the laboratory fall short in expectation when used in practice. Research requires pure cases, while the reality of our patients is that of comorbidity. So while we are still absorbing the first of these two *E*s, why am I introducing *efficiency,* the final and perhaps the most controversial of our three *E*s?

The answer is straightforward: The most widely debated word in healthcare today is cost. How is cost managed in the face of its relentless escalation? Beginning with psychoanalysis, with its years of couch therapy, to today's psychotherapy that grinds out a succession of 50-minute hours in offices apart from mainstream healthcare, psychology has not been heralded by the public for its efficiency. In the meantime, medicine has introduced remarkable advances reflecting all three of our *E*s.

Consider as just one example the stent, an innovation that has reduced dramatically the number of invasive cardiac procedures that not only are expensive in their application, but also are followed by a lengthy and costly recovery period. With the stent, the patient walks out of the hospital the next day. Do we have that kind of dramatic efficiency in behavioral healthcare? Perhaps not to the drama of our example, but there is a surprising array of efficiencies that are not only overlooked, but also often shunned by practitioners who remain mired in the 50-minute hour. Ten highly diverse examples have been chosen from several times that number as representative of uniqueness, unexpectedness, and effectiveness. Let us look at these, keeping in mind that this is only a sampling.

EXAMPLE 1: JUMP DOOR FEVER: EFFICIENCY IN AN UNEXPECTED PLACE

In the early part of World War II, William Menninger was appointed chief psychiatrist for the military. This renowned psychotherapist who, with his brother, Karl, had founded the famed Menninger Clinic in Topeka, Kansas, took advantage of the open-ended opportunities accorded him by the War Powers Act of 1942. He created the School of Military Neuropsychiatry on Long Island, New York, where he assembled the greatest names in our profession for that time and sent hand-picked contingencies of "students" from the military. I was one of these.

The problem we faced was that 40% of the casualties among paratroopers were what was called "jump door fever," or freezing at the jump door and being unable to jump in the cadence required to prevent bunching in midair or overshooting the target. There was a superstition among paratroopers based on a misunderstanding of the law of averages that showed that the average life of a trooper was three combat jumps (two for an officer). From this stemmed the belief that was actually facilitating: Facing a jump, the soldier could say that this was not his or her fourth, but the first (second, third) combat jump and it was not time to die. But eventually came the fourth jump and some paratroopers would freeze at the jump door. The jump sergeant would count to 10 and then, with his boot in the back of the paratrooper, he would push him out the door. Invariably this resulted in a number 10 panic attack, causing the trooper to forget all training, and death most often followed.

Frieda Fromm-Reichmann was placed in charge of solving this problem. She reasoned that although love is the strongest human emotion, it involves time, while rage is immediate. She taught us to talk the paratrooper within 10 seconds into jumping voluntarily by so enraging him that he jumped in defiance. After receiving this training, I never lost another trooper to jump door fever. It was also the briefest psychotherapy I have ever done.

Today, psychotherapists are not called upon to save a paratrooper's life, but there are many effective, efficient interventions that skillfully employ rage in the service of the ego (for descriptions of these, see Cummings, 2006; Cummings, 2000; Cummings & Sayama, 1995). They are swift and lasting, but how many psychotherapists today receive any such training? Because we are paid by the hour (as are plumbers), efficiency is counterproductive, and the 50-minute hour can unfortunately be extended to weeks beyond what otherwise would have been efficient. There is a lesson to be learned: Efficiency is often the product of necessity.

EXAMPLE 2: FRIEDA FROMM-REICHMANN ON ACCESSING A PSYCHOTIC PATIENT'S INNER WORLD IN 5 MINUTES

Currently, psychotic patients are treated almost exclusively with antipsychotic medications with varying degrees of effectiveness. I lived through the "bedlam" era of state mental hospitals preceding the introduction of Thorazine, and there is no arguing that antipsychotic medication has improved the treatment of schizophrenia, so much so that it has all but eliminated behavioral interventions. Thorazine was heralded at first as not only effective but also efficient; however, we have now become aware of the consequent limitations of such exclusivity. These medications do not eliminate delusions and hallucinations; rather, they make them tolerable for the patient, but only as long as the patient continues the medication regimen. However, the long-term side effects are such that patients do go off their meds, the psychosis once again becomes flagrant, and the patient is rehospitalized; this costly, inefficient sequence can be repeated over and over. What is missing is behavioral management of the psychosis, but few psychotherapists today receive training in or are even aware of effective behavioral interventions in schizophrenia.

This was not always so and need not be so now. In the premedication era, chronic hospitalized schizophrenics were frequently seen smearing their own feces. Instead of avoiding them and allowing the attendants to clean up the mess, Fromm-Reichmann (1950) would sit down on the floor with the patient. Putting on surgical gloves, several pairs of which she kept in the pocket of her smock, she would join the patient in the smearing process for about 5 minutes. Then, removing and discarding the soiled gloves, she would pull out a candy bar from the supply in the other pocket and offer it to the patient, saying, "Here is a candy bar. You might like it better than the feces. If you do, when I come by again tomorrow morning you will not be smearing your feces and I will have another candy bar for you." Invariably the patient was clean and awaiting the candy bar the next day: simple, effective, efficient.

The author observed this a number of times as he accompanied Dr. Fromm-Reichmann on her rounds. She taught him that just because a schizophrenic talks to us does not mean that he has let us into his world. Only after we have joined the patient's delusion are we admitted and accepted into that world—a necessary forerunner to effective behavioral intervention with psychosis. Joining the patient's delusion is still a remarkably effective treatment, but it is now known to only a few highly skilled psychotherapists. This does not, of course, involve fecal smearing, but techniques for joining various delusions abound (Cummings & Sayama, 1995). As Fromm-Reichmann poignantly demonstrated in only 5 minutes, there is "psychic" room in a delusion for one person, and once the therapist has joined the delusion, it is abandoned and the patient becomes accessible to continued behavioral interventions that markedly improve efficiency in the management of psychosis.

EXAMPLE 3: THE IMMEDIATE GROUP ILLUSTRATIVE OF THE THREE *E*S

Returning now to the present era, providing coverage 9:00 to 5:00 so that patients in crisis can be seen immediately is a costly and inefficient procedure that is regarded by almost all treatment centers as inevitable. Some clinics have one person covering the entire day, while others rotate therapists so that a different one is present from hour to hour. The inefficiency occurs when an hour or more pass without a need to be seen, with nary a complaint from psychotherapists, who are delighted to have a free hour. An effective and efficient response is to tell all patients who call wanting to be seen immediately to come in at 3:00 p.m. Called the "immediate group," the patients are not directly told that they will be seen in a group, but this is implied in the statement, "Three in the afternoon is when we see all patients who need to be seen today." This is repeated when the group assembles.

The characteristics of the immediate group are that (a) one professional sees all the patients in a group session, (b) by meeting from 3:00 to 5:00 there is still time to hospitalize a patient who might need it, and (c) attendees are encouraged to return the next day should they wish to. Thus, along with persons who are there initially, the group is composed of those who are returning the second, third, or fourth time. Rarely will there be a fifth time.

Because of its uniqueness, for 12 months patients who called were randomly assigned to the traditional mode or the immediate group. The results showed the superiority of the immediate group over the traditional method in that only 23% of those attending the immediate group needed to go on to specialty mental healthcare versus 68% for the traditional method. As for total sessions required (crisis plus follow-up), those in the immediate group averaged 2.8 sessions, while those assigned to the traditional mode averaged 7.4 (crisis plus follow-up). The cost of the immediate group was less than one third that of the traditional approach and it was made a standard procedure at Kaiser Permanente in San Francisco in 1967 (Cummings & Cummings, 2000). Its resurrection and use in behavioral care today would constitute a decided efficiency reform.

EXAMPLE 4. HIGH UTILIZERS OF MEDICAL CARE: SAVING DOLLARS WHILE PROVIDING APPROPRIATE PATIENT CARE

There probably does not exist a more effective cost-saving intervention than the outreach program for high utilizers of medicine and surgery, and its inclusion in health reform has the potential to save billions of dollars. At the same time, patients who are translating psychological problems and emotional distress into physical symptoms (called "somatization") will finally receive the appropriate treatment through behavioral services. Widely known for over 40 years, somatization is the subject of over 300 published studies and is definitively explicated in an edited volume by Cummings, O'Donohue, and Ferguson (2002).

Beginning as early as the mid-1960s, it was shown that (1) 60–70% of patients seen in primary care are either somatizing or have psychological issues that are impeding the healing of an actual physical disease, and (2) outreaching these patients, who comprise 15% of the highest utilizers of medicine and surgery, and providing appropriate behavioral services reduce overall health costs (after deducting for the cost of the behavioral care) by a total of as much as 40%. So impressed was the National Institute of Mental Health (NIMH) that it named the methodology *medical cost offset*. The outreach is performed by a trained professional who does not challenge the patient's belief that all of his or her problems are physical. In other words, care is taken not to label the patient a somatizer. A simple message that invites the patient to come in on the basis that "someone who is having as many medical issues as you are having must surely be upset about it" is sufficient to bring in 11 or 12% of this 15%—enough to result in the substantial medical cost offset. Other techniques have been developed to gain the cooperation of most of the remaining 3–4%.

Medical utilization is a straightforward tabulation of all physician and physician ancillary visits, laboratory and imaging tests, emergency room or drop-in clinic visits, hospital days, and issued prescriptions. The creation of a weighted system for the various services did not in any way improve the accuracy of the findings and was abandoned as too cumbersome. The reason usually given why this method is not universally deployed is that, in all but a few health systems, the medical and psychiatric databases are not compatible and the appropriate tracking of behavioral interventions on medicine and surgery is not possible. True health reform would necessitate revamping of databases into combined electronic systems so that ultimate health reform would make medical cost offset routine.

EXAMPLE 5. OUTPATIENT THERAPY IN THE HOSPITAL EMERGENCY ROOM: TURNING A PARADOX INTO EFFICIENT TREATMENT

Emotionally distressed patients often find themselves in the emergency room (ER) late at night, usually brought there by family or referred from evening drop-in medical care. The sequence of events usually follows a pattern. A psychiatrist is called, and over the telephone the patient is admitted to a mental care ward overnight; the psychiatrist arrives to evaluate the patient the following morning. By that time, the patient has spent the night in a "crazy place" and decides, "I must be sicker than I thought," and reflects that conclusion. So the patient is invariably admitted to the psychiatric unit or hospital as a psychiatric patient. Psychiatric hospitalization is costly, upward of thousands of dollars a day. Over a period of 10 years with 25 million covered lives, a simple efficiency was shown to reduce inpatient psychiatric admissions by as much as 90%.

The prepaid behavioral health plan known as American Biodyne sent to the ER a specially trained behavioral provider (a specially trained clinical psychologist or social worker), who began *outpatient* treatment right there during the night. If the patient responded to outpatient intervention, the same as she or he might have done in a psychotherapy outpatient office during the day, the patient was sent home with family and seen in the outpatient behavioral care service the next morning, and for several consecutive mornings if this was deemed appropriate. This needed reform enabled American Biodyne to reduce its inpatient psychiatric costs by over 90%, offset by far less expensive (thus efficient) but also effective brief outpatient care (Cummings, Cummings, & Johnson, 1997).

EXAMPLE 6. ENFORCED HOMEWORK: EXTENDING TREATMENT AND DENYING TREATMENT ARE ALL IN A DAY'S EFFICIENT WORK

Psychotherapists are always looking for a way to bridge the treatment hiatus between sessions, and they usually resort to scheduling two and even three sessions a week. Ever since Budman and Gurman (1988) showed this could be done effectively by assigning homework after each session, this practice has become somewhat common among psychotherapists. However, these same psychotherapists did not enforce the homework, and because it was often not performed by the patient, homework was deemed ineffective and was largely abandoned. On the other hand, it was demonstrated that when the homework is enforced, it extends the effect of the session through the following week to the next session: It is as if the patient had been in continuous treatment (Cummings & Cummings, 2000; Cummings & Sayama, 1995).

At the outset, the patient agrees that if the weekly homework is not completed, the patient forfeits that session in which the homework is due. This may sound harsh, but seldom does the therapist have to send the patient home more than once, while the positive effect of a session extended throughout the week is rewarding. Progress accelerates and the therapy is concluded in a much shorter time than if the sessions had not been extended through enforced homework. In my years of supervising all kinds of psychotherapists, it is apparent that "therapeutic drift" characterizes much of psychotherapy. Little is happening, but since a third-party payer is footing the bill, there is drift session after session in the rationalization that something therapeutic one day may happen. Efficient therapy requires the therapist to be firm and stop coddling the patient, who really is not helpless. Health reform must include a shift from well-meaning, but misguided, compassion by subjecting practitioners to retraining so that they will be more like doctors than nuns.

EXAMPLE 7: THE HALLWAY HANDOFF

Primary care physicians (PCPs) are scheduled with just 15 minutes for each patient to be seen. This is a far cry from the 50-minute hour. Much to the consternation of most practitioners, the behavioral care provider also works effectively within a 15-minute session when responding to what is called in integrated behavioral/primary care the "hallway handoff." Michael Balint (1957) stated presciently half a century ago that "physicians must become more like psychologists while psychologists must become more like physicians." The integration of behavioral health into primary care is perhaps the most ambitious and rewarding of all possible healthcare reforms, spanning physical as well as mental health and eliminating the two silos of physical health versus mental health.

For far too long, mental health has been outside mainstream healthcare, resulting in the inefficiencies of higher cost of physical health and inadequate delivery of behavioral health. The primary care physician learned long ago that patients referred for psychotherapy are angered that their doctor thinks that "it's all in my head." Even if they do not express their anger, they feel the stigma that still exists, and only a few ever go across town to the private psychotherapist's office. With the newer psychotropic medications now available, the PCP finds it simpler to write out a prescription, even though antidepressants have been shown to be relatively ineffective with all but the most serious depressions. Consequently, 80–85% of mental health counseling, as well as medication, is dispensed by the PCP, making primary care the de facto mental health system of America.

In the hallway handoff, a PCP who is confronted with a patient whose problems are largely emotional or psychological only needs to walk the patient down the hall to the behavioral care provider (BCP) colocated within the primary care setting. In such instances and because behavioral care is a seamless part of the healthcare setting, up to 90% of patients in the hallway handoff will engage in the process and follow through with psychotherapy.

Much has been written about the hallway handoff (e.g., Blount, 1997; Cummings, O'Donohue, & Cummings, 2009; Cummings, O'Donohue, Hayes, & Follette, 2001; Robinson & Reiter, 2007) and integrated primary behavioral care, but as it is more feasibly accomplished in staff model delivery systems, it is found mostly in the military, TriCare, the Veterans Administration, and only a few notable private sector systems such as Cherokee Health Service. It is lagging behind in the giant managed care companies that are proceeding with caution as they wait to see how the recently enacted health reform is implemented.

But it needs to become an integral part of health reform. A bureaucratic impairment to implementing the hallway handoff is a well-meaning restriction intended to save money. Found in a number of health plans and in Medicare and Medicaid, it forbids a mental health appointment on the same day as a medical appointment. Once in place, such outdated restrictions assume a life of their own, but in health reform they have no meaningful place.

EXAMPLE 8. WHEN IRISH NUNS ARE SMILING: THE PSYCHOTHERAPY OFFICE GOES INTERNATIONAL

There are times when a mini-epidemic overloads a delivery system and the answer may lie outside the office or even outside the delivery of psychotherapy. Such a problem arose in one prepaid healthcare setting when several dozen women all presented with a variety of vague complaints, ranging from tension headaches to depression. A happenstance observation by one of the receptionists revealed that all these mothers had something in common: All had a son in a Catholic grammar or junior high school. Targeted inquiries were made by their various psychotherapists; these revealed that all their sons had lost interest in school and were doing poorly. Further inquiry also revealed that the local Catholic school district had exchanged nuns with a contingent of Irish nuns; the American nuns were spending the year teaching in Ireland while the Irish nuns were doing the same here in this community.

It was time for the author to meet with the monsignor who was superintendent of Catholic instruction. Over lunch he stated he had already incurred dissatisfaction, and he conjectured that the strictness and authoritarian attitude of the nuns from Ireland were not suitable for the American classroom. It was near the end of the semester and the monsignor arranged to return the nuns to Ireland as the American nuns returned to the community.

Overnight, the "epidemic" of anxious, depressed mothers abated. Had the emphasis remained in the treatment room, undoubtedly the clinic overload would have persisted the entire year. This is only one of many instances in which efficiency requires stepping aside from the traditional role and outside the office of the psychotherapist. Yes, this is far from the 50-minute hour for which we were trained.

EXAMPLE 9. YOUR OFFICE ON THE FREEWAY AND IN THE SUBWAY: IT DOES MORE THAN JUST SAVE RENT

There are many behavioral interventions that, by the very nature of the conditions they address, cannot be conducted in the treatment room or office. Among these are behavioral interventions in phobias that require desensitization in the environment in which they occur. For example, for a house-bound agoraphobic, they must start in the home where the patient is emotionally imprisoned. Desensitization of a freeway phobia catapults the therapist into a car on the freeway; likewise, phobias for subways, bridges, tunnels, elevators, and such put the behavioral provider in these very locations.

Phobic patients learn to avoid situations that invoke a panic attack, but this is not always possible. Their lives become more and more restricted, so often they inadvertently find themselves in a situation that precipitates a panic attack. Their symptoms resemble a heart attack, and because these phobic persons are loathe to admit their phobias due to their fear of being found to be really mentally ill, they say nothing and allow themselves to be rushed to the emergency room. Desensitization in the field (i.e., in natural phobic environments) is remarkably effective, but this, too, takes the psychotherapist out of the office as well as changes the entire concept of the 50-minute hour.

The author and his colleagues conduct these programs with as many as six to eight phobic patients in a group, except for freeway and other such phobias that would comfortably limit three and no more than four patients in an auto. In order to avoid leaving their offices, psychotherapists often misquote ethics code restrictions on dual relationships. However, desensitization in the field can be and is conducted in a professional and ethical manner, much to the benefit of the patient and the healthcare system.

EXAMPLE 10. A THERAPEUTIC SHOPPING "SPREE": THIS ONE IS LONGER THAN THE 50-MINUTE HOUR, BUT EFFICIENT

Chronic schizophrenics can often be helped to make an adjustment to daily living if they can avoid crises that result in their rehospitalization. It is through repeated, yet often avoidable hospitalizations that costs mount in the treatment of this population. A crisis to a schizophrenic is not the same as what most people would think of as a crisis. It can involve just buying a pair of socks or ordering something to eat.

In their childhoods, chronic schizophrenics learned to be intimidated by people without knowing why. Their mannerisms, often peculiar speech patterns, and the fact that they did not grasp things like most children singled them out for ridicule. They developed a shyness and avoidance pattern that followed them into adulthood and even grew in severity. Confronted now with buying a pair of socks, the chronic schizophrenic is fearful in the bustling department store.

While in line approaching the cashier, he or she feels as if everyone is staring at and about to make fun of him or her. The intimidation grows by the minute, and soon the feeling of fright is producing mannerisms in speech, walk, and general demeanor. Other customers notice this behavior and move farther and farther away from the schizophrenic. Adults do not ridicule as do children; they shy away. They become concerned when odd speech mannerisms commence and often the store security detail is called. Misunderstandings escalate and the schizophrenic is whisked off to the hospital, where his or her record of previous hospitalizations results in a speedy admission, often in restraints (medicinal and physical).

Programs in daily living for schizophrenics, conducted in groups, can teach chronic but otherwise stabilized patients to purchase clothes or a meal, ask directions on public transportation, check out a library book, and the myriad day-to-day activities that seem so simple but are terrifying to these patients. The author and his colleagues, who conducted such groups for years, found stores, restaurants, and public transit remarkably understanding when they were informed in advance and their cooperation solicited. Such outings are usually 2 or 3 hours in length, and although this exceeds the 50-minute hour in length, as many as six patients can participate at one time.

The patients who have already let the psychotherapist into their inner world and trust him or her through techniques previously described are emboldened through learning simple everyday behaviors, and the therapist finds it rewarding. In my experience, however, chronic schizophrenics are more willing to work within such a field program than psychotherapists are willing to leave their entrenched offices. In health reform, such effective and efficient programs should become standard, saving tens of millions of healthcare dollars.

SUMMARY AND CONCLUSIONS

The practice of psychotherapy has only recently begun to emphasize the importance of efficacy, or evidence-based treatment (EBT), and it is in the earliest stages of addressing effectiveness (i.e., whether and how well these EBTs work outside the laboratory). It has not yet scratched the surface of efficiency, and competing EBTs are equally adopted in spite of huge variations in length, cost, practicality, and other factors that dictate cost. This deficiency has strong implications for health reform, where cost is of prime importance and behavioral care has shown itself to be among the most, if not the most, inefficient of all healthcare delivery systems.

This chapter has discussed 10 examples out of dozens of efficient behavioral interventions that are illustrative of all three Es: efficacy, effectiveness, and efficiency. All require that we traverse our slavishness to the 50-minute hour, maintaining it when useful, but abandoning it when efficient alternatives exist. Because cost is at the top of the list in discussing health reform, the future—if not the continued existence of behavioral health—is dependent upon our successfully addressing the third E: efficiency.

REFERENCES

APA (American Psychological Association), Presidential Task Force on Evidence Based-Practice. (2006). Evidence-based practice in psychology. *American Psychologist, 61,* 271–285.

Balint, M. (1957). *The doctor, his patient and the illness.* New York, NY: International Universities Press.

Barlow, D. H. (2004). Psychological treatments. *American Psychologist, 59,* 869–878.

Blount, A. (Ed.). (1997). *Integrated primary care: The future of medical and mental health collaboration.* New York, NY: Norton.

Budman, S. M., & Gurman, A. S. (1988). *Theory and practice of brief therapy.* New York, NY: Guilford.

Chambless, D. L., & Honlon, S. D. (1998). Defining empirically supported therapies. *Journal of Consulting and Clinical Psychology, 66,* 7–18.

Cummings, N., & Sayama, M. (1995). *Focused psychotherapy: A casebook of brief, intermittent psychotherapy throughout the life cycle.* New York, NY: Brunner Mazel (now Routledge).

Cummings, N. A. (2006). Resistance as an ally in psychotherapy. In W. O'Donohue, N. A. Cummings, & J. L. Cummings (Eds.), *Clinical strategies on becoming a psychotherapist* (pp. 129–145). New York, NY: Elsevier.

Cummings, N. A., & Cummings, J. L. (2000). *The essence of psychotherapy: Reinventing the art in the era of data.* San Diego, CA: Academic Press.

Cummings, N. A., Cummings, J. L., & Johnson, J. N. (Eds.). (1997). *Behavioral health in primary care: A guide for clinical integration.* Madison, CT: Psychosocial Press.

Cummings, N. A., O'Donohue, W. T., & Cummings, J. L. (2009). The financial dimension of integrated primary care. *Journal of Clinical Psychology in Medical Settings, 1*(2), 11–20.

Cummings, N. A., O'Donohue, W. T., & Ferguson, K. E. (Eds.). (2002). *The impact of medical cost offset on practice and research: Making it work for you.* Vol. 5, Foundation for Behavioral Health: Healthcare Utilization and Cost Series. Reno, NV: Context Press.

Cummings, N. A., O'Donohue, W. T., Hayes, S. C., & Follette, V. (Eds.). (2001). *Integrated behavioral healthcare: Positioning mental health practice with medical/surgical practice.* San Diego, CA: Academic Press.

Fromm-Reichmann, F. (1950). *Principles of intensive psychotherapy.* Chicago, IL: University of Chicago Press.

Norcross, J. C., Klonsky, E. D., & Tropiano, H. L. (2008). The research-practice gap: Clinical scientists and independent practitioners speak. *Clinical Psychologist, 61*(3), 14–17.

Reisman, J. M. (1976). *A history of clinical psychology.* New York, NY: Irvington Press.

Robinson, P. J., & Reiter, J. T. (2007). *Behavioral consultants and primary care: A guide for integrating services.* New York, NY: Springer.

Three

The Financial Dimension of Integrated Behavioral/Primary Care

NICHOLAS A. CUMMINGS, WILLIAM T. O'DONOHUE, AND JANET L. CUMMINGS

> Very few people do anything creative after the age of 35. The reason is that very few people do anything creative before the age of 35.
>
> Joel Hildebrand (2008)

INTRODUCTION

There are two reasons why mental health, now more appropriately termed behavioral healthcare, is declining: (a) a lack of understanding among psychotherapists of healthcare economics, particularly the intricacies of medical cost offset; and (b) our failure as a profession to see the importance of behavioral interventions as an integral part of the healthcare system inasmuch as the nation pays for healthcare, not psychosocial care. In recent years, we have relied on parity legislation, which ostensibly mandates equal importance between physical and mental health, and have spectacularly enacted it in 44 states as of this writing. However, lacking the appreciation that economics always trumps legislation, the profession is startled that the percentage of the mental health portion of the nation's total health budget has declined from 8% before parity legislation to 4.5% (Carnahan, 2002; Forbes, 2004). Economists are well aware of such an untoward relationship, pointing, for example, to rent controls, which invariably result in drastic reductions of available low-cost housing (Sowell, 2003).

This chapter will briefly describe the rapid changes in the economics of healthcare during the past 75 years, including the post-World War II enthusiastic espousal of psychotherapy by the American public. This was followed by a precipitous decline as our outcomes research in behavioral care remained ignorant of financial outcomes, leaving it to the government and managed care to curtail escalating mental health costs arbitrarily. Preceding this drastic economic shift, time-limited (brief) psychotherapy was developing, encouraged by financially sensitive outcomes research.

Unfortunately, psychology fiercely resisted these trends and scoffed at the harbingers that the delivery of behavioral care was about to industrialize and that financial considerations would usurp the decision-making process. At the present time, psychology is on the cusp of becoming part of the healthcare system through integrated behavioral/primary care, renewing the primacy of financial considerations such as return on investment (ROI) and medical cost offset, as well as an urgency that we avoid the mistakes emerging in some flawed implementations of integrated care (Cummings, O'Donohue, & Ferguson, 2003).

A BRIEF HISTORY OF HEALTHCARE ECONOMIC DEVELOPMENTS: 1929–2009

When the Great Depression (1929–1941) engulfed the United States, medicine had come of age, transitioning from an often apprentice-trained profession to accredited medical schools and state laws with licensure governing its practice. Essentially, medicine was all of healthcare, with everything else (e.g., nursing) being ancillary. Before World War II, there were about 200 psychologists in the private practice of psychotherapy scattered about the nation, most of whom were women practicing with a master's degree who saw children. These were tolerated by the 5,000 psychiatrists in existence at the time—most practicing without board certification.

Physicians were far from wealthy in spite of a shortage. They were dedicated, often working long hours because they were determined to see every patient who wanted to be seen; never refusing a house call, even at night; and never remanding an unpaid bill to a collection agency because that was considered unethical and unprofessional. There was no healthcare insurance; few patients could pay in those economically depressed years, and those who could pay would be charged double to make up for the destitute majority. This was the era of "Robin Hood medicine," with tired, overworked, and underpaid physicians looking old by their 50s and dying at an early age.

Patients were grateful and saw doctors only when absolutely necessary; they often paid in kind (bushels of corn, dressed chickens, handyman services, even housecleaning). Physicians continued to treat patients, no matter how large the unpaid bill. Hospitals were all nonprofit, were often religiously affiliated, and held annual charity drives to make up huge shortfalls because they treated everyone in spite of inability to pay. It was the avowed responsibility of religious and charitable groups to see to it that everyone, especially children and the elderly, received at least the minimum in healthcare. Then came prepaid healthcare—very little at first, but once it took hold, the doctor–patient relationship would never be the same.

First on the scene were the so-called "Blues." To create a much needed revenue stream, hospitals organized into an organization named Blue Cross. For those who could afford a monthly premium (small by today's standards), any needed inpatient services were prepaid. In defense, physicians organized into a parallel organization named Blue Shield that prepaid most outpatient services. In the 1930s, the need for prepaid care was so intense that special laws were created for "medical services corporations" that enabled their success by exempting the Blues from the rigorous regulations and large reserves required of full-fledged insurance companies. This special legislation was later used to keep out other forms of prepaid healthcare. It should also be noted that mental healthcare was a stated exclusion.

During World War II, when both goods and labor were in short supply, the government imposed ceiling prices on all commodities and wages. The newly created war industries needed to recruit tens of thousands of workers from the farm belt, whom they would train for such purposes. Unable to use the inducement of higher wages, Henry J. Kaiser, in his shipyards, as well as other industrialists in their aircraft and other war industries, hit upon the option of providing healthcare for workers and their families. Because healthcare was difficult to obtain in rural areas, the inducement worked; hundreds of thousands of farmers, especially from the economically depressed "dust bowl" (Oklahoma, Arkansas, Texas), moved to the industrial North and West. Employer-paid healthcare was born and soon became a standard in the United States.

Amid accusations of "socialized medicine" by both the Blues and the American Medical Association, after World War II Kaiser brought his previously in-house health plan to the general public. Beginning in Northern California, prepaid healthcare purchased by employers or labor unions was based on capitation: Each month, the Permanente Medical Group received a set fee for each enrolled member, in advance; in return, it provided all the care, both outpatient and inpatient, with no further fee or copayment from the patient treated. As the first health maintenance organization (or HMO, even before the name had been coined), Kaiser-Permanente so impressed the federal government in its delivery of quality care at efficient cost that, in the mid-1970s Congress passed the HMO Enabling Act. Heretofore, HMOs had been California and Minnesota phenomena, but soon there were HMOs in all parts of the country; they were the precursors to managed care.

Little noticed by the health professions, in the mid-1980s the U.S. Supreme Court ruled that healthcare was subject to antitrust and restraint of trade laws. This nullified state laws forbidding the corporate practice of medicine. Almost simultaneously, the Congress enacted DRGs (diagnosis-related groups), which defined the maximum number of hospital days for which the federal government would pay for over 400 diagnoses. These two developments made possible and ushered in managed care and the rapid tethering of the spiraling healthcare rate of inflation.

However, because DRGs could not be written for psychiatry, the problem of out-of-control costs for mental health was turned over to the private sector, and managed behavioral health organizations (MBHOs) were created almost overnight. Foreseeing the birth of MBHOs, Cummings (1986; see also Cummings & Fernandez, 1985) created a model whereby practitioners rather than "bean counters" would still determine the course of behavioral care. Called American Biodyne, its tremendous success as a practitioner-driven MBHO was rejected as unnecessary by psychology and psychiatry. Furthermore, these professions ignored the need as well as their responsibility to contain runaway mental health costs (Fox, 2004), and soon the practice lost control of its own destiny. Perpetuating this antibusiness bias and economic illiteracy (Cummings & O'Donohue, 2008), psychotherapists have seen a precipitous decline in their practices and in their incomes. Psychology is now the lowest paid doctoral health profession.

AFTER WORLD WAR II: THE BIRTH OF NONPSYCHIATRIC PSYCHOTHERAPY

General William (Will) Menninger, chief psychiatrist for the U.S. Army during World War II, introduced many innovations, including the effective use of young, specially trained psychologists who rendered immediate behavioral interventions in the battalion aid stations (tent-style movable medical facilities just behind the battlefront). To Menninger, the need for immediate behavioral interventions was necessary to prevent onset of chronic mental states. Thus, he implemented the world's first integration of behavioral health into a primary care setting, a fact that has been lost in history. Nonetheless, this and other mental health innovations were widely heralded in books and movies, and there arose a tremendous interest in psychotherapy. The demand far exceeded the supply of psychotherapists, and the Veterans Administration and the National Institute of Mental Health (NIMH), reasoning there would never be enough psychiatrists, created student stipends and educational funding, not only for psychiatrists but also for psychologists and social workers.

The combination of intense societal interest and public funding launched nonpsychiatric psychotherapy, but it was not easy at first. Organized psychiatry opposed the private practice of psychology, fought its efforts toward licensure, and was joined, paradoxically, by the then academically controlled American Psychological Association. A 30-year battle ensued (chronicled in Wright and Cummings, 2005), but as soon as doctoral psychology won the intense struggle, social work on a master's level followed in psychology's footsteps, soon to be joined by such newly spawned master's professions as marriage and family therapy (MFT) as well as counselors.

Soon there was an oversupply of psychotherapists—over 700,000 as of this writing (Hogan, 2003); although authorities recognize a great need in society for behavioral interventions, need does not necessarily translate into demand. The golden age of psychotherapy was over by the mid-1990s, done in by our insistence on long-term (largely psychoanalytically oriented) psychotherapy, as well as the profession's refusal to address out-of-control mental health costs that, for a time, exceeded a 16% inflation rate. Controls were foisted upon the economically helpless psychotherapy practitioners—often arbitrarily, but ever so drastically.

THE BIOMEDICAL REVOLUTION

In the mid-1980s, psychiatry began "medicalizing," a term denoting that it had now become essentially a prescribing and hospitalization profession. Psychotherapy, disdainfully referred to as "talk therapy," is essentially lacking in current psychiatric residencies; the relatively few psychiatrists who still perform psychotherapy tend to be over age 50 and practice largely in the northeastern part of the country. DSM diagnostic categories have been reformulated so that they resemble syndromes for which medication is the preferred treatment (Mojtabal & Olfson, 2008).

However, it is interesting that up to 80% of psychotropic medications are prescribed by nonpsychiatric physicians—a practice predicted two decades ago. The ever prescient editor of the *American Journal of Psychotherapy* (Lesse, 1985) foresaw not only that medications would replace much of psychotherapy, but also that computers and a new, more easily prescribed generation of psychotropic drugs with fewer side effects would make it possible for primary care physicians to issue most of these medications. The past 10 years have seen referrals by physicians to psychotherapy fall by almost 50%. Where once 95% of patients discharged from psychiatric hospitals were referred to outpatient psychotherapy, by 2005 the figure had fallen to only 10% (Cummings & O'Donohue, 2008).

The ever present seeking of the quick fix is now bolstered by primary care physicians who find the prescribing of these medications easy and lucrative and avoid the angry confrontation of patients who resent being told they need to see a "shrink." A mounting number of studies reveals serious psychotropic drug side effects and even death, suicide, or violence—especially among children, teenagers, and the elderly (U.S. Department of Health and Human Services, 2008; Wiggins & Cummings, 1998). However, it is anticipated that medication will continue to replace behavioral interventions until psychologists become an integral presence in the healthcare system.

WHERE ARE OUR PATIENTS?

In the decades of insistence that psychotherapy is not an integral part of the medical system, we created two silos: a huge silo called physical health, which gets the lion's share of funding (about 95%), and a tiny, perpetually underfunded silo called mental health. In our paranoia that psychotherapy is not medicine, we failed to appreciate what dentistry, nursing, optometry, podiatry, and all other healthcare professions knew decades ago: It is healthcare that gets funded—not the esoteric mental health silo that suffers from stigma, quality concerns, and lack of access. It insists on solo practices across town, while healthcare has become essentially group practices congregating in convenient, easily accessible health centers near hospitals where all other healthcare professionals practice (Cummings, 2007).

An early, large-scale collaborative model research was the 7-year Hawaii Medicaid Project (Cummings, Dorken, Pallak, & Henke, 1991), an extensive demonstration that recouped its funding investment within 18 months. A congressionally mandated three-way contract among the Health Care Financing Administration, the State of Hawaii, and the nonprofit Biodyne Institute launched an entirely new mental healthcare delivery system in which the Medicaid ($N = 36,000$) and federal employee ($N = 93,000$) populations of Hawaii were randomized into the control group, which received the extant health system, and the experimental group, which was treated in the innovative delivery system.

The Biodyne model was 68 targeted, evidence-based behavioral interventions; working closely with physicians, the highest 15% of utilizers of healthcare were outreached. The purpose of the experiment was to test in a prospective, controlled setting the results of previous nonrandomized research that revealed the medical cost offset effect: Brief, targeted behavioral interventions resulted in reduction of medical and surgical costs far beyond the cost of providing the behavioral interventions (Cummings & Follette, 1968; Follette & Cummings, 1967). The NIMH had already conducted 28 replications (Jones & Vischi, 1980), but they, too, were retrospective studies.

Estimates are consistent for decades (see, for example, Follete & Cummings, 1967, to Kroenke & Mangelsdorf, 1989): 60–70% of visits to primary care reflect psychological issues and emotional distress through physical symptoms that mimic physical disease or have psychological and lifestyle problems that are interfering with medical treatment or contribute to noncompliance with the medical regimen. Primary care physicians (PCPs) are constantly confronted with such patients, and they respond with medication and counseling to the extent that 85% of psychological problems are addressed by these PCPs. This makes the primary care system the de facto mental health treatment system in the United States. This is where our patients are!

INTEGRATION, NOT JUST COLLABORATION

Recognizing this, there is an increasing effort in health psychology to increase collaboration between physical and mental health (Peek & Heinrich, 1995), but this falls short inasmuch as it retains two silos and only seeks to increase the amount of communication and cooperation between the two. Beginning in 1997, however, a system emerged that would integrate behavioral health into primary care by placing behavioral care providers (BCPs) into the primary care setting, working side by side with PCPs. A growing number of textbooks have emerged, along with training programs that would train psychologists working in the primary care setting (chronologically, some of these textbooks are Blount, 1997; Cummings, Cummings, & Johnson, 1997; Cummings, O'Donohue, Hayes, & Follette, 2001; Cummings et al., 2003; O'Donohue, Cummings, Hayes, & Follette, 2005; O'Donohue, Byrd, Cummings, & Henderson, 2005; O'Donohue, Cummings, Cucciare, Runyan, & Cummings, 2005; Robinson & Reiter, 2007).

One of the earliest demonstrations in which especially trained BCPs were colocated with PCPs in the primary care setting was the Hawaii Integrated Healthcare Project II (Laygo et al., 2003), which was funded by the federal government. At about the same time, the U.S. Air Force integrated its medical system worldwide (Runyan, Fonseca, & Hunter, 2003). There have been a number of successful examples of the integration of behavioral health into primary care in TriCare, the Cherokee Health System, the Veterans Administration, and the U.S. Navy, but until Kaiser Permanente in Northern California retooled its delivery system accordingly, the private sector had lagged behind.

As the data emerge, a number of characteristics are attributable to appropriately conducted integrated behavioral/primary care. Unfortunately, some examples of so-called integrated primary care fall far short of adequate delivery of care because of insufficient training of the BCPs or the lack of orientation of PCPs in the effective use of the system. Furthermore, there exists a widespread lack of appreciation by administrators of the complexity of the system. The attitude, "Oh, this is simple to do," results in a system that simply is not!

Integrated Care and Medical Cost Offset

When fully and effectively implemented, there is a 20–30% reduction in overall medical and surgical costs. Since it was first discovered 40 years ago, there have been extensive replications of the medical cost offset effect (see first the summary by Jones & Vischi, 1979). A composite visualization is seen in Figure 3.1, which shows a steady decline of medical and surgical costs from the year previous to the behavioral interventions through the succeeding 5 years. This resulted in a 65% decrease in the treated population. With integrated behavioral and primary interventions fully implemented, this translates to a 20–30% medical cost offset to the covered population.

These studies were all retrospective in design, raising questions as to the validity of the findings. The aforementioned Hawaii Medicaid study not only was prospective, but it also randomized a very large population ($N = 130,000$) into an experimental group (the new model delivery system) and a control group (the traditional but very liberal Medicaid/federal employees benefit in Hawaii). It was conducted over a 3-year period with a 7-year follow-up and further delineated both the experimental and control groups into those who were chronically ill and those who were not.

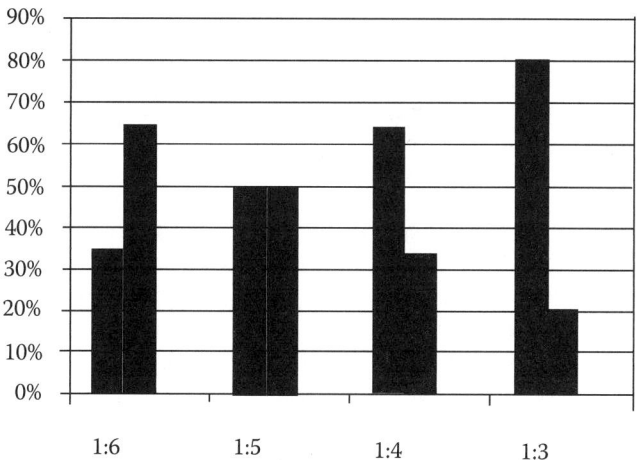

Figure 3.1 Composite schematization of the increases in the percentages of psychiatric/psychological treatment that can be conducted in primary care as a function of the ratio of BCPs to PSPs, whether it is 1:6, 1:5, 1:4, or 1:3. Compiled 2008 by the Cummings Foundation for Behavioral Health from data reported by family medical practices in Arizona and California. The second bar in each subset indicates the declining percentage of such patients that remain to be referred to specialty psych care (e.g., only 20% with the 1:3 ratio).

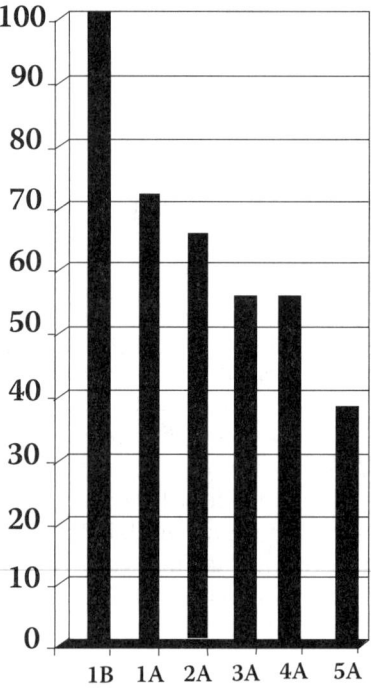

Figure 3.2 Nonchronic group. Average medical utilization in constant dollars for the Hawaii Project nonchronic group for the year before (1B) for those receiving targeted and focused treatment, other mental health treatment in the private practice community, and no mental health treatment the five years after (1A, 2A, 3A, 4A, and 5A). (From Cummings, N. A., Dorken, H., Pallak, M. S., & Henke, C. J. 1991. The impact of psychological intervention on health care costs and utilization: The Hawaii Medicaid Project. HCFA contract report #11-C-983344/9.)

The results of the nonchronically ill population are shown in Figure 3.2. Those treated in the new delivery system revealed within 18 months a 35% reduction in medical and surgical costs, while those receiving traditional treatment in the community *increased* these costs by 25% during the same period. Better off were those patients receiving no mental health treatment, who revealed only a 15% increase.

The results with the chronically ill population revealed similar results, as shown in Figure 3.3, but with the costs and subsequent savings (or increases as in the group treated with traditional services) substantially higher. It is apparent that not only do chronically ill patients cost the system significantly more, but the potential cost savings is also over twice as much as in the nonchronic population.

Financial Dimension of Integrated Behavioral/Primary Care

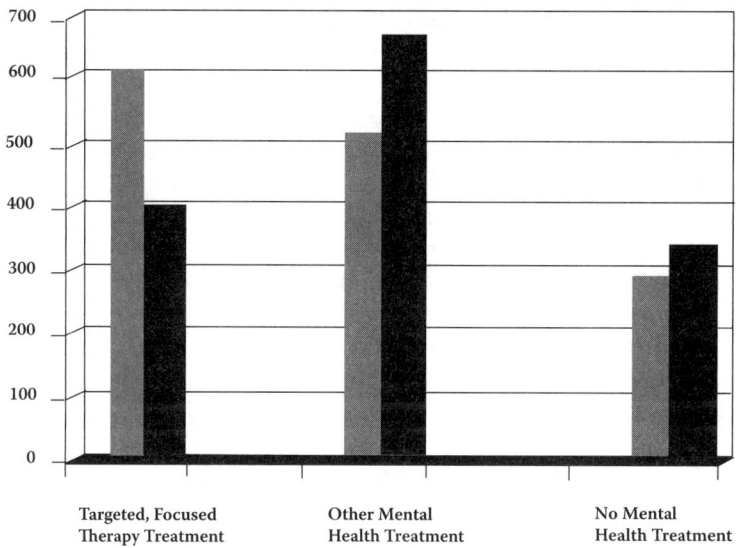

Figure 3.3 Chronically ill group. Average medical utilization in constant dollars for the Hawaii Project chronically ill group for the year before (lightly shaded columns) and the year after (darkly shaded columns) for those receiving targeted and focused treatment in the private practice community, and no mental health treatment. (From Cummings, N. A., Dorken, H., Pallak, M. S., & Henke, C. J. 1993. In N. A. Cummings & M. S. Pallak (Eds.), *Medicaid, managed behavioral health and implications for public policy* (pp. 3–23), vol. 2, Healthcare Utilization and Cost Series. San Francisco, CA: Foundation for Behavioral Health.)

The startling finding that traditional therapy increases costs is further explained within an inadvertent design of this study. To fulfill the many issues of diversity so important in Hawaii required a larger staff than was otherwise needed to deliver the services. This was fulfilled by hiring twice as many providers, but for half the time. The other half of their time was a continuation of their private practices in their offices. The medical cost offset obtained reflects their functioning in the new delivery system. However, in their individual private practices, where they were not involved in constant monitoring, clinical case conferencing, and other quality measures, they reverted to traditional treatment in spite of their having been extensively trained in the new behavioral model. This serendipitous finding stresses the importance of continued supervision and quality assurance procedures in integrated behavioral/primary care to prevent regression to the mean of traditional practice.

Effect of Traditional Therapy on Costs

The fear that traditional psychotherapy increases costs is disturbing, but justified. Ten years later, at the urging of the American Psychological Association, the Congress approved the Fort Bragg Champus Study, ostensibly to demonstrate that nontethered (i.e., unsupervised or unmanaged) traditional psychotherapy would dramatically decrease costs. The underlying belief was that third-party payer restrictions on practice were the high-cost culprit in mental health. The results were a disaster. An $8 million program increased 10-fold to $80 million without, as the researchers admitted, any demonstrable improvement in the well-being of the population treated (Bickman, 1996).

Leveraging Physicians' Time

The cost savings do not stop there. Physicians' time is leveraged, releasing them to perform procedures more in keeping with their medical training. In private group practices, this most often means time to perform more income-generating medical procedures. An oft repeated exclamation is that, with a BCP present for the hallway handoff, "I no longer have to worry when a patient might unexpectedly break down in my office, absorbing 45 minutes while I have a waiting room full of patients."

COST SAVINGS AS A MARKETING TOOL

From either lack of information or distaste for sound business principles, psychologists seldom invoke the medical cost offset effect when they are marketing their services to the public. When they do, they are remiss in not having a full grasp of when it works and when it does not; a blanket statement that psychological treatment ipso facto reduces medical and surgical costs turns off industry actuaries, who are far more knowledgeable. Most are well aware, for example, of the Fort Bragg Champus Study.

Until integrated behavioral/primary care impacts their services, psychologists are even less aware that it reduces specialty psychiatric and psychological costs. The need to refer patients to specialty psych care depends upon the intensity of the integrated system—often measured by the ratio of BCPs to PCPs, which may range from a minimum of 1:6 to as high as 1:3. At the Kaiser Permanente Health Plan, specialty psychiatry

Financial Dimension of Integrated Behavioral/Primary Care

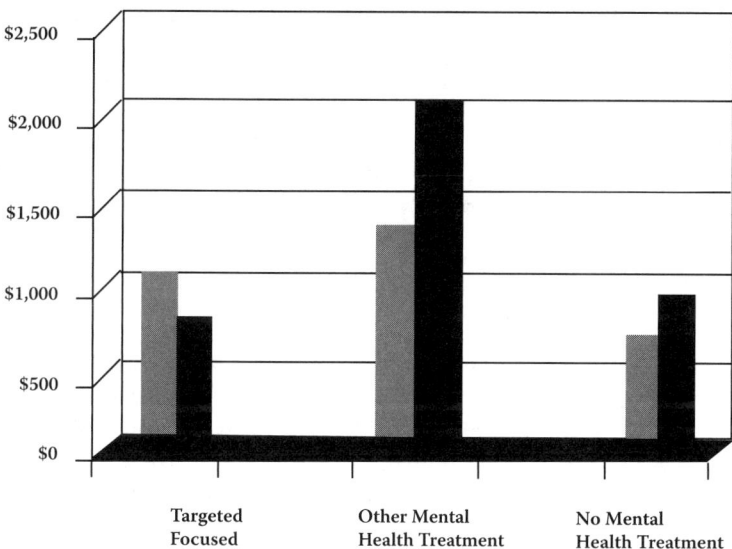

Figure 3.4 Composite schematization of the increases in the percentages of psychiatric/psychological treatment that can be conducted in primary care as a function of the ratio of BCPs to PCPs, whether it is 1:6, 1:5, 1:4, or 1:3. (Compiled in 2008 by the Cummings Foundation for Behavioral Health from data reported by family medical practices in Arizona and California.) The second bar in each subset indicates the declining percentage of such patients that remain to be referred to specialty psych care (e.g., only 20% with the 1:3 ratio).

has been reduced in size by 60% because it now treats only chronic psychiatric and psychological conditions.

Figure 3.4 shows the decline in specialty psychiatry with the increase in BCP/PCP ratios and the corresponding percentage of psychological conditions that can be handled more effectively and efficiently in the less costly primary care setting. It will be noted that up to 80% of these patients can be so treated, but it is imperative that while behavioral interventions are going on there is always at least one BCP available for the hallway handoff.

It is important to note that the reduction in referrals to specialty psych does not translate into a diminution of psychotherapy. To the contrary, there is an astounding increase in the number of patients who engage in follow-up treatment with the BCP after the hallway handoff. In the nonintegrated primary care setting, of the 40% of the emotionally distressed patients identified by PCPs, only 10% ever accept a referral and actually enter psychotherapy. The others are given a prescription or they simple ignore the referral. In the integrated primary care system, where there is no stigma or other resistances because it is a seamless "healthcare" process (as differentiated from "mental health") in which the patient always feels comfortable, 85–90% of those hallway handoffs will engage in subsequent behavioral interventions. This finding is generally consistent in all integrated settings offering sufficient follow-up services.

QUALITY ASSURANCE

In the delivery of mental and behavioral care services, too often the need for quality assurance is neglected, resulting in needless substandard care and even questionable interventions. At American Biodyne, even after the rigorous retraining affectionately dubbed the "Biodyne Bootcamp," fully 15% of clinicians' time was spent in quality assurance. This included a 3-hour case conference each Friday morning, in which the staff eagerly presented their failures or near-failures; one-on-one supervision; and group supervision.

Such an expenditure of time was and continues to be startling to the practitioners and the industry, but recent extensive research by Scott Miller (2008) and his colleagues demonstrates that the one feature that determines the master psychotherapist (defined as effectiveness) is constant evaluation and feedback. This investment at Biodyne was reflected in the total absence of malpractice claims: In 10 years with 25 million enrollees and 10,000 psychotherapists, there was not a single malpractice claim or a patent complaint that had to be adjudicated. When Biodyne passed into new hands in 1992, one of the first features eliminated was the 15% of time devoted to quality assurance. Within months, malpractice suits began to appear.

Quality can be defined as "exceeding your customer's expectations." Quality improvement should be continuous; the bar is always moving higher. Quality always requires consistent measurement to determine the extent to which these objectives are being achieved. Because behavioral health has not embraced the quality ethic, there are precious few data to determine the extent to which we even come close to our customers' expectations. However, there are plenty of reasons to be concerned.

We also have to be careful to define who our customers are. Clearly, one focus has to be on the patient. If patients do not like what we are providing, then they simply will not show up in the first place (e.g., they will go to their primary care physicians for their problems), or they can simply stop attending (the modal number of psychotherapy sessions is one). Many health professionals now have

- created wonderful waiting rooms (e.g., pediatric dentists have high-quality arcade games and flat-screen TVs)
- developed incentive systems for compliance (the orthodontist of the second author's children rents the swimming park the last day of the season exclusively for compliant patients)
- developed additional services and procedures that customers want (teeth whitening, sealants)
- invested in electronic medical records that vastly decrease errors (the saying now in medicine is that "paper kills")
- promoted evidence-based practice to decrease unwanted variability in practice patterns

All these actions have created more satisfied patients.

However, another customer is the third-party payer. In behavioral health there is actually a stream of payers, usually consisting of care management organizations such as Magellan, Value Options, Cigna, etc., who often have contracts with an HMO (such as United or Blue Cross/Blue Shield) that, in turn, contracts with an employer, union, or federal government agency (e.g., the Department of Defense). Each of these payers cares about the value it receives for its dollar (i.e., has expectations that we, in taking a quality perspective, try to exceed). As a profession, we have not understood what the expectations of these organizations are, have not innovated in trying to meet these expectations, and have not measured on dimensions that might impress them.

Instead, we have vilified our payers, spent a lot of money suing the folks who write our paychecks (APA has spent over $10 million in such lawsuits). When we do measure, our efforts often fall short of what might interest the payer, especially if it is an employer. Typically, for example, our outcomes research, if any, might focus on BDI (Beck's Depression Inventory) scores, but not measure anything related to missed workdays or medical utilization, which are vital to our customer.

The quality problem in behavioral care services is often the "elephant in the room" when business decisions are being made. Part of the reason why people may go to their primary care physician is that this individual is more trusted than the mental health practitioner. Surveys of patients have revealed that they are concerned about the effectiveness of mental health interventions as well as the "normality" of mental health practitioners. We are too often seen as strange and ineffective—a perception that may not be all that delusional. It is important that integrated care does not adopt this same quality problem, for integrated care is doomed if it merely colocates something resembling a Rorschach-administering, rebirthing psychotherapist who is simultaneously dealing with his or her own issues.

Such a flaky, non-evidence-based, ineffective, and even deleterious practitioner invokes in the patient what economists call the "lemon problem." Value of a product (astonishingly, psychotherapists still do not see their services as a product) determines the price the customer is willing to pay, while the consistency of the quality is directly related to price. A customer will pay the price, for example, for milk that has value: consistently high quality, absence of contamination, curdling, or skimming. If two thirds of the time the milk manifests lowered quality in the form of one or more of these quality problems, the price will drop dramatically, or the customer may switch to soy milk. When the latter occurs, the price may drop below the cost of producing the milk, and it might disappear from the store shelves altogether.

Consider, then, if the public perception is that psychotherapy is effective only occasionally, or not at all, or that the practitioner suffers from psychological issues of greater magnitude than the patient. The demand for such services diminishes while at the same time our educational system has produced a glut of psychotherapists (Cummings & O'Donohue, 2008).

As a profession, we have conveniently blamed price depression on the greed of managed care. Some of this is true because there are good- as well as bad-quality managed care companies, but it is not clear what we can do about this. We can, however, address the factors under our control. We have ignored quality factors, and our several national mental health organizations have neglected to adopt and enforce quality improvement practices that are substantive. Only then can we reverse the price depression in psychotherapy (see O'Donohue & Fisher, 2007, for more on quality improvement in mental health).

FUNDING OF INTEGRATED CARE

Integrated behavioral/primary care is like a pomegranate: Overwhelmingly, people say they like it, but few buy it. It has often been pointed out that, in healthcare, it is 20 years after the proven effectiveness of a treatment before it is fully adopted. In this point of view, it will be 10 more years before integrated care is mainstream. Aside from this, however, what are some of the impediments?

Public Funding

The military, TriCare, and the Veterans Administration have been at the forefront in funding demonstration projects. This has been made possible through top-down decisions, and it has been facilitated by the fact that all of these demonstrations are in staff model delivery systems rather than networks. Invariably, these demonstration projects have been showered with high praise and general satisfaction, but when the funding dries up, the heretofore successful delivery system is allowed to wither and dry up. Even in the one extensive private system in which integrated care has been acknowledged and mandated, some of the scores of Kaiser Permanente medical centers have been allowed to opt out or lag behind.

Private Funding

In the 1990s, the managed care organizations, including the managed behavioral health organizations (MBHOs, commonly referred to as "carve-outs"), began to morph out of *managed care*, in which they took an active part in the delivery of services and even made service decisions, and into *care management*, in which they manage the benefit but do not tell the doctors how to practice in their offices. Much of this was in response to an outcry from both the practitioners and the public

The current care management organizations like and support the concept of integrated behavioral/primary care, would welcome the effectiveness of such an innovation, and would be willing to create payment mechanisms through which BCPs could be reimbursed. However, they cannot direct professionals to practice in this manner. The question then arises: How is this to be funded? It is time for practitioners to rise to the occasion, paying attention to the following considerations.

Every industry attempts to become more efficient. Competition is a key driver in this pursuit, for if a competitor can provide the same or higher quality service (or product) at a lower price than you can, you will soon be driven out of business. Customers enjoy more for less and will not be dissuaded by your poor value proposition; in spite of your pain, this is a good thing because value continues to increase. Economists call this process in the competitive marketplace "creative destruction," and it behooves our profession to become more productive and efficient. In the current marketplace, the majority of the American public is not convinced that psychotherapy is of greater value (cost, time expended, outcomes) than psychotropic medication, so how is this to be done?

Integrated care as a model of service delivery achieves increased efficiencies because it places service where folks seem to want it: one stop shopping in their primary care physician's office. It also allows the practitioner to be more productive by adopting a number of practice standards that differ from standard mental health specialty care (whether in private offices or mental health clinics and centers):

- Brief, evidenced-based assessment (not utilizing MMPIs, Rorschach tests, or extensive histories)
- Consultation liaison models (the BCP is seen as an extender of the physician and augments the PCP's treatments without taking over the patient and starting anew)
- Focused, evidence-based interventions saving time and money over the non-evidence-based interventions
- Evidence-based groups possible because of the large number of patients with a particular behavioral problem (e.g., obesity, chronic pain, depression, noncompliance with medical regimen)
- The standard of restoring functioning rather than completely curing or personality restructuring
- A wider scope of practice—the BCP is not just a specialist in DSM problems but also effectively treats subclinical problems and pathways to medical utilization (e.g., stress, noncompliance), as well as behavioral medicine interventions (e.g., chronic pain, obesity)

Integrated care is based on the premise that has generally been supported by data that reveal that clinicians practicing in this way can decrease overall medical costs. Behavioral care costs rise slightly due to provision of behavioral/primary care services, but more expensive medical and surgical costs decline to a much greater extent. The net savings have often been in the range of 20–30%, which is staggering (see Cummings et al., 2003, for a review). Thus, payers can see that the more productive, efficient system is integrated behavioral/primary care.

Therefore, the premise for arguing for integrated care is not, "We will help you find more money," but rather, "The money is already there if you rearrange the way funds are being spent now. You will have healthier patients demanding fewer medical services, as well as extra funds left over."

The "Laboratory Model" of Integrated Care

Most practicing psychotherapists see patients who belong to a variety of third-party payers. Consequently, BCPs are economically unable to contract directly in a special network with one carrier because the patient flow would probably not be sufficient. Medical laboratories faced this same problem and solved it decades ago by locating in the midst of existing medical centers, enabling them to serve many surrounding physicians' offices as well as health plans. Physicians are "herd animals": They congregate in medical centers. The key is proximity and immediate accessibility—a successful model that a number of psychologist groups practicing integrated care have replicated. One such group, which began with 3 psychologists, now has grown to 23, while another went from 5 to 42. They belong to all networks, but the reason for their success is the appreciation by the independent physicians for their remarkable adaptation of the hallway handoff.

BCPs in Physician Group Practices

A number of psychologists in scattered locations around the country have persuaded family medical group practices to include one or more BCPs. When the group practice is large, it is easy to have more than one BCP, but economics limits a group of five or six physicians to just one BCP. This precludes the ability to have one BCP always available for the hallway handoff while the other is doing the treatment. Through accommodated scheduling, however, these limitations can be largely overcome.

DIFFICULTIES, PERVERSE INCENTIVES, AND INADEQUATE IMPLEMENTATION

The road to integrated behavioral/primary care has not been and will not be easy. There are a number of key difficulties and even perverse incentives (economists call them "moral hazards") in the field. Here is a brief listing of the major financial difficulties:

- Chief financial officers (CFOs) require a fairly sophisticated return on investment (ROI) analysis that will compare this proposal to all other possible investments. Integrated care is competing for scarce dollars against such alternative investments as disease management programs, hiring more employees who can bill additional amounts, or even new information systems such as electronic medical records—all of which presuppose savings. Promoting integrated care needs to generate clear and credible financial data that can be compared to these alternative investments. Currently, there is a paucity of such data. These data need to show that in population X (e.g., urban Medicaid), an investment of Y will produce an ROI of Z (usually a return of 5:1—a difficult goal to achieve in the 12-month period favored by CFOs).
- The outcome data that exist for integrated care are often missing key financial outcomes. We find that BDI scores decrease, but we know nothing about the impact on medical utilization, disability payments, or absenteeism.
- Perverse incentives abound. Healthcare budgets are usually constructed from that of last year. If integrated care decreases costs, a smaller budget next year may result. In federal funding, the government often demands that any savings be sent back to Washington, removing local incentives to save money.
- A lot of innovation is going on in healthcare, often producing "innovation fatigue": Management does not want to administer one more innovation.
- One of integrated care's competitors is the nurse-driven disease management that has proliferated into a several billion dollar industry. These programs appear to be less risky to managers, they often have impressive ROI data, and they do have some positive clinical impact. However, they are not a panacea. They can be useful in the easiest cases but are no substitute for astute clinicians dealing with the complex cases found in integrated care (see Cummings, O'Donohue, & Naylor, 2005). However, comparative studies are

needed to show the relative advantages and disadvantages of these programs. Ideally, they should complement each other.
- Many insurers will not pay for behavioral health consultation codes. In fee-for-service environments, these are essential in supporting integrated care because they allow the BCP reimbursement for non-DSM problems (e.g., chronic pain, treatment compliance).
- Medicaid does not allow for medical and behavioral billing on the same day—an archaic regulation unsuccessfully intended to prevent fraud that essentially stops the hallway handoff in its tracks.
- Although there are now a number of large-scale integration systems (e.g., the U.S. Air Force, Veterans Administration, U.S. Army and Navy, TriCare, Cherokee Healthcare, Kaiser Permanente), there is perhaps even a larger number that are poorly constructed and are jeopardizing the concept by predictably poor and even negative results. These range from collaborative models that maintain the two silos or employ poorly trained personnel who lack training in such imperatives as neurology, clinical medicine, medical psychology, and pharmacology to a lack of appreciation of how the medical system works and the lingo that accompanies it.

SUMMARY AND CONCLUSIONS

The recent precipitous decline in referrals for psychotherapy has rekindled the need for reevaluation of psychology's longstanding and self-defeating stance that we are not part of the healthcare system. America pays for healthcare, not psychosocial care; all other professions rendering treatment (e.g., dentistry, nursing, osteopathy, optometry, podiatry) have taken advantage of the nation's evolution from a medical system to a healthcare system. As part of this healthcare system, they are prospering, while psychotherapy is languishing.

The integration of behavioral health into primary care, in which BCPs are colocated in the primary care setting alongside PCPs, has evolved in the last decade as a successful, viable method of bridging this gap. Many impediments to successful implementation persist. These range from the reluctance of mental health practitioners to give up solo practice, the 50-minute hour, and their traditional mode of practice to the fact that our current third-party payer system is not constructed to meet the funding of this evolving system. Henry J. Kaiser, the industrialist hero of World War II who built the Victory ships (often in 5 days from keel to launch) and saved Great Britain and who, through Dr. Sidney Garfield, founded the Kaiser Permanente system, would admonish, "Find a need and fill it." The need has been found, but filling it will require boldness and innovation from psychological practitioners.

Generally speaking, psychology training programs have been predictably unresponsive, but there are now a few with state-of-the-art programs about to debut by 2009. It is the strong belief of the authors that these will more appropriately emerge from the health sciences divisions of medical schools than through traditional clinical psychology doctoral programs.

REFERENCES

Bickman, L. (1996). A continuum of care: More is not always better. *American Psychologist, 51,* 689–701.

Blount, A. (Ed.). (1997). *Integrated primary care: The future of medical and mental health collaboration.* New York, NY: Norton.

Carnahan, I. (2002, January 21). Asylum for the insane. *Forbes,* 33–34.

Cummings, N. A. (1986). The dismantling of our health system: Strategies for the survival of psychological practice. *American Psychologist, 41,* 426–431.

Cummings, N. A. (2007). Treatment and assessment take place in an economic setting, always. In S. O. Lilienfeld & W. T. O'Donohue (Eds.), *The great ideas of clinical science* (pp. 163–184). New York, NY: Routledge (Taylor and Francis Group).

Cummings, N. A., Cummings, J. L., & Johnson, J. N. (Eds.). (1997). *Behavioral health in primary care: A guide for clinical integration.* Madison, CT: Psychosocial Press.

Cummings, N. A., Dorken, H., Pallak, M. S., & Henke, C. J. (1991). The impact of psychological intervention on health care costs and utilization: The Hawaii Medicaid Project. HCFA contract report #11-C-983344/9.

Cummings, N. A., Dorken, H., Pallak, M. S., & Henke, C. J. (1993). The impact of psychological intervention on health care cost and utilization. In N. A. Cummings & M. S. Pallak (Eds.), *Medicaid, managed behavioral health and implications for public policy* (pp. 3–23), vol. 2, Healthcare Utilization and Cost Series. San Francisco, CA: Foundation for Behavioral Health.

Cummings, N. A., & Fernandez, L. (1985). Exciting new opportunities for psychologists in the market place. *Independent Practitioner, 5,* 38–42.

Cummings, N. A., & Follette, W. T. (1968). Psychiatric services and medical utilization in a prepaid health plan setting: Part 2. *Medical Care, 6,* 31–41.

Cummings, N. A., & O'Donohue, W. T. (2008). *Eleven blunders that cripple psychotherapy in America: A remedial unblundering.* New York, NY: Routledge (Taylor and Francis Group).

Cummings, N. A., O'Donohue, W. T., & Ferguson, K. E. (Eds.). (2003). *Behavioral health in primary care: Beyond efficacy to effectiveness.* Cummings Foundation for Behavioral Health: Health Utilization and Cost Series, vol. 6. Reno, NV: Context Press.

Cummings, N. A., O'Donohue, W. T., & Ferguson, K. E. (Eds.). (2005). *Psychological approaches to disease management.* Cummings Foundation for Behavioral Health: Healthcare Utilization and Cost Series, vol. 8. Reno, NV: Context Press.

Cummings, N. A., O'Donohue, W. T., Hayes, S. C., & Follette, V. (Eds.). (2001). *Integrated behavioral healthcare: Positioning mental health practice with medical/surgical practice.* San Diego, CA: Academic Press.

Cummings, N. A., O'Donohue, W. T., & Naylor, E. (2005). *Psychological approaches to chronic disease management.* Reno, NV: Context Press.

Follette, W. T., & Cummings, N. A. (1967). Psychiatric services and medical utilization in a prepaid health plan setting. *Medical Care, 5,* 25–35.

Forbes, S. (2004, September 20). Insuring healthcare coverage. *Forbes,* 32.

Fox, R. E. (2004). It's about money: Protecting and enhancing our incomes. *Independent Practitioner, 24*(4), 158–159.

Hildebrand, J. (2008). As quoted in "The Business of Life," *Forbes,* September 1, p. 120.

Hogan, M. F. (2003). New Freedom Commission report: The president's New Freedom Commission—Recommendations to transform mental health care in America. *Psychiatric Services, 54,* 1467–1474.

Jones, K. R., & Vischi, T. R. (1979). The impact of alcohol, drug abuse, and mental health treatment on medical care utilization: A review of the research literature. *Medical Care, 17*(Suppl.), 43–131.

Kroenke, K., & Mangelsdorf, D. (1989). Common symptoms in ambulatory care: Incidence, evaluation, therapy and outcome. *American Journal of Medicine, 86,* 262–286.

Laygo, R., O'Donohue, W., Hall, S., Kaplan, A., Wood, R., Cummings, J.,...Shaffer, I. (2003). Preliminary results from the Hawaii Integrated Healthcare Project II. In N. A. Cummings, W. T. O'Donohue, & K. E. Ferguson (Eds.), *Behavioral health as primary care: Beyond efficacy to effectiveness* (pp. 11–143). Cumming Foundation for Behavioral Health, Healthcare Utilization and Cost Series, vol. 6. Reno, NV: Context Press.

Lesse, S. (1985). *The future of the health sciences: Anticipating tomorrow.* Northvale, NJ: Jason Aronson.

Miller, S. D. (2008). www.BaloneyWatch.comn

Mojtabal, R., & Olfson, M. (2008). National trends in psychotherapy by office-based psychiatrists. *Archives of General Psychiatry, 85*(8), 41–49.

O'Donohue, W. T., Byrd, M. R., Cummings, N. A., & Henderson, D. A. (Eds.). (2005). *Behavioral integrative care: Treatments that work in the primary care setting.* New York, NY: Brunner-Routledge.

O'Donohue, W. T., Cummings, N. A., Cucciare, M. A., Runyan, C. N., & Cummings, J. L. (Eds.). (2005). *Integrated behavioral health care: A guide to effective intervention.* Amherst, NY: Humanity Books (Prometheus).

O'Donohue, W. T., Cummings, N. A., Hayes, S., & Follette, V. (2005). *Integrated behavioral healthcare: Positioning mental health practice with medical/surgical practice.* San Diego: Academic Press.

O'Donohue, W. T., & Fisher, J. E. (Eds.). (2007). *Practitioners guide to evidence-based psychotherapy.* New York, NY: Springer.

Peek, C. J., & Heinrich, R. L. (1995). Building collaborative healthcare organizations: From idea to innovation. *Family Systems Medicine, 13,* 327–342.

Robinson, P. J., & Reiter, J. T. (2007). *Behavioral consultants and primary care: A guide to integrating services.* New York, NY: Springer.

Runyan, C. N., Fonseca, V. P., & Hunter, C. (2003). Integrating consultative behavioral healthcare into the Air Force medical system. In N. A. Cummings, W. T. O'Donohue, & K. E. Ferguson (Eds.), *Behavioral health in primary care:*

Beyond efficacy to effectiveness (pp. 145–163). Cummings Foundation for Behavioral Health: Healthcare Utilization and Cost Series, vol. 6. Reno, NV: Context Press.

Sowell, T. (2003). *Applied economics.* New York, NY: Basic Books.

U.S. Department of Health and Human Services. (2008). Antipsychotic medications linked to deaths in elderly patients. DHHS news release, August 23. Author.

Wiggins, J. G., & Cummings, N. A. (1998). A national study of the experience of psychologists with psychotropic medication and psychotherapy. *Professional Psychology, Research and Practice, 29*(6), 549–552.

Wright, R. H., & Cummings, N. A. (Eds.). (2005). *Destructive trends in mental health: The well-intentioned path to harm.* New York, NY: Routledge (Taylor and Francis Group).

Four

Mental Health Informatics

BRUCE LUBOTSKY LEVIN AND ARDIS HANSON

INTRODUCTION

Health information technology (HIT) promises new possibilities in the delivery of healthcare and mental healthcare. Although President Bush set a goal to have electronic health records (EHRs) for the majority of Americans by 2014, only a quarter of physicians use EHRs in ambulatory settings and 5% of hospitals use computerized physician order entry (Jha et al., 2006). The Centers for Medicare & Medicaid Services (2010), or CMS, has instituted e-prescribing and EHR programs to increase the adoption and use of HIT in the United States. However, many healthcare and safety net providers feel there are significant gaps in their understanding of how implementation of HIT and EHR will improve healthcare and behavioral healthcare. This perception of the value of HIT and the EHR creates critical challenges for the development of policies aimed at speeding adoption.

PURPOSE OF THE CHAPTER

The authors of this chapter will first describe problems in the use of electronic health information in decision making, focusing on historical perspectives, program evaluation, outcomes assessment, and implementation of evidence-based practices. They will then review federal reforms that assist in the implementation of HIT and its use in decision making. Finally, the authors will conclude with recommendations to assist in the adoption, implementation, and utilization of EHR in the decision-making process.

HISTORICAL PERSPECTIVES

The idea of a national mental health database using health records in concert with decision-making tools to determine performance, utilization, and outcomes is not new. In the early 1970s, the Mental Health Statistics Improvement Program, or MHSIP, was created "to develop rules for collecting mental health data, to advise the federal government on data issues, and to develop and implement projects to improve mental health data nationwide" (Mental Health Statistics Improvement Program, n.d., p. 1). Members included state and local governments, public and private nonprofit service providers, and mental health researchers. Almost a decade later, this initiative culminated in the design of a national mental health statistics system (Patton & Leginski, 1983).

In 1989, the National Institute of Mental Health (NIMH) published *Data Standards for Mental Health Decision Support* (Leginski & Croze, 1989), which became the de facto reference document for much of the subsequent public mental health data system development. Also of significance were the federal grant initiatives of NIMH and the Center for Mental Health Services (CMHS) to help states and treatment agencies develop mental health data systems and use the data collected in those systems in decision-making activities.

During the last two decades, a number of additional HIT initiatives have emerged. Title II of the Health Information Portability and Accountability Act (1996), or HIPAA, known as the administrative simplification provisions, required the establishment of national standards for electronic healthcare transactions and national identifiers for providers, health insurance plans, and employers.

In 2003, the President's New Freedom Commission on Mental Health (2003) urged the use of technology to speed adoption and implementation of evidence-based practices in mental health. By 2004, President George W. Bush directed the U.S. Department of Health and Human Services (HHS) to create a national health information technology coordinator.

In 2009, President-elect Obama announced that large-scale adoption of HIT was a priority and that all U.S. residents were to have electronic health records within 5 years (Jones, 2009). This would be accomplished through an economic stimulus plan, P.L. 111-5 (American Recovery and Reinvestment Act [ARRA], 2009). Specifically, the ARRA created the Health Information Technology for Economic and Clinical Health

(HITECH) Act, which promotes the widespread adoption of HIT to support the electronic sharing of clinical data among healthcare stakeholders (U.S. House of Representatives Ways and Means Committee, 2009). The central feature of this data sharing is the electronic health record also known as an electronic medical record, EMR), "a longitudinal electronic record of patient health information generated by one or more encounters in any care delivery setting" (Healthcare Information and Management Systems Society [HIMSS], 2010, p. 1).

The use of the EHR is particularly troublesome for mental health practitioners. Mental health data are often not composed of medical test results. Although medical tests are important information for mental health practitioners, mental health data often comprise handwritten notes by practitioners that may or may not be fully transcribed into electronic text. In addition, mental health data include prior diagnoses, assessment reports, and termination summaries, which may only appear in handwritten formats transferred from office to office. Further, the notes may be converted into diagnostic or administrative categories, such as DSM or ICD codes, or into minimal record formats created for use by a solo practitioner, office staff, or small group practice. This creates a problem of successfully integrating EHRs from one practitioner with the paper-based records of another practitioner. Records are printed and incorporated into the paper-based system or paper records are scanned and appended to electronic files, creating additional work for both practitioners and office staff.

One of the major reasons the electronic record format was created was to provide a legible, quickly accessible record, even if much of the handwritten detail is lost, and to make mental health data quantifiable across an individual or group practice, as well as for managed care organizations and state and federal programs (Greenfield & Wolf-Branigin, 2009; Meredith, 2010).

Mental illnesses are often difficult presentations to diagnose. Primary care physicians may have difficulties in distinguishing between distress and disorder, severity and impairment—much less determining social problems from medical problems (Gask, Klinkman, Fortes, & Dowrick, 2008). Unlike paper records, an EHR would help standardize assessment and diagnostic criteria by establishing parameters and a common language in mental health (Gask et al., 2008; Jablensky, 1978). However, the importance of including anecdotal descriptions of illness in medical records should not be overlooked or ignored, especially in determining nosological and syndromatological classifications (Fox & Scherl, 1984; Freer, 1980; Moller, 2005).

APPLICATIONS IN HEALTH AND BEHAVIORAL HEALTH

There are many unsolved problems related to healthcare and information technology. Perhaps the most confounding problem is how to manage the complexity and magnitude of personal and public health information for millions of individuals over their lifetimes within the context of rapidly evolving scientific, medical, and technological innovation. Data are gathered in many formats. They can be textual, visual, spatial, and numeric as well as primary or secondary data. Federal agencies collect data in numeric form. Through analysis, numeric data become statistical data. There are three main issues in the use of data in the move toward a national EHR: (1) the range of data necessary for decision making, (2) the complexity of data in decision making, and (3) adoption and implementation of EHR in decision making.

The Range of Data Necessary for Decision Making

Each behavioral health agency, organization, and delivery system has its own health information systems, databases, formatting structure, data collection, and reporting requirements. These systems may or may not be transparent to users and data repositories across the variety of healthcare and mental healthcare organizational settings either regionally or nationally. Further, each of these entities has its preferred distribution or communication channels, its preferred formats, and its preferred schedules. For example, states have developed highly decentralized information management, infrastructure, technology, and operations to meet the needs of state agencies independent of one another (Hanson & Levin, in press). Furthermore, health and mental health data are combinations of numerous agency, regulatory, administrative, oversight, and financial data sets. These data are required by each state or federal agency and then are reported to other state and federal agencies as required for Medicaid, Medicare, and other public entitlement programs (Hanson & Levin, in press).

In addition to local, county, state, and federal health and mental health agencies, academic researchers create multiple proprietary data sets. Their data sets are often amalgams of original, private, or public data sets comprising primary and secondary data that address patient outcomes and treatment effectiveness. Primary data are often obtained through clinical studies, controlled trials, or case studies. Data are collected by numerous agencies, private and public providers, and academics and can be retrospective (data about past conditions), interventional (what happens during the time the intervention is delivered), or observational (case studies).

Data can be quantitative or qualitative. For example, mental health and substance abuse statistics from primary data include (but are not limited to) the estimated number of adults with serious mental disorders, the estimated number of children and adolescents with serious emotional disturbance, sources of funding for treatment of individuals with mental and substance use disorders, state per-capita expenditures, and the number of publicly funded state and county inpatient beds. However, there are problems with primary data: There can be significant random errors in rates based upon small numbers of health events or errors in the inputting or scanning of data.

Secondary data have many advantages as a primary resource for population-based behavioral health research, including easier access, less expensive than collecting original data, more readily available, and the preselected population (e.g., all members of the Federal Employees Benefit Plan). However, secondary data may be problematic regarding their origins or data set limitations, which may or may not be clearly stated. Although there is an interesting potential to combine primary and secondary data, substantial challenges remain in the integration of such data for comparative effectiveness research (CER) in population-based behavioral health, especially with the inclusion of epidemiologic and surveillance data.

The dual challenges of the rapidly changing demographics in the United States and concurrent rising costs in healthcare and mental healthcare have created a greater interest in the epidemiology of behavioral healthcare, especially in the areas of capacity, demand, and quality. In addition, policy makers, state and local public health agencies, and behavioral health program administrators often use surveillance data on injury and disease for resource allocation, planning, and program evaluation.

One emerging and critical aspect of epidemiology is its contribution to the development, implementation, and evaluation of evidence-based behavioral health interventions as they relate to the current federal focus on CER. By comparing treatments and strategies to improve health, clinicians and patients are best able to decide on the most appropriate treatment approach.

CER also has the potential to contribute information for improving the health of communities and the performance of health and mental health systems. As a basic component of the ARRA, over $1.1 billion has been allocated to support research on CER in two areas:

1. Conduct, support, or synthesize research that compares the clinical outcomes, effectiveness, and appropriateness of items, services, and procedures that are used to prevent, diagnose, or treat diseases, disorders, and other health conditions
2. Encourage the development and use of clinical registries, clinical data networks, and other forms of electronic health data that can be used to generate or obtain outcomes data (U.S. Department of Health and Human Services, 2010a, p. 1)

Complexity of Data and Decision Making

Decision making in behavioral health must deal with complex overlays of directives at the state and federal levels. The federal agenda for behavioral health, established by the NIMH (1999), focuses on a decision-making model for interventions that uses a micro- to macroperspective linking patient-level variables to services-level variables. The NIMH has established three goals for this initiative. First, NIMH hopes to improve its understanding of characteristics in the decision-making process. Second, NIMH sees this model as viable to test decision aids in effectiveness research across diverse populations and treatment settings. Finally, NIMH hopes to illustrate and incorporate preference concepts in the design of behavioral interventions (NIMH, 1999). Linking the decision-making processes of the patient and the provider should afford better outcomes in treatment initiation and adherence, patient outcomes, and system outcomes at both individual and population-based levels. In addition to the NIMH agenda, there is an overlay of CER in decision making.

CER has minimum threshold criteria that must be met. Of these, the "potential to inform decision making by patients, clinicians, or other stakeholders" and its "responsiveness to expressed needs of patients, clinicians, or other stakeholders" are two critical components in the adoption of the EHR. In addition, any CER will be judged on its potential impact to decrease prevalence and burden of disease, variability in patient outcomes, treatment and utilization costs, and the potential for increased patient benefit or decreased harm. CER will also address uncertainty and risk in treatment management decisions and practice variability. Finally, CER would assist in the development of data infrastructure, methods development, and training (U.S. Department of Health and Human Services, 2010b).

There are numerous clinical behavioral health questions that come up daily. For example, when are the atypical antipsychotics not recommended for certain disorders? Is brief cognitive therapy as efficacious in treating severe anxiety disorder as a joint medication and therapeutic model? Wang, Ulbricht, and Schoenbaum (2009) view CER as helping to inform decisions for treatments that improve outcomes under practice conditions and offering choices on alternative treatments. Further, CER should use a blend of randomized clinical trials, practical clinical trials, or alternative methods, such as clinical epidemiology, quasi-experimental studies, and simulation studies (Wang et al., 2009). However, there is a knowledge gap between evidence-based interventions and effective delivery and adoption by behavioral healthcare delivery systems.

Adoption and Implementation of EHR in Decision Making

There are many reasons why widespread adoption and implementation of EHR have not occurred, including related costs, resistance to change, fear or avoidance of technology, and patterns of day-to-day work behaviors. Because most organizational routines are followed at a subconscious level, any new *and* sustainable change requires effort on the part of both the individual and the organization. In addition, the consideration of both the *context* of care and the *content* of care is a challenge in change implementation.

The National Research Council suggests that today's clinical systems provide poor support for the cognitive tasks and work flow of clinicians (Stead & Lin, 2009). Further, developers of clinical systems may often have poorly defined requirements or poor development processes. More importantly, they may fail to adopt iterative, evolutionary, or consumer-centered approaches in their designs (Stead & Lin, 2009).

Usability has become an increasingly important topic in the HIT literature, with many HIT professionals examining problems of user adoption and implementation (Armijo, McDonnell, & Werner, 2009; Campbell, Guappone, Sittig, Dykstra, & Ash,

2009; Campbell, Sittig, Guappone, Dykstra, & Ash, 2007; Chaffee & Zimmerman, 2010; Coons et al., 2009; Walker, 2005). Using data from the National Ambulatory Medical Care Survey, Hing and Hsiao (2010) surveyed a national probability sample of physicians on their use of the electronic medical record (EMR). The study defined a basic EMR system as having the following features: patient demographic information, clinical notes, prescription orders, laboratory tests, and patient problem lists. Fully functional EMR systems also included medical history and follow-up, orders and status for tests and prescriptions, status of orders sent electronically, warnings of drug interactions or contraindications, electronic images of test results, warnings for out-of-range test levels, and reminders for guideline-based interventions (Hing & Hsiao, 2010).

Solo or single specialty practices ranged from approximately 20–74% of physicians having any types of an EMR to approximately 5–33% having a basic EMR to approximately 2–12% having fully functional systems. Although 25% of medical practices (excluding radiologists, anesthesiologists, and pathologists) sampled had any type of an EMR system, approximately 7% had a basic EMR (as defined previously), while approximately 2% had a fully functional EMR (Hing & Hsiao, 2010). EMR use also was related to practice characteristics. Use of an EMR by solo or group physician-owned practices and community health centers was lower than that by HMOs (86%). EMR use was also higher in practices of 11 physicians or more or in multispecialty practices.

One of the challenges of evaluating usability in EHRs is the complexity of user tasks, work flows, and the user environment. For example, alerts and reminders may help or hinder a clinician. To be effective, alerts would need to increase clinician efficiency, be useful in the decision-making process, have relevant information, be in an easily understood interface, and be integrated into the work flow (Krall & Sittig, 2002). The interrelatedness of how decision making, preferences, and behaviors are influenced and influence each other is critical in the effectiveness of an intervention prescribed by a clinician for a patient. Although formal decision analysis models have proved successful in high-risk acute situations, such as emergency and intensive care settings (Ji, Smith, Huynh, & Najarian, 2009), decision making in chronic disease management in nonacute settings may be decontextualized (Mysore, Pluye, Grad, & Johnson-Lafleur, 2009). Further, effects on patient outcomes remain largely understudied (Garg et al., 2005).

Problematic design aspects for computerized provider order entry systems, for example, include documentation and data entry options, screen display and layout, selection lists and menus, log in and log out procedures, clues and guidelines, and timing of alerts (Khajouei & Jaspers, 2008). Consider the request: "I need to refill an antipsychotic medication." From an actual clinical work flow, the clinician needs to consider, at a minimum, the following pieces of information (i.e., data elements):

- Patient history (including clinical notes, medication history, visit dates, lab results)
- Future appointments
- Clinical outcomes (e.g., what the goal is for this patient)
- Monitoring (e.g., frequency of labs)
- Patient-identified outcomes
- Task of formally creating the refill
- Task of formally approving the refill
- Cost and formulary coverage
- Communicating with support staff or the pharmacy

In addition, the display screens may be different for physicians, pharmacists, nurses, and other support personnel as well as for the patient. These usability issues can adversely affect a clinician's use of a system based upon how easy it is for him or her to use the system, if the system mirrors or is similar to current task behaviors, and how the system enhances patient safety and quality of care.

Systematic reviews on interactive health information systems show mixed methodological results. Summative studies comprise the majority of the research and address barriers to adoption issues (Peute, Spithoven, Bakker, & Jaspers, 2008). Formative usability studies fail to have a uniform format describing iterative development research (Peute et al., 2008). In one systematic review of 256 studies, the authors determined that few individual studies or collections of studies allowed readers to generalize a study's reported benefit (Shekelle, Morton, & Keeler, 2006).

O'Malley, Grossman, Cohen, Kemper, and Pham (2009) identified several issues in adoption and implementation. Although EMRs can facilitate care coordination within offices, they are less able to support coordination between clinicians and settings. This is due, in part, to current design and data element standardization problems. In addition, information overload is a challenge for clinicians because filters for data contained in EMRs are problematic. Further, there is a prevailing belief by clinicians that EMRs cannot do justice to the medical decision-making process, much less provide assistance in future care coordination (O'Malley et al., 2009).

However, in another scenario, the EHR is not problematic. Instead, it is seen as a single point of entry into a longitudinal review of a patient, with its history of

> patient demographics, progress notes, problems, medications, vital signs, past medical history, immunizations, laboratory data and radiology reports. The EHR automates and streamlines the clinician's workflow. The EHR has the ability to generate a complete record of a clinical patient encounter, as well as supporting other care-related activities directly or indirectly via interface, including evidence-based decision support, quality management, and outcomes reporting. (Healthcare Information and Management Systems Society [HIMSS], 2010, p. 1)

Exemplary Programs

With more than 1,300 facilities, the United States Veterans Administration (VA) is the largest healthcare system in the country, annually serving millions of veterans. An early adopter of technology, the VA began using computerized patient records in the mid-1990s. Today, its patient records system has expanded into an interoperable nationwide HIT system: the Veterans Health Information Systems and Technology Architecture (VistA). The VA is seen as an exemplary model for HIT implementation and quality of care (Kizer & Dudley, 2009). VistA has extensive capabilities for administrative and clinical work by providing, for example, patient records to VA healthcare workers 24/7, utilizing clinical reminders, and increasing coordination of care (http://www.virec.research.va.gov/DataSourcesName/VISTA/VISTAdocumentation.htm). A recent study comparing the quality of VA healthcare with that of care in a national sample demonstrated that the VA outperformed all other sectors of U.S. healthcare across 294 measures of quality in disease prevention and treatment (Asch et al., 2004).

The Department of Defense's military electronic health record, AHLTA, is found in over 100 U.S. military treatment facilities worldwide, ranging from hospitals to medical and dental clinics, with a daily average of 140,000 clinical encounters (Bohnsack, Parker, & Zheng, 2009). Operationalized in 2004, AHLTA helps provide coordination of care and benefits administration to over nine million military personnel and their families. Designed for healthcare practitioners, administrators, clerical, and support staff, the newest version of AHLTA includes a health assessment management tool, a tasking module that allows work flow to be assigned and tracked, and developmental tracking modules.

In 2009, a pilot program was started between the U.S. Department of Veterans Affairs, Kaiser Permanente, and the U.S. Department of Defense that will allow the exchange of EHR information utilizing the NHIN standards created by the U.S. Department of Health and Human Services (Kaiser/VA/DoD Partnership Piloting a Nationwide EHR Network, 2010).

Currently, the VA is creating a health data repository (HDR) with highly structured reference terminologies that will derive data from legacy systems, transaction-oriented systems, and free-text records into clinical decision-making protocols. The equivalent of the legal medical record, the HDR is compatible with the VA IT architecture. This is similar to the DoD AHLTA's clinical data repository (CDR) and health data dictionary (HDD), which uses commercially available products, a health data dictionary, and standardized medical terminology. This enables the capture of structured computable data (Benge, Beach, Gladding, & Maestas, 2008). AHLTA and VistA share data through the DoD/VA Bi-Directional Health Information Exchange (BHIE).

RECOMMENDATIONS

Trabin (2004) argues that the role of biostatistics and health informatics will evolve significantly based upon the financial and political support provided to the behavioral health field. This remains a very complex issue. It encompasses federal, state, and local rules and requirements as well as requirements, responses, and uses at the organizational and individual levels. Thus, any review must accommodate macro-, meso-, and microperspectives in framing problems as well as making recommendations. Three major areas must be addressed in suggested recommendations: (1) demonstration of a return on investment (ROI) for health information technology, (2) integration of primary and secondary health and mental health data, and (3) training and workforce development initiatives.

The Demonstration of an ROI for Health Information Technology

Clarification of the value of health information exchange is critical in terms of costs savings, improved efficiencies, and enhanced quality of care. However, clinicians may hesitate to adopt EHRs due to initial start-up costs, developmental funding, delays in ROI, and the difficulty of HIT as a sustainable business model (Balfour et al., 2009; eHealth Initiative, 2009). To avoid these issues, there need to be improved documentation and methodological designs of HIT studies. Shekelle and colleagues (2006) recommend more complete descriptions of both the intervention and the organizational and economic environment in which HIT is implemented. The eHealth Initiative (2009) suggests careful scrutiny of disbursement of funds and projects. Such scrutiny should lend itself to clear documentation of projects that are generalizable, are replicable across settings, and result in best practices, thereby encouraging adoption and implementation of HIT.

Organizations should be required to collaborate in standards development. The Nationwide Health Information Network (NHIN), for example, is a collection of standards, protocols, legal agreements, specifications, and services that enables the secure exchange of health information over the Internet. As part of the federal HIT Policy Committee, NHIN started development of HIT prototype architectures in 2004, developing specifications, services, and working constructs. HIMSS is a membership organization comparable to the National Information Standards Organization, which develops standards for the information industry. The stimulus legislation also establishes a Federal Coordinating Council for Comparative Effectiveness Research. The $1.1 billion-funded council will examine the effectiveness of pharmaceuticals and medical devices.

The authors suggest these groups examine ROI and HIT as part of their role in measuring and documenting improvements in healthcare. Further, the council should ensure that any review addresses HIT elements in the deliberation of appropriateness of care coordination from both the patient and clinician perspectives. Finally, behavioral health interventions are considered "soft" technology. We would recommend that studying behavioral health interventions be included in the council's scope of review.

As prototype architectures are developed, it is critical to consider the numerous types of practices in healthcare and behavioral healthcare, including practice groups and individual practitioners, large healthcare organizations, and local, state, and national healthcare systems. An HIT system designed for a hospital practice will not suit the needs of a solo practitioner. Work-flow processes and cognitive decision making may be mirrored in both small and large practices; however, the length of time to develop an HIT varies. Studies on usability and work-flow design can be completed more rapidly in small-scale practice settings and may have implications for scaling to larger group practices, hospitals, or health systems at a county, state, or national level. However, iterative process improvement and small-scale optimization are areas neglected in the literature and in healthcare and mental healthcare. Furthermore, there is a lack of agreement in the research literature on usability, process design, and scalability.

We suggest using summative evaluation to promote adoption and use, the use of formative evaluation research for design, and use of CER to identify technologies that are most likely to be effective in the future. For example, Peute and colleagues (2008) found that most usability studies addressed summative issues. Not only did formative usability studies lack uniformity in their description of results, but there was also little attempt to explain how the study improved a system's iterative development cycles. Further, whether or not a system is adopted depends upon the degree of its usability. The more complex the process being created is, the more important adoption, implementation, and sustainability concerns become.

By including usability at the beginning of the design process, the length of time for iterative system designs may shorten significantly, especially if insights into the clinical decision-making and outcomes process can be improved (Peute et al., 2008). Finally, because usability studies depend heavily upon qualitative methods to determine effectiveness and adoption, minimum guidelines should be implemented to ensure more consistency in qualitative usability studies. Such guidelines would have an emphasis on the end product of clinical performance.

Successful urban, rural, and frontier demonstration projects funded by CMS as well as other federal and national participants in HIT would show how to achieve improved quality of care, care coordination, and lower costs. Iterative projects in smaller practices are accomplished more quickly and more easily. Further, multiple small iterative projects, run in parallel, increase the possibility of successful design and outcomes and allow unsuccessful approaches to be discarded quickly in favor of new iterations and designs (Stead & Lin, 2009).

Balancing small-scale efforts with large-scale efforts seems the best path to show ROI to private, group, community-based, and system levels. This would provide opportunities for healthcare professionals and the healthcare industry to encourage further adoption of HIT in clinical practices, regardless of practice size or geographical location. The CMS and the Office of the Inspector General are revising existing regulations that may affect HIT adoption to remove barriers and encourage provider collaboration in the development of effective HIT systems.

Finally, defining a clear role for health information exchange in the phrase "meaningful use" is a step forward in having HIT seen as a core requirement for effective clinical practice. Currently, there is significant uncertainty as to what is "meaningful use," what steps are necessary to qualify for funds, and what impact there is for clinicians and staff. Stead and Lin (2009) suggest that the incentive should be placed upon clinical performance gains, rather than simply on the acquisition of technology.

There are numerous studies on adoption and implementation of HIT in clinical and community settings (Chaffee & Zimmerman, 2010; Chaudhry et al., 2006; Chen & Skinner, 2008; O'Malley et al., 2009; Wang et al., 2009; Wiljer et al., 2008); however, there are few studies on HIT acquisition processes and subsequent deployment of these systems. For example, changing operational processes is a key aspect for clinicians and staff to realize the potential that EMR has to facilitate the coordination of care. However, the focus for EMR use is on documenting billable events, such as office visits and procedures (O'Malley et al., 2009). We also suggest restructuring reimbursement models to recognize care coordination as a billable activity.

Integration of Primary and Secondary Health and Mental Health Data

Stead and Lin (2009) suggest that government actively encourage efforts to aggregate the numerous data sources with adequate safeguards and protections for patient privacy and confidentiality. Creating a national data infrastructure is not an allowable expense in current reimbursement schedules. Changing data aggregation to a priority and an allowable expense under reimbursement will help build the data infrastructure, which currently is highly fragmented and isolated. This will not happen quickly. Such an infrastructure requires time to establish a critical mass of private and public data, ensure data quality, and create core systems and work-flow processes to handle integrity in data transmission and receipt.

Another important component is the decoupling of data from software. Each software application has its own data formats, servers have their own transmission protocols, and organizations establish their priorities on working with data. One suggestion is to provide reimbursement for healthcare practices, organizations, and systems that are able to export data using homogeneous standards rather than numerous heterogeneous formats. For example, a hospital HIT may use the latest relational database management technology with all of the same hardware and software in all of its units. However, a solo practitioner may use older hardware and older versions of software of the same technology, which does not allow certain data collection activities, such as long text notes, or data export capacity without complex translation algorithms or protocols. With the work of the HIMSS and the NHIN to establish standard formats, guidelines for reimbursable data activities could be established.

From academic and research perspectives, the government should encourage transdisciplinary research that can lead to translational research, allowing innovative ways for examining and solving the complexity of clinical decision making in a computer-assisted environment. A translational perspective would provide new ways of visualizing and modeling healthcare work flows, rethinking scalability and distributive decision making, and how technology facilitates cognitive, performance, and work-flow practices of health practitioners, patients, and organizations. New languages to describe work roles and routines would assist researchers and developers to create care and coordination guidelines as well as new "inferential" systems that can abstract treatment suggestions based upon mapping patient information to clinical conditions.

Stead and Lin (2009) describe clinically oriented computer systems that can assist in differentiating clinically relevant information and uncertainty models that assist in cognitive understanding by the practitioner and reduce risk to patient care. In addition, these systems would have appropriate interfaces for the numerous audiences working in healthcare: healthcare practitioners, administrative staff, insurance companies, and patients, their caregivers, and their relatives. Each group would receive the relevant information in a usable format that may contain tables, graphs, text, and test results or images to increase the quality of care and improve patient and practice outcomes.

Training and Workforce Development

Changing work routines is more than just a matter of training on systems that promise cost savings and subsidies for adoption. It is critical that clinicians and support personnel be able easily to adapt and sustain work flows that integrate HIT. If the focus is on clinical performance gains rather than simple acquisition of HIT, then HIT automates current and redesigned work-flow processes that support the staff and workplace environment. This is particularly true in the shift from task-specific capabilities to more effective cognitive capability and decision making by healthcare personnel. The National Research Council suggests that standards oriented toward cognitive support and comprehension should be developed within the context of the work environment (Stead & Lin, 2009).

Increased adherence to guidelines or protocols, improved medication safety, and enhanced surveillance and monitoring using HIT can be effected through implementation assistance and technical assistance services to clinicians and support personnel (eHealth Initiative, 2009). Further, vendors should be required to supply healthcare IT systems that provide meaningful cognitive support for healthcare professionals. Practice is not always a strict, linear progression that follows the identical motivation, path, interaction, and information to the identical outcome by each and every practitioner in his or her decision-making process. Therefore, inherent differences in organizational work processes may demand divergent levels of formalization, especially in issues of scalability, transportability, and generalizability.

Education and training issues are vital from preservice and in-service perspectives. In addition to the traditional discipline areas, there will be a need to merge informatics with clinical care, administration, services delivery, and outcomes evaluation. Experts will be needed with comparable knowledge in informatics *and* in health and behavioral health services. Opportunities such as the National Institutes of Health career development programs and the National Library of Medicine informatics programs should be expanded to other academic institutions in the United States.

Recommendations for Solo Practitioners and Small Group Practices

For solo practitioners and small group practices or clinics, it is important to take time and determine what the critical elements are for an individual practice. There are literally hundreds of vendors that have EHR applications, ranging from "free" application to $50,000 fees. When selecting an HIT vendor, consider talking with a consultant funded by the CMS to determine the best solution for a practice. An HIT vendor will require a long-term partnership, so product, service, and standards/certifications (e.g., the Certification Commission for Health Information Technology, or CCHIT) are critical elements.

In automating a paper-based office, there are four key workflow areas to consider: office communication, patient contact process, patient–provider interaction, and medical records. For example, office communication among staff and to patients may move to increased electronic messaging. Scheduling appointments will no longer be done on paper calendars, but rather will be incorporated into an electronic calendar. This may require more than just a single dedicated scheduling workstation. Patient–provider interactions may still include handwritten notes, but the notes may be scanned and attached to the patient record or recoded into appropriate diagnostic or billing categories by the practitioner at the end of each session to facilitate patient departure at the service desk. The medical record may be modified to include scanned documents and e-mail notifications among staff and to patients. Clearly, it is not just a matter of incorporating new software but also of significant cultural changes in how work is accomplished by each member of the staff and among the members of the healthcare and mental healthcare practice.

It is critical to establish a realistic budget, a plan, and a team to address hardware, software, services, maintenance, and transition issues. EHRs for behavioral health may include templates for evaluation and progress notes, automated coding of E/M codes, and medication and prescription management tools, such as e-prescribing to generate prescriptions electronically and a laboratory request interface to track patient lab results. Other administrative features may include additional applications, such as patient scheduling, a quick-retrieval notes feature for use during patient appointments, and extensibility as new applications are created. Because it is unlikely that one can purchase a complete and ready solution that is perfect for a practice, keep in mind that one is selecting a partner, *not* a product, especially as EHR implementation may take 18 months or longer. In summary, it is recommended that one use functionality, usability, support, and costs as the criteria for reviewing EHRs.

It may also be a good strategy to speak with consultants, who can walk solo practitioners and small-group practitioners through over 300 EHRs currently on the market. Consultants range from Software Advice (www.softwareadvice.com), which matches health practitioners with vendors who focus in specialty areas, to BuyerZone (http://www.buyerzone.com), which focuses on the healthcare market.

In addition, the National Council for Community Behavioral Healthcare (http://www.thenationalcouncil.org/cs/consulting_referrals) provides consulting referrals in the area of EHRs and HIT. Organizations such as the American Psychiatric Association (http://www.psych.org/MainMenu/PsychiatricPractice/QualityImprovement/ElectronicHealthRecords.aspx) and the American Health Information Management Association (http://www.ahima.org/e-him/) provide practical guides to assist healthcare professionals in their transition to EHR systems (Amatayakul, 2009). In its buyer's guide for small medical practices, for example, the California HealthCare Foundation (http://www.chcf.org/) evaluated eight EHRs, ranging from good to better to best, based upon 15 key EHR functions identified in the report (Barrett, Holmes, & McAuley, 2003).

IMPLICATIONS FOR MENTAL HEALTH INFORMATICS

The President's New Freedom Commission on Mental Health (2003) concluded that the nation's mental health service delivery system is ill equipped to meet the complex needs of persons with serious mental illnesses. This service quality crisis is attributed to the long-standing divergence of research efforts and clinical programs, which is often between 15 and 20 years for actual implementation (President's New Freedom Commission on Mental Health, 2003). Further, the rapid change in health and mental health technology over the past decade has brought even more volatility to research and practice settings. Mental health services technologies, such as evidence-based practice, are considered "soft" technologies and are particularly vulnerable to problems with fidelity in implementation (Aarons, 2005) theoretically. This can be prevented with effective communication among the organizations, teams, or groups working with these technologies.

Currently, there is a lack of understanding and research related to factors critical for implementation, and organizational culture, structure, climate, and work attitudes are believed to affect the adoption of evidence-based practices and adherence to treatment protocols, which in turn affect therapeutic alliances and services delivery. Layers in health information technology and the challenges grow exponentially when considering the need to incorporate both the *context* and the *content* of care in a national, broad-based technology implementation. The approach to procedural development within mental healthcare settings is generally one of establishing a framework for accepted execution of tasks, a formal identification of task process, or an outline for operating requirements, policy, or modus operandi.

For organizations, practitioners, and patients to transition to a technology-intensive environment that will drive treatment and coordination of care in their decision making, there needs to be reflection on how decision making occurs, how practices work, and how to make the transition economically and organizationally feasible. This is critical in behavioral health, where numerous clinical, professional, and allied health professionals may comprise a team or be a part of a larger group of teams across governmental, organizational, agency, community, and home health and mental health settings. Thus, understanding the complexity of health technology adoption and implementation from numerous perspectives may lead to recommendations that, as a whole, provide insights into health and behavioral health practice, decision making, and patient–practitioner relationships from the individual practitioner and patient level to the national systems-wide and population-based level.

REFERENCES

Aarons, G. A. (2005). Measuring provider attitudes toward evidence-based practice: Consideration of organizational context and individual differences. *Child and Adolescent Psychiatric Clinics of North America, 14*(2), 255–271.

Amatayakul, M. K. (2009). *Electronic health records: A practical guide for professionals and organizations* (4th ed.). Chicago, IL: American Health Information Management Association.

American Recovery and Reinvestment Act (ARRA). (2009). Pub.L. 111-5. Retrieved from http://frwebgate.access.gpo.gov/cgi-bin/getdoc.cgi?dbname=111_cong_public_laws&docid=f:publ005.111

Armijo, D., McDonnell, C., & Werner, K. (2009). *Electronic health record usability: Evaluation and use case framework* (AHRQ Publication No. 09(10)-0091-1-EF). Rockville, MD: Agency for Healthcare Research and Quality. Retrieved from http://healthit.ahrq.gov/portal/server.pt/gateway/ PTARGS_0_1248_907504_0_0_18/09(10)-0091-1-EF.pdf

Asch, S. M., McGlynn, E. A., Hogan, M. M., Hayward, R. A., Shekelle, P., Rubenstein, L., et al. (2004). Comparison of quality of care for patients in the Veterans Health Administration and patients in a national sample. *Annals of Internal Medicine, 141*(12), 938–945.

Balfour, D. C., III, Evans, S., Januska, J., Lee, H. Y., Lewis, S. J., Nolan, S. R., et al. (2009). Health information technology: Results from a roundtable discussion. *Journal of Managed Care Pharmacy, 15*(1 Suppl A), 10–17. Retrieved from http://www.amcp.org/data/jmcp/Jan09a%20Suppl_S10-S17.pdf

Barrett, M. J., Holmes, B. J., & McAuley, S. E. (2003). *Electronic medical records: A buyer's guide for small physician practices* (ihealth reports). Oakland, CA: California HealthCare Foundation. Retrieved from http://www.chcf.org/~/media/Files/PDF/F/ForresterEMRBuyersGuideRevise.pdf

Benge, J., Beach, T., Gladding, C., & Maestas, G. (2008). Use of electronic health record structured text and its payoffs. The approach and barriers to using structured text in EHR to document care encounters. *Journal of Healthcare Information Management, 22*(1), 14–19.

Bohnsack, K. J., Parker, D. P., & Zheng, K. (2009). Quantifying temporal documentation patterns in clinician use of AHLTA-the DoD's ambulatory electronic health record. *AMIA... Annual Symposium Proceedings/AMIA Symposium. AMIA Symposium, 2009,* 50–54.

Campbell, E. M., Guappone, K. P., Sittig, D. F., Dykstra, R. H., & Ash, J. S. (2009). Computerized provider order entry adoption: Implications for clinical workflow. *Journal of General Internal Medicine, 24*(1), 21–26.

Campbell, E. M., Sittig, D. F., Guappone, K. P., Dykstra, R. H., & Ash, J. S. (2007). Overdependence on technology: An unintended adverse consequence of computerized provider order entry. *AMIA...Annual Symposium Proceedings/ AMIA Symposium. AMIA Symposium,* 94–98.

Centers for Medicare & Medicaid Services. (2010). *Federal Register, 75*(8), 1850–1870. Retrieved from http://edocket.access.gpo.gov/2010/pdf/E9-31217.pdf

Chaffee, B. W., & Zimmerman, C. R. (2010). Developing and implementing clinical decision support for use in a computerized prescriber-order-entry system. *American Journal of Health-System Pharmacy, 67*(5), 391–400.

Chaudhry, B., Wang, J., Wu, S., Maglione, M., Mojica, W., Roth, E., et al. (2006). Systematic review: Impact of health information technology on quality, efficiency, and costs of medical care. *Annals of Internal Medicine, 144*(10), 742–752.

Chen, L.-W., & Skinner, A. M. (2008). *Electronic health records adoption: Rural providers' decision-making process* (Rural Policy Brief No. 4). Omaha, NE: RUPRI Center for Rural Health Policy Analysis. Retrieved from http://www.unmc.edu/ruprihealth/Pubs/pb2008-4.pdf

Coons, S. J., Gwaltney, C. J., Hays, R. D., Lundy, J. J., Sloan, J. A., Revicki, D. A., et al. (2009). Recommendations on evidence needed to support measurement equivalence between electronic and paper-based patient-reported outcome (PRO) measures: ISPOR ePRO Good Research Practices Task Force report. *Value in Health: Journal of the International Society for Pharmacoeconomics and Outcomes Research, 12*(4), 419–429.

eHealth Initiative. (2009). *Migrating toward meaningful use: The state of health information exchange*. Washington, DC: eHealth Initiative. Retrieved from http://www.ehealth-initiative.org/sites/default/files/file/2009%20Survey%20Report%20FINAL.pdf

Fox, S. S., & Scherl, D. J. (1984). Recovering the past: Patient and family review of children's old mental health treatment records. *American Journal of Orthopsychiatry, 54*(2), 290–297.

Freer, C. B. (1980). Description of illness: Limitations and approaches. *Journal of Family Practice, 10*(5), 867–870.

Garg, A. X., Adhikari, N. K., McDonald, H., Rosas-Arellano, M. P., Devereaux, P. J., Beyene, J., et al. (2005). Effects of computerized clinical decision support systems on practitioner performance and patient outcomes: A systematic review. *Journal of the American Medical Association, 293*(10), 1223–1238.

Gask, L., Klinkman, M., Fortes, S., & Dowrick, C. (2008). Capturing complexity: The case for a new classification system for mental disorders in primary care. *European Psychiatry: Journal of the Association of European Psychiatrists, 23*(7), 469–476.

Greenfield, L., & Wolf-Branigin, M. (2009). Mental health indicator interaction in predicting substance abuse treatment outcomes in Nevada. *American Journal of Drug and Alcohol Abuse, 35*(5), 350–357.

Hanson, A., & Levin, B. L. (In press). The complexity of mental health services research data. In B. L. Levin, K. D. Hennessey, & J. Petrila (Eds.), *Mental health services: A public health perspective* (3rd ed.). New York, NY: Oxford University Press.

Healthcare Information and Management Systems Society (HIMSS). (2010). EHR: Electronic health record. Web site: URL http://www.himss.org/ASP/topics_ehr.asp

Health Information Portability and Accountability Act. (1996). Pub. L. No. 104-191. Retrieved from http://www.gpo.gov/fdsys/pkg/PLAW-104publ191/pdf/PLAW-104publ191.pdf

Hing, E., & Hsiao, C.-J. (2010). *Electronic medical record by office-based physicians and their practices: United States, 2007* (National Health Statistics Report No. 23). Hyattsville, MD: National Center for Health Statistics.

Jablensky, A. (1978). The need for standardization of psychiatric assessment. The epidemiological point of view. *Acta Psychiatrica Belgica, 78*(4), 549–558.

Jha, A. K., Ferris, T. G., Donelan, K., DesRoches, C., Shields, A., Rosenbaum, S. et al. (2006). How common are electronic health records in the United States? A summary of the evidence. *Health Affairs, 25*(6), 496–507.

Ji, S. Y., Smith, R., Huynh, T., & Najarian, K. (2009). A comparative analysis of multi-level computer-assisted decision-making systems for traumatic injuries. *BMC Medical Informatics and Decision-making, 9*, 2.

Jones, K. C. (2009 January). Obama wants e-health records in five years. *InformationWeek* [HTML]. Retrieved from http://www.informationweek.com/news/healthcare/showArticle.jhtml?articleID=212800199

Kaiser/VA/DoD partnership piloting a nationwide EHR network. (2010). *Healthcare Benchmarks and Quality Improvement, 17*(2), 13–15.

Khajouei, R., & Jaspers, M. W. (2008). CPOE system design aspects and their qualitative effect on usability. *Studies in Health Technology and Informatics, 136*, 309–314.

Kizer, K. W., & Dudley, R. A. (2009). Extreme makeover: Transformation of the veterans health care system. *Annual Review of Public Health, 30*, 313–339.

Krall, M. A., & Sittig, D. F. (2002). Clinicians' assessments of outpatient electronic medical record alert and reminder usability and usefulness requirements. *Proceedings of AMIA Symposium,* 400–404.

Leginski, W. A., & Croze, C. (1989). Data standards for mental decision support systems: A report of the Task Force to Revise the Data Content and System Guidelines of the Mental Health Statistics Improvement Program. Rockville, MD: U.S. Dept. of Health and Human Services, Public Health Service, Alcohol, Drug Abuse, and Mental Health Administration, National Institute of Mental Health.

Mental Health Statistics Improvement Program. (n.d.). *What is MHSIP?* Alexandria, VA: The Program. Retrieved from http://www.mhsip.org/whatis.html

Meredith, J. (2010). Electronic patient record evaluation in community mental health. *Informatics in Primary Care, 17*(4), 209–213.

Moller, H. J. (2005). Problems associated with the classification and diagnosis of psychiatric disorders. *World Journal of Biological Psychiatry: Official Journal of the World Federation of Societies of Biological Psychiatry, 6*(1), 45–56.

Mysore, N., Pluye, P., Grad, R. M., & Johnson-Lafleur, J. (2009). Tensions associated with the use of electronic knowledge resources within clinical decision-making processes: A multiple case study. *International Journal of Medical Informatics, 78*(5), 321–329.

National Institute of Mental Health. (1999). *Bridging science and service: A report by the National Advisory Mental Health Council Clinical Treatment and Services Research Workgroup.* Washington, DC: National Institute of Mental Health.

O'Malley, A. S., Grossman, J. M., Cohen, G. R., Kemper, N. M., & Pham, H. H. (2009). Are electronic medical records helpful for care coordination? Experiences of physician practices. *Journal of General Internal Medicine, 25*(3), 177–185.

Patton, R. E., & Leginski, W. A. (1983). *The design and content of a national mental health statistics system.* Rockville, MD: U.S. Dept. of Health and Human Services, Public Health Service, Alcohol, Drug Abuse, and Mental Health Administration, National Institute of Mental Health.

Peute, L. W., Spithoven, R., Bakker, P. J., & Jaspers, M. W. (2008). Usability studies on interactive health information systems; where do we stand? *Studies in Health Technology and Informatics, 136,* 327–332.

President's New Freedom Commission on Mental Health. (2003). *Achieving the promise: Transforming mental health care in America: Final report* (DHHS publication no. SMA-03-3832). Rockville, MD: President's New Freedom Commission on Mental Health. Retrieved from http://purl.access.gpo.gov/GPO/LPS36928

Shekelle, P. G., Morton, S. C., & Keeler, E. B. (2006). Costs and benefits of health information technology. *Evidence Report/Technology Assessment, 132,* 1–71.

Stead, W. W., & Lin, H. S. (2009). *Computational technology for effective health care: Immediate steps and strategic directions.* Washington, DC: The National Academies Press. Retrieved from http://www.nap.edu/catalog.php?record_id=12572

Trabin, T. (2004). *Burden and hope: The value of statistics and informatics in mental health.* Rockville, MD: Mental Health Statistics Improvement Program (MHSIP). Retrieved from http://www.mhsip.org/library/pdfFiles/burdenandhope.pdf

U.S. Department of Health and Human Services. (2010a). *Comparative effectiveness research funding.* Washington, DC: USDHHS. Retrieved from http://www.hhs.gov/recovery/programs/cer/

U.S. Department of Health and Human Services. (2010b). *Report to the President and the Congress on comparative effectiveness research.* Washington, DC: USDHHS. Retrieved from http://www.hhs.gov/recovery/programs/cer/exec-summary.html

U.S. House of Representatives Ways and Means Committee. (2009, January 16). Title IV—Health Information Technology for Economic and Clinical Health Act: Health Information Technology for Economic and Clinical Health (HITECH) Act. Vol. http://waysandmeans.house.gov/media/pdf/110/hit2.pdf

Walker, J. M. (2005). Usability. In J. M. Walker, E. J. Bieber, & F. Richards (Eds.), *Implementing an electronic health record system* (pp. 47–59). New York, NY: Springer.

Wang, P. S., Ulbricht, C. M., & Schoenbaum, M. (2009). Improving mental health treatments through comparative effectiveness research. *Health Affairs (Project Hope), 28*(3), 783–791.

Wiljer, D., Urowitz, S., Apatu, E., DeLenardo, C., Eysenbach, G., Harth, T., et al. (2008). Patient accessible electronic health records: exploring recommendations for successful implementation strategies. *Journal of Medical Internet Research, 10*(4), e34.

Five

E-health and Telehealth

ANTHONY PAPA AND CRISSA DRAPER

PROBLEMS IN MENTAL HEALTH DELIVERY IN THE UNITED STATES

There are significant challenges in delivering mental healthcare in the United States. Many people who would benefit from mental health treatment do not seek it due to cost or stigma or geographical barriers (Mojtabai, 2005, 2007). Others do not have access to appropriate mental health resources or information (Dumesnil & Verger, 2009). Many who do seek out treatment receive therapy that is not based on empirical research (e.g., Lovell & Richards, 2000; Westen, 2005). Moreover, the logistics of delivering empirically based practices via traditional delivery systems (i.e., clinic/practice-based face-to-face services) do not add up because the number of people who would benefit from treatment for mental illness far outstrips the number of practitioners offering empirically based services (e.g., Westen, 2005). Given this, there is an enormous demand for interventions that are less resource intensive, less stigmatizing, and more widely accessible (Schopp, Demiris, & Glueckauf, 2006).

One solution to these difficulties is the systematic integration of e-health and telehealth into the mental health delivery practice. While the use of these interventions has limitations, integrating e-health and telehealth has the potential to deliver empirically based care that obviates many barriers to seeking care by providing a safe and anonymous environment for people who do not seek treatment due to stigma, by allowing practitioners to treat more patients with less face-to-face time, by providing access to those who cannot otherwise access treatment due to geographical limitations or physical disability, or by providing affordable care for those who do not seek mental healthcare due to cost. It can even help individuals who just cannot take an hour out of their day plus the time needed to drive across town, park, wait, and then spend an hour face to face with a therapist before being able to get back to their car and drive back to work.

E-health, particularly, has the potential to promote the use and dissemination of evidence-based practice. A growing literature now suggests that empirically based interventions for problems ranging from depression to posttraumatic stress disorder (PTSD) to trichotillomania potentially could be delivered via the Internet to people anywhere (Christensen, Griffiths, & Jorm, 2004; Litz, Engel, Bryant, & Papa, 2007; O'Donohue, & Draper, 2010; Mouton-Odum, Keuthen, Wagener, Stanley, & DeBakey, 2006). With such programs, individuals comfortable with seeking therapy in this type of environment could potentially take their "therapist" with them on a weekend getaway for little to no cost. Moreover, adjunctive use of empirically based e-health programs can potentially be used as a training tool for practitioners looking to learn new or better therapies (Draper, Hall, & O'Donohue, 2008; Marks, Cavanagh, & Gega, 2007). This chapter will look at e-health and telehealth and the potential of these different ways of delivering therapy to address many difficulties that our current healthcare system faces.

WHAT ARE E-HEALTH AND TELEHEALTH?

Given the myriad difficulties in getting evidence-based care to those who need it, and in getting those who need mental healthcare to engage in treatment, new approaches for expanding access to and delivery of mental health treatments are emerging. Telehealth mainly refers to use of telephone or videoconferencing technology for treatment or assessment of patients in remote areas or in need of specialized attention. It also potentially involves using this technology for the training and supervision of therapists. This could include the use of mobile devices or short message service (SMS) text messaging as adjunctive, aftercare, or self-monitoring tools (e.g., Bauer, de Niet, Timman, & Kordy, 2010). E-health treatments involve such approaches as cognitive-behavioral therapy (CBT) delivered via a specially designed Web site, e-mail, or a CD-ROM.

For example, Wagner, Knaevelsrud, & Maercker (2005, 2006) report the use of a therapist-interactive, e-mail-based therapeutic writing intervention for those who experienced mostly traumatic loss and who evidenced critical levels of posttraumatic stress symptoms. The intervention had large effect sizes on the brief symptom inventory depression subscale ($d = 1.74$ from pre- to posttreatment, $d = 1.27$ from pretreatment to 3-month follow-up, and $d = 1.96$ from pretreatment to 1.5-year follow-up), the impact of events scale intrusion ($d = 1.52$ from pre- to post-t, $d = 1.63$ from pre- to 3-month follow-up, and $d = 1.96$ from pre- to 1.5-year follow-up), and avoidance scales ($d = 1.25$ from pre- to post-t, $d = 1.26$ from pre- to 3-month follow-up, and $d = 1.53$ from pre- to 1.5-year follow-up) (see Wagner & Maercker, 2007).

Of those surveyed, 83% rated the contact as personal, 73% did not miss face-to-face contact, and 85% found that contact exclusively by e-mail was pleasant (Wagner et al., 2006). Similar ratings for the quality of the therapeutic alliance were found when this protocol was applied to the treatment of PTSD (Knaevelsrud & Maercker, 2007). Moreover, this study found that working alliance ratings by therapists and patients on the working alliance inventory (Horvath & Greenberg, 1989) were high and inversely related to outcomes on symptom measures. E-health treatments can be completely self-guided or completed with a professional. However, for the most part, they are designed to be minimal therapist contact, self-management approaches where a therapist may monitor and guide a patient at various intervals—on the phone, in person, or via e-mail. However, in between meetings, the patient is largely responsible for his or her own progress.

These treatment delivery options have several potential advantages over face-to-face therapies. Given that many people do not seek treatment or delay treatment for over a decade (Hoge, Auchterlonie, & Milliken, 2006; Lovell & Richards, 2000; Wang, Berglund, et al., 2005; Wang, Lane, et al. 2005), the Internet, videoconferencing technology, and e-mail can provide ready access to mental health information and treatment to underserved populations and those who may not have the resources, access, or inclination to seek specialty care (e.g., Glueckauf, Pickett, Ketterson, Loomis, & Rozensky, 2003; Kenwright, Marks, Gega, & Mataix-Cols, 2004; Lorig & Holman, 2003; Luce, Winzelberg, Zabinski, & Osborne, 2003; Ritterband et al., 2003). The greater privacy and convenience of accessing an intervention from one's home is particularly beneficial for those who believe that a social stigma is associated with visiting a therapist, those with busy schedules, or those who are homebound, disabled, or without readily available or reliable transportation (e.g., Heckman et al., 2004; McKay et al., 2004).

The added benefits are that self-disclosure can be facilitated by the anonymity of the computer (Barak & Gluck-Ofri, 2007; Joinson, 1999, 2001, 2004). In addition, telephone- and Internet-delivered therapy may be more cost effective than traditional face-to-face therapy (Griffiths & Christensen, 2007; Vergara Rojax & Gagnon, 2008). Development and equipment costs can be significant, but access can be widely disseminated, ameliorating the cost per user.

Another benefit for therapist-supported treatment delivered by Internet or computer is that it requires less professional time because therapists' commitment usually involves ad hoc support for emergencies or implementation questions, monitoring user progress and symptoms, and/or brief check-ins. In addition, developing a standardized Internet delivery mechanism for treatments can allow a much greater number of individuals to receive standardized, evidence-based interventions. This ability to deliver standardized, evidence-based interventions widely is an important strength of this modality because evidence-based treatment methods are not widely used outside specialty clinics and research settings (e.g., Rosen et al., 2004), despite often being rated as the most credible and desirable treatment (Zoellner, Feeny, Cochran, & Pruitt, 2003). For example, despite the Institute of Medicine's (2008) report that exposure therapy is the strongest evidence-based treatment for PTSD, only 17% of psychologists who treat psychological trauma report using exposure therapy for PTSD, though 56% reported training in the technique (Becker, Zayfert, & Anderson, 2004).

A number of professional barriers to implementing specialty care exist, including a lack of training and supervision, a lack of familiarity or comfort with systematic treatment procedures, and beliefs that using delineated treatment plans is too mechanistic and may be overly intrusive and invasive (Astin & Rothbaum, 2000). These are obstacles that an Internet-based self-management intervention can ameliorate. For example, DESTRESS (https://www.destresstraining.org/) is a self-guided, Internet-based CBT program for PTSD that was designed to help users manage their reactions to stimuli that trigger recall of traumatic experiences using a skills-building approach. Skills taught include stress management strategies and self-monitoring, among others, and users are guided in graduated in vivo exposure exercises to practice these skills (Litz et al., 2007).

In an 8-week, randomized controlled trial, military service members with PTSD were assigned to either DESTRESS or an Internet-delivered, nondirective, supportive counseling program. Results indicated that participants in DESTRESS had greater reductions in PTSD (d =.95), depression (d =1.03), and anxiety symptoms (d =1.01) at 6-month follow-up than the supportive counseling condition. In terms of clinically significant change, a greater percentage of those in the DESTRESS group than those in the supportive counseling condition no longer met criteria for PTSD (25 vs. 3%) and could be classified as high-end state functioning (25 vs. 0%; Beck depression inventory-II and Beck anxiety inventory scores < 12 and PTSD symptom scale-interview version scores < 6). The intervention was well tolerated and the dropout rate was similar to that of face-to-face therapy. This intervention has since been standardized and is being further tested in a variety of settings, including as an adjunctive service in a primary healthcare setting to access the large population of returning combat veterans.

Given an unmet demand for empirically validated treatments, the promise of minimal contact therapies to make mental healthcare widely accessible has made them a hot research topic in healthcare policy (e.g., Marks & Cavanagh, 2009), and evidence is accumulating to support the efficacy of these interventions in multiple domains (e.g., Lange, Van de Ven, & Schrieken, 2003; Litz et al., 2007; Cuijpers et al., 2009). In the medical field, self-management interventions have been found to be an effective means to aid in management of chronic health conditions such as diabetes, cardiovascular disease, stroke, arthritis, and asthma (e.g., Dodge, Janz, & Clark, 2002; Lorig et al., 1999, 2001; Lorig & Holman, 2003; Lorig, Ritter, Villa, & Armas, 2009). Integration of these interventions into standard medical care for chronic illness has been associated with improvements that include improved health status as well as lower healthcare costs via reduction in service utilization and intensity of care (e.g., Bodenheimer, Lorig, Holman, & Grumbach, 2002; Wheeler, 2003).

One of the main barriers to integration of self-management programs has been lack of training in provision of self-management programs (Bodenheimer et al., 2002). Self-management programs delivered via the Internet have demonstrated similar benefits in terms of lowered healthcare utilization and overall cost of management of illness, but also obviate the need for extra staff or training to provided self-management education and follow-up (e.g., Lorig et al., 2008, 2010; Lorig, Ritter, Laurent, & Plant, 2006, 2008). In the mental health field, Internet self-management has demonstrated initial efficacy as a secondary prevention (Kenardy, McCafferty, & Rosa, 2003) and tertiary intervention for anxiety disorders (Newman, Erikson, Przeworski, & Dzus, 2003).

For example, a 10-session Internet-based treatment of panic disorder with therapist support via e-mail was as effective as an equivalent 10-session in-person CBT (Calbring, 2005). Internet-delivered prevention has also been demonstrated to be as effective as a group therapy in reducing risk for body image dissatisfaction in eating disorders (e.g., Celio et al., 2000; see also Luce et al., 2003) and a viable method of providing standardized, evidenced-based, self-management treatment for depression (Christensen et al., 2004), panic and phobic disorders (e.g., Schneider, Mataix-Cols, Marks, & Bachofen, 2005), chronic headaches (e.g., Devineni & Blanchard, 2005), and PTSD (Lange, Rietdijk, et al., 2003; Litz et al., 2007).

Cuijpers and colleagues' (2009) meta-analysis of the efficacy of computer-aided therapy looked at 13 randomized controlled trials for anxiety that compared a computer-based delivery of treatment (Internet based, computer based—i.e., DVDs, etc.— and handheld/palmtop based) to face-to-face therapy and found that treatment effects did not differ between groups and that dropout rates did not differ (see also Reger & Gahm, 2009, for similar findings). A comparison of effects sizes in an additional meta-analysis of 23 studies of computer-aided treatment for anxiety found no difference between self-guided therapies and face-to-face treatment at posttreatment or follow-up (Cuijpers et al., in press).

Looking at 12 studies of only Internet-delivered treatment for depression and anxiety, Spek et al. (2007) found that Internet-based interventions showed different levels of efficacy based on diagnosis (anxiety > depression), focus (tertiary interventions > primary prevention), and therapist involvement (therapist assisted > nonassisted). Barak, Hen, Boniel-Nissim, and Shapira's (2008) review suggested that computer-based treatment is more effective for some disorders than for others (see also Griffiths, Farrer, & Christensen, 2010, and Newton & Ciliska, 2006) and that the effects of treatments may be influenced by factors like interface design and access, symptoms and therapeutic goals targeted (psychoeducation, behavior, cognition, etc.), type of therapist contact (audio, e-mail, chat, etc.), and age of users—in addition to timing of therapist contact (Kenwright et al., 2005) and quality of therapeutic alliance (Knaevelsrud & Maercker, 2007).

These initial findings are promising, but research on the effectiveness of computer-based interventions is still in its infancy. Being able to draw strong conclusions based on the meta-analyses described earlier has been hampered by the limited amount of research, small sample sizes in studies, lack of independent verification, lack of consistent inclusion criteria, and unblinded assessment found in many of the studies included in these analyses (see Marks et al., 2009, for detailed discussion). This is despite the fact that the medium allows for strong research designs.

E-health sites have several advantages to traditional psychotherapy research. First, tight internal control easily lends itself to component studies, studies on dosing effects, order effects, or on identifying moderators and mediators. Researchers do not have to be concerned with fidelity or training issues that come with face-to-face therapist interactions or allocating the time and resources for large-scale randomized controlled trials. In addition, e-health programs have excellent external validity; they can be tested in the exact form in which they would be delivered in the real world. Despite the research possibilities inherent within the medium and initial findings of efficacy, lack of targeted funding in the area has limited development mainly to small-scale studies.

An area that has seen a strong resurgence in interest has been telehealth, given the growing affordability and reliability of videoconferencing technology. Historically, controlled effectiveness research was sparse and plagued by small sample sizes, but the last few years have shown a rapid increase in well-controlled studies favorably comparing the efficacy of psychotherapy delivered face-to-face to therapy delivered via videoconferencing technology. In these studies, psychotherapy delivered via videoconferencing has been found to demonstrate similar levels of efficacy for the treatment of PTSD (Frueh et al., 2007; Germain, Marchand, Bouchard, Drouin, & Guay, 2009), panic disorder (Bouchard et al., 2004), substance use (Frueh, Henderson, & Myrick, 2005; McKay et al., 2004), depression (e.g., Elliott, Brossart, Berry, & Fine, 2008; Nelson, Barnard, & Cain, 2006; Ruskin et al., 2004), insomnia (Bastien, Morin, Ouellet, Blais, & Bouchard, 2004), and mixed outpatient populations (Day & Schneider, 2002; O'Reilly et al., 2007). A significant body of case studies and single case designs supports the utility of videoconferencing-delivered therapy for PTSD from motor vehicle accident (Hassija & Gray, 2009), bulimia (Bakke, Mitchell, Wonderlich, & Erickson, 2001; Simpson et al., 2006), and obsessive-compulsive disorder (Himle et al., 2006).

Use of videoconferencing technology is a cost-effective and easily tolerated means for neuropsychological and psychiatric assessment (e.g., Baer, Brown-Beasley, Sorce, & Henriques, 1993; Baer et al., 1993; Glueckauf, Ketterson, Loomis, & Dages, 2004; Greist, 1998; Hildebrand, Chow, Williams, Nelson, & Wass, 2004; Hockey, Yellowlees, & Murphy, 2004), providing follow-up care (Mermelstein, Hedeker, & Wong, 2003), and supervision and training of therapists (e.g., Heckner & Giard, 2005; Hilty et al., 2006; Walter, Rosenquist, & Bawtinhimer, 2004). As a result it has been increasingly adopted by the Federal Bureau of Prisons (e.g., Magaletta, Fagan, & Ax, 1998) and the U.S. Veterans Administration in order to provide specialty care and assessment for geographically remote patients (e.g., Godleski, Nieves, Darkins, & Lehmann, 2008; Tuerk, Yoder, Ruggerio, Gross, & Acierno, 2010). It also has been used to access rural Native American populations (e.g., Oliveira et al., 2006; Savin, Garry, Zuccaro, & Novins, 2006), as well as populations in remote northern Canada (e.g., Crossley, Morgan, Lanting, Bellow-Haas, & Kirk, 2008; O'Reilly et al., 2007).

HOW DO E-HEALTH AND TELEHEALTH ADD TO OUR CURRENT HEALTHCARE SYSTEM?

Stepped Care and Adjunctive Services

Given evidence that telehealth and e-health can be effective interventions for certain disorders for many people and that traditional face-to-face empirically supported treatments do not work for everyone (see Davison, 2000; Newman, 2000), an important use of e-health and telehealth interventions can be as adjunctive therapies, possibly to increase the efficacy of face-to-face protocols for nonresponders or as one of the first modalities in a stepped-care model for treatment designed to reduce the need for therapist contact hours. For example, Greist et al. (2002) found that 62% of participants assigned to a telephone-based, computer-guided interactive treatment for OCD were responsive to treatment and those who did not respond were helped by subsequent face-to-face therapy, reducing the total number of therapist direct contact hours necessary to achieve positive outcomes across the study sample.

Stepped care is a model in which individuals are provided a continuum of care intensities based on severity of presentation. Given that the majority of individuals who need mental healthcare can be successfully treated with low-intensity care and only a small volume of individuals need intensive treatment (e.g., Gellatly et al., 2007; Katon et al., 1999), stepped care is designed so that individuals start at the lowest level of intensity of care feasible for the given presentation and move to a more intensive level of care (in cost, time, professional expertise, or other resources) in the event that the lower level is not effective for the individual (see Bower & Gilbody, 2005, and O'Donohue & Draper, 2010, for reviews).

In this model, triage weighs the balance between the least restrictive therapy and the therapy most likely to help an individual, making it a time- and cost-efficient model to meet mental healthcare needs (Bower & Gilbody, 2005; Espie, 2009). For example, a stepped-care model providing CBT for insomnia (Espie, 2009) may start with self-management options delivered by book, CD and DVD, or Internet, and followed by group therapies. Only then does it move to the traditional face-to-face, 1 hour per week session model with paraprofessionals; an individual moves up to individual treatment with a specialist only as needed. These face-to-face therapies can be delivered via videoconferencing technology as feasible. For other mental health needs, steps may include watchful waiting such as is necessary for the recently bereaved (Papa & Litz, in press) and may include inpatient treatments.

Marks et al. (2003) created a free clinic consisting of four different, previously validated computer-delivered, therapist-supported and -monitored therapies to address phobias, panic, depression, general anxiety, and obsessive-compulsive disorder in a major metropolitan area. Patients were referred by local primary care and mental health clinics where approximately 50% received face-to-face treatment in addition to participating in the e-clinic. This had an overall effect of reducing waiting lists for most of the referral sources by providing those with lower levels of severity adequate care and allowing therapist resources to be devoted to those in the greatest need. The clinic employed the equivalent of one full-time therapist and was open for 15 months. This full-time therapist-equivalent addressed 335 referrals during this time period; of those referred for treatment within the clinic, the full-time therapist-equivalent had an average of 1 hour of patient contact after a 30-minute screening.

Contrast this to an average of 50 referrals per year per therapist for a typical CBT clinic with 8 hours of patient contact per 12-week period. Of the 210 who were offered services, 42 (20%) refused computer-based therapy, highlighting the potential need to embed these therapies within a stepped-care model. It should be noted that the e-clinic was free and the cost of face-to-face therapies was not reported, suggesting that, in some cases, participants could have chosen e-health out of cost consciousness alone. In addition, of the 210 individuals offered services, an additional 60 (29%) dropped out during service provision or did not give follow-up data (a percentage comparable to face-to-face CBT; see Bados, Balaguer, & Saldaña, 2007; Hembree et al., 2003) and 108 completed treatment and provided outcome data. On the whole, users of the clinic were mainly satisfied with their experience and treatments had medium to large effects on outcomes across outcome indices.

In addition to reducing the demand for therapist time, inclusion of e-health within a stepped-care model also has the potential to allow the provision of an increased range of specialized services and thus the development of more tailored individualized treatment plans for more people in need (see Green & Iverson, 2009; Lovell & Richards, 2000). Indeed, allowing the option of minimal contact therapies within an integrated-care delivery model has the potential to impact the whole process of provision of services.

This can range from allowing wait list clients to begin supportive services immediately, giving therapists access to closer monitoring of changes in symptom levels in wait list groups (as well as ongoing patients), and providing support for face-to-face therapy by allowing attending therapists to provide specialized adjunctive treatments that they may not have the requisite expertise to provide to potentially increasing compliance with homework assignments because these technologies can provide a more interactive experience between sessions (Green & Iverson, 2009; Williams & Martinez, 2008). Finally, use of minimal contact therapies in a stepped-care approach has the potential to provide an initial positive experience for those reluctant to engage in traditional forms of psychotherapy as well as increase the likelihood of engaging in more intensive treatments as needed (e.g., Draper & Papa, in preparation).

Reducing Barriers to Seeking Treatment

Over a quarter of the population of the United States is estimated to suffer from some form of diagnosable mental illness in a given year (National Institute of Mental Health, 2008). Of these, an overwhelming number never seek treatment; numbers of those not seeking or receiving treatment range from about 50%, (Kohn, Saxena, Levav, & Saraceno, 2004) to over 60% (Kessler et al., 2001). Those who do seek treatment generally wait over a decade before their first appointment and typically consist of the most severe cases (Carragher, Adamson, Bunting, & McCann, 2010; Wang, Berglund et al., 2005).

This finding is attributed to various reasons, but fear of social stigma is a primary one (Brown et al., 2010; Carragher et al., 2010; Raylu, Oei, & Loo, 2008). However, as noted previously, seeking treatment through technological means may overcome stigma as a barrier to care. Many have postulated that the anonymity and portability provided by these types of treatment may minimize fears of social stigma, thereby increasing individuals to seek treatment (Green & Iverson, 2009; Heckman et al., 2004; Young, 2005). While few studies have directly tested this face-valid claim, there is evidence that the anonymity of the computer facilitates self-disclosure (Joinson, 1999, 2001, 2004) and that people tend to be more honest or more willing to endorse stigmatizing behaviors in computer-based assessments (Gribble et al., 2000).

Preliminary data from the authors of this chapter suggest a significant increase in willingness to seek treatment when e-health is presented as an option. This finding is consistent with evidence that the ability to utilize an Internet intervention at home helps increase utilization of face-to-face care (e.g., Glueckauf et al., 2003; Kenwright et al., 2004; Lorig & Holman, 2003; Luce et al., 2003; Ritterband et al., 2003).

Expanding Access to Care

Approximately 50 million people in the United States currently live in rural areas (USDA Economic Research Service, 2008). Individuals in rural populations are less likely to have health insurance, are likely to stay uninsured for longer periods of time, and are more likely to suffer from chronic disorders with behavioral health components, such as heart disease and diabetes (Kaiser Commission on Key Facts, 2003). Moreover, people living in rural areas are up to 53% less likely than those in metropolitan areas to access mental health services, even though individuals in these settings are found more commonly to suffer from mental health difficulties (Hauenstein et al., 2007).

This may in part be due to stigma, but an insufficient number of rural practitioners represents a significant barrier to accessing mental healthcare for individuals with mental health issues in rural settings (American Psychological Association, 2010).

Limited mental health resources in rural areas may mean that, even when mental health resources are available, specialized care may not be available for all disorders (Schopp et al., 2006; American Psychological Association, 2010). In these cases, telehealth and e-health have the potential to provide specialized services as the primary means to deliver care to remote persons in areas where specialized care is unavailable (Green & Iverson, 2009; Griffiths & Christensen, 2007; Hauenstein et al., 2007; Jackson et al., 2007). For example, empirically based treatment is available via the Internet for trichotilomania (Mouton-Odum et al., 2006) or tinnitus (Andersson & Kaldo, 2004). Furthermore, use of these technologies can provide training for rural practitioners faced with a case outside the scope of their training or experience (e.g., Oliveira et al., 2006).

For example, studies have indicated that individuals returning to the United States after serving in the military in Iraq and Afghanistan evidence substantial mental health problems, including depression, substance abuse, and PTSD, that are associated with substantial functional impairments and social costs (Hoge et al., 2006; Wright et al., 2009). The Veterans Administration, tasked with providing care for this large, widely scattered population, has increasingly turned to e-health and telehealth to meet this need. Morland and colleagues (2010) recently found that a treatment protocol for PTSD-related anger delivered to veterans via videoconferencing technology was equivalent to the same therapy delivered in face-to-face therapy in a randomized clinical trial.

Tuerk and colleagues (2010) report a pilot study in which prolonged exposure therapy for PTSD was effectively delivered to veterans at rural VA satellite clinics via videoconferencing technology. As Hassija and Gray (2009) noted in their successful case study providing exposure therapy for a rural individual with PTSD, "When these technologies are provided to connect rural clients with distant specialists, the relevant comparison is not telehealth services relative to traditional face-to-face service. The relevant comparison is telehealth services relative to no services at all" (p. 93). This is true for any population that does not currently have access to treatment. Although the long-distance treatments discussed generally have success on par with face-to-face services, it is important to recall this distinction when analyzing results of long-distance therapies for people who would otherwise have nothing.

Beyond access difficulties for rural populations, other populations may also have barriers to seeking care related to issues such as lack of transportation or childcare, or other logistical reasons (i.e., McKay et al., 2004). For example, those experiencing disability might find it difficult to make it across town, find handicapped parking, and/or sit in a waiting room before then having to sit in the consulting room for an hour. These practical barriers may be heightened for the newly disabled, who might still be adjusting to new limitations, and put them at high risk for experiencing mental health difficulties as well as in a position whereby accessing psychotherapy in a traditional sense could be daunting. In all cases, the use of technology within the mental health delivery system can provide part of the solution for providing individuals the help they may need.

Reducing Cost

In a typical outpatient center, full-time psychotherapists may be expected to have 30 or more hours of direct clinical contact per week. Based on our experience with a Web site designed to provide therapist-supported and -monitored self-exposure for PTSD, it requires a psychotherapist about 2 hours per day to monitor, follow up, and respond to a running "caseload" of 30–40 intervention users, leaving approximately 30 hours per week for other duties; this represents the potential for significant cost savings. Few studies have reported the actual cost benefits associated with the use of minimal-contact therapies. Those that do note that these technologies require a number of up-front costs that can reduce the potential savings, such as fees for licensing or hosting Internet-delivered treatment on HIPAA-compliant servers and the need to buy video conferencing equipment or computers (e.g., Marks et al., 2003, reviewed previously).

Another is the potential need to pay computer programmers to develop interventions as well as design secure portals to access these treatments. This is particularly important as quality and usability of Internet-based interventions are not often assessed or maximized for the target population, but these extratherapeutic factors may significantly affect therapeutic efficacy (e.g., Bellazzi, Montani, Riva, & Stefanelli, 2001; Demiris, Finkelstein, & Speedie, 2001). On the whole, though, the cost minimization potential in the use of these technologies is based on a financial model that includes higher up-front variable costs but lower fixed costs over time. Profitability increases based on virtually unlimited potential throughput in service provision after the upfront costs are offset, as opposed to face-to-face therapy with high, constant fixed costs and limitations on how many services can be provided.

Given the number of potential mediators of the effectiveness of e-health interventions (e.g., Barak et al., 2008), the variability in effectiveness of e-health interventions (e.g., Spek et al., 2007), and lack of computer expertise in mental health professionals, along with the easy proliferation and distribution of e-health content, it is necessary to use the services of professional Web developers in the development and validation of computer-based interfaces. It is particularly important to complete development within a formative evaluation framework that includes a strong participatory design focus (i.e., Carter, Buckey, Greenhalgh, Holland, & Hegel 2005; Darin & Kurniawan, 2000; Flagg, 1990; Furstenberg, Carter, Henderson, & Ahles, 2002). This involves developing prototypes, eliciting feedback from experts and target users, and implementing changes. This iterative testing and refinement of intervention interfaces focuses on (1) readability, (2) usability, (3) credibility, and (4) functionality:

- Readability refers to two issues. First, is the text presented accessible to potential users with lesser reading skill but still engaging to those who are better educated? The second is related to reading text on a computer screen. For example, font size is an important consideration for older adults in Web-based utilities (Darin & Kurniawan, 2000; Demiris et al., 2001). One solution in text-heavy protocols is to provide connections to printer-friendly pages. Another is to embed voice-over audio so that users have the option to listen rather than read information.
- Usability refers to whether or not participants find the Internet interface intuitive and easy to navigate. As noted, the effectiveness of Internet interventions may also be dependent on the users' perceptions about the expertise of the developers, which is, in part, based on the content.
- Credibility may directly affect expectancies of change and significantly influence responsiveness to treatment (see Carlbring et al., 2005; Kenardy et al., 2003).
- Functionality refers to whether the software portions of the program are sufficiently developed and flexible enough to deliver the intervention effectively, do not require extensive therapist support to communicate

ideas and skills, allow for easy and immediate access to and reporting of individual user data for monitoring therapists, can provide sufficient alerts if a user indicates need of immediate clinical attention, and (related to clinical monitoring) allow for easy data capture and integration with statistical software for evaluation purposes.

While this process may be necessary to ensure that any e-health program is maximally effective, too often it is not done because it can be expensive in terms of time and overall development costs.

These up-front costs represent a significant limitation for the development and dissemination of these therapies; as a result, development and implementation of these therapies within clinic settings remain largely dependent on federally funded grant programs that can assist with the costs of development (e.g., NIMH) or implementation (e.g., congressionally mandated health information technology grants, telehealth resource center grants, telehealth network grants). However, the combination of demand and academic researchers' lack of access to capital investment is an opportunity for entrepreneurs (e.g., meyouhealth.com, New England Research Institutes, archimageonline.com, prochange.com, rippleeffects.com) because these costs are minimal compared to start-up costs of many businesses and can be further offset with small business innovation research program/small business technology transfer grant support (see http://grants.nih.gov/grants/funding/sbir.htm).

Other ways to reduce the up-front costs of development include the creation of new tools that make creating such sites relatively inexpensive and easy even for people without extensive computer training. For example, LifeGuide, a program developed in the UK, provides people with a user-friendly Web-building tool geared specifically to the needs of the mental health field (e.g., allowing easily created forms that gather data, generating tailored information to clients in the form of skip logic, and integrating automated text messages for generalizability). This may assist in reducing programming costs during development (Hare et al., 2009).

In addition to costs associated with programming and formative evaluation, other costs may add to the overall bottom line in widely integrating e-health programs in mental health delivery. The Food and Drug Administration (FDA) considers software used for the diagnosis or treatment of a medical disorder to fall under its regulatory mandate under the Federal Food, Drug and Cosmetic Act (FDAC; see also FDA Center for Device and Radiological Health [CDRH] White Paper on Telemedicine-Related Activities, 1996). As such, the FDA requires premarket notification, scientific review by a panel of experts and subsequent approval, and postmarket data collection, reporting, and monitoring (www.fda.gov/RegulatoryInformation/Legislation/FederalFoodDrugandCosmeticActFDCAct/SignificantAmendmentstotheFDCAct/FDAMA/FullTextofFDAMAlaw/default.htm) (FDA, 1997).

While the up-front costs can be somewhat daunting, the potential for Internet and telehealth interventions to reach a large number of people can ameliorate the per-patient cost as the number of users increases. Again, as with efficacy data for Internet-based therapies, few studies have reported the actual costs of providing treatment. One of the few examples is Marks et al. (2003), which was reported earlier. After factoring in overheads and licensing costs for the Internet-based therapies, Marks and colleagues estimated a 15% savings per patient for 350 patients and estimated that the savings would have risen to 41% at 1,350 patents.

Kaltenthaler and colleagues' 2006 review of 20 studies reporting cost effectiveness of mainly CD-ROM-based interventions—that is, "Beating the Blues" (Proudfoot et al., 2004), "Cope" (Gega, Marks, & Mataix-Cols, 2004), "Overcoming Depression" (Whitfield, Hinshelwood, Pashely, Campsie, & Williams, 2006), "Fear Fighter" (Hayward, MacGregor, Peck, & Wilkes, 2007), and "BT Steps" (Marks et al., 1998)—concluded that the costs of computerized therapy versus treatment as usual was equivocal, based on the uncertainty that a typical clinic would have sufficient patient throughput to ameliorate these costs. However, this conclusion was based on existing licensing structures that charged a licensing fee per clinic site for a CD-ROM.

The licensing fee and throughput ratio can be much more favorable for Internet-delivered therapies. Sites like MoodGym have done cost analyses to show that their Internet-delivered treatment for depression is significantly cheaper than (both to provider and consumer) and equally effective as face-to-face therapy for mild to moderate depression that does not include the success of the site's prevention program (Calear, Christensen, Mackinnon, Griffiths, & O'Kearney, 2009; Christensen et al., 2004; Christensen, Griffiths, & Korten,

2002). What is more, the site is free to consumers and available to anyone with an Internet connection.

In addition to savings related to reduction of face-to-face care, other savings exist. The Centers for Disease Control estimated that 14% percentage of Americans took an antidepressant medication in 2004. This figure is more than double the percentage of Americans estimated to meet diagnostic criteria for major depressive disorder in a given year (6.7%) and almost 30% higher than the lifetime prevalence of subclinical depression (10%; Kessler, Zhao, Blazer, & Swartz, 1997; NCHS Pressroom, 2004; National Institute of Mental Health, 2008). Research has suggested that psychopharmacology is among the most expensive long-term treatment for depression as well as the most often utilized (Antonuccio, Thomas, & Danton, 1997; Bosmans et al., 2008; Heuzenroeder et al., 2004; Vos, Corry, Haby, Carter, & Andrews, 2005). This is despite evidence that psychosocial treatments for depression have comparable short-term results and more favorable long-term results in terms of decreased relapse rates (e.g., Dimidjian et al., 2006).

There are a number of reasons for the potential over-reliance upon psychopharmacology. Receiving psychotropic medication from one's primary care physician is less stigmatizing and is easier than educating oneself when seeking care from a mental health provider—given a general lack of information on or understanding of psychosocial interventions (Dumesnil & Verger, 2009; Pietrzak, Johnson, Goldstein, Malley, & Southwick, 2009). Easily accessible sites like MoodGym can reduce the reliance on psychotropic medication in these cases by providing education about depression as well as care that does not entail weekly trips to a mental health provider's office.

In addition, there is significant evidence that integration of psychosocial services within primary healthcare settings can reduce utilization, improve outcomes, and thus reduce overall costs of healthcare per patient (e.g., Chiles, Lambert, & Hatch, 1999). However, if mental health providers were to become embedded within primary care settings tomorrow, this would likely contribute only to the situation where the demand for psychosocial services often outstrips the supply; again, e-health offers a solution. Cavanagh and colleagues (2006) have developed a site for depression and anxiety called "Beating the Blues" and have found that the integration of this site in routine care settings has been effective in reducing these symptoms, thereby likely creating a medical cost offset for clinics prescribing care from these sites. Other sites have been created that would lend particularly well to use in these settings—such as Buhrman, Fältenhag, Ström, and Andersson's (2004) site with telehealth support for individuals suffering from chronic back pain, which showed significant increase in control over pain and decrease in pain. However, these sites have not yet been tested in integrated-care settings or medical cost offset data reported.

In contrast to the limited economic data for e-health interventions, there is a larger body of literature examining the use of telehealth technologies. For example, Shore, Brooks, Savin, Manson, and Libby (2007) compared the use of videoconferencing for psychiatric diagnostic interviewing to service a rural Native American population versus in-person interviews. The costs associated with in-person interviewing consisted of psychiatrists' salaries as well as the costs associated with travel to remote clinics (food, lodging, transportation). Shore and colleagues report the original costs of providing telehealth services based on the technology available in 2003 and their costs based on use of new technologies and services used in 2005.

In 2003, costs included salaries, monthly fees for long-distance and integrated services digital network, and port fees. They found that the cost of in-person diagnostic services was $31,475, while that telehealth services was $33,240. However, in 2005, due to market-driven decreasing costs of long-distance and videoconferencing transmission rates and the conversion to digital technology that eliminated port fees, use of telehealth technology provided an average savings of 39%. These or greater cost benefits have been found consistently across studies that have evaluated cost when the utilization is high enough as a result of community need as well as sufficient institutional support, and/or the distances covered by telehealth providers are geographically broad enough (see Richardson, Frueh, Grubaugh, Egede, & Elhai, 2009; Schopp, Johnstone, & Merrill, 2000; Simpson, 2009). In addition, the growing distribution of voice over Internet protocols (VoIP) and Internet-based services such as Skype have had the continued effect of driving down videoconferencing fees for closed communications systems; as security protocols for Internet-based services are improved, they may obviate the need for these extra fees, reducing these costs even further.

Disseminating Evidence-Based Care

Although our field has been looking more and more toward the use and dissemination of evidence-based practice, it remains a fact that many such practices still do not make their way to the offices of private practitioners (Aarons, Wells, Zagursky, Fettes, & Palinkas, 2009). There may not be a great incentive for practitioners to learn and practice evidence-based therapies; there is no accountability for doing so, no agency to oversee the appropriateness of treatment, and no economic push-back from an uninformed public. As previously noted, although the use of exposure therapy has long been determined to be the gold standard in treatment for posttraumatic stress disorder, the majority of practitioners still do not use this therapy in their practice—even those who reportedly specialize in treating PTSD (Becker et al., 2004).

Practitioners are often hard pressed to take time out of their busy practices to find the right training tool for the right new therapy that is offered at the right time and the right location. Even when practitioners make such efforts, it is unclear that continuing education workshops provide enough in-depth information to allow them to do the actual therapy they have just been taught, instead of just some translation of the topography of the therapy. For example, whereas behavioral activation is a therapy well based in research, even a weekend workshop may be remembered over time as simply telling individuals to increase pleasurable activities rather than implementing the subtleties of the contextual behavioral change model described by Jacobson, Martell, and Dimidjian (2001). These concepts, easily forgotten through brief or long past workshops, may translate the idea that dissemination of evidence-based therapies can be problematic. Typically, very little follow-up examines how useful most dissemination attempts turn out to be because the standard for evaluating such attempts is generally a brief memory questionnaire given in close temporal proximity to the workshop (e.g., Corrigan, McCracken, & Blaser, 2003). As research has repeatedly shown, attitudes for engaging in behaviors and actually behaving in these ways are very different things.

Use and dissemination are ever changing problems with ever changing solutions, but the use of e-health may provide some answers to some of these problems. For example, looking back at the problem of disseminating evidence-based practices for PTSD (see also Litz & Salters-Pedneault, 2007), Web sites such as Interapy, a Web-based intervention, have been developed and tested for individuals suffering from this disorder and use writing-based exposure exercises to bring them empirically derived treatment in the comfort of their own homes. DESTRESS is a therapist-supported, self-guided exposure to trauma triggers that implements best practices for the treatment of PTSD (see Foa, Keane, & Friedman, 2008) in an Internet-based framework which has been garnering empirical support (Litz et al., 2007). These sites bring evidence-based practices to individuals and potentially allow therapists to extend their range of practice.

Moreover, adjunctive use of empirically based e-health programs can facilitate practitioners' use of evidence-based practice as a training tool for practitioners looking to learn new therapies (Draper et al., 2008; Marks et al., 2007). This might be as a result of the need for practitioners to support the use of empirically based therapies as adjunctive therapies (Joseph Ruzak, personal communication) or via specifically designed therapist-based trainings. In this sense, e-health could be among the most useful tools in bringing training of evidence-based programs into the homes or offices of those who might benefit. What is more, because there is no added cost to the creators of such training for additional usage, individuals may then be given lifetime access to updates as science progresses or to refresh their memories.

Though this section has focused mainly on e-health and dissemination, it should be noted that videoconferencing technology has long been used in postgraduate education, to provide continuing education units for established practitioners, and in provision of clinical supervision for rural healthcare providers and empirically supported care to geographically isolated persons (Curran, Fleet, & Kirby, 2006; Greenwood & Williams, 2008; Heckner & Giard, 2005; Hilty et al., 2006; Magaletta et al., 1998; Wood, Miller, & Hargrove, 2005).

Walter and colleagues (2004) report the use of videoconferencing technology in psychiatric training programs across a number of medical schools around the United States to provide residents with specialized training by experts outside the specified geographical areas. Residents accessed these seminars in real time via an integrated systems digital network (ISDN) videoconferencing technology at 384 kbps or via video streaming at 80 kbps. As in a study by Lewis, Bredfeldt, Strode, and D'Arezzo (1998), they found that residents' ratings of their experience were limited by the quality of the connection and the ease of use of the technology, highlighting the need for continued investment in high-speed communications infrastructure in order for this technology to become widely useful.

BARRIERS TO USE OF E-HEALTH AND TELEHEALTH

Despite the strong potential contribution that integration of e-health and telehealth technologies may have in expanding access and utilization of empirically based mental health interventions, a number of significant barriers to the widespread use of these technologies remains. As previously noted, the up-front costs of development for Internet-based therapies and the cost of equipment for videoconferencing may represent the most significant barriers for the widespread integration of these treatment delivery modalities into existing mental healthcare systems. However, there are a number of other barriers to development of e-health interventions and in the integration of these solutions in the current healthcare system. These barriers fall into four broad categories: empirical, financial, legislative, and dissemination barriers.

Empirical barriers include lack of adequately powered clinical trials; lack of attention to individual differences (i.e., age, income), diagnostic types (e.g., anxiety vs. depression), and nonprogrammatic issues (e.g., usability, readability) that may moderate treatment effectiveness; and lack of extensive research looking at the integration of these technologies into existing mental healthcare delivery systems and within a stepped-care model—particularly the characteristics that are indicative of success in lower levels of a stepped-care model beyond symptom severity (e.g., Green & Iverson, 2009; Marks et al., 2009; Shafran et al., 2009). At this juncture, though, probably the most pressing concern is efficacy. As previously noted, empirical support for e-health and telehealth interventions is hampered by small sample sizes in studies and lack of consistent inclusion criteria, among other limitations.

Given the lack of strong empirical evidence at this time, ethical concerns have been raised about the use of Internet-based interventions about privacy, scope of practice, use of unvalidated interventions, and crisis intervention responsivity, among others (Alleman, 2002; Childress, 2000; Midkiff & Wyatt, 2008). If these technologies are to be integrated into mental healthcare, an equally pressing related issue is the unique moderators of efficacy of e-health and telehealth to assist practitioners in determining the appropriate level of care in a stepped-care delivery model (see Shafran et al., 2009).

Financial barriers include the potential for significant start-up costs reviewed earlier. However, many financial barriers have legislative roots or solutions, such as lack of adequate resources to reduce start-up costs for practitioners, clinics, and hospitals and a lack of reimbursement mechanisms and financial incentive for the use of these treatment modalities. The Department of Health and Human Services' contracted report from the Institute of Medicine (2004) emphasized the need for integrated telehealth and e-health as a key part of meeting the expanding demand for services throughout the United States. However, despite the IOM's recommendations, one of the primary hurdles to implementation is legislative. Legislative barriers are a category that overlaps with the previous barriers encompassing how research dollars will be spent or what services will be covered by Medicare, and how licensing and scope of practice will be handled at state levels. Other legislative issues include investments in updated telecommunications infrastructure in rural areas.

Many issues around licensing and reimbursement for services have yet to be addressed adequately at either the state or federal level. For the most part, incorporating telehealth or e-health interventions into clinical practice requires limiting the geographic area covered to the state or states in which that the provider is licensed, though a small number of states provide limited licenses for the practice of telemedicine within their jurisdiction (Chamberlin, 2010). In terms of reimbursement, Medicare currently limits payment only to telehealth services delivered by real-time video conferencing in a clinician's office, clinic, or hospital or in a service area of less than 50,000 people.

Private insurers and state Medicaid programs have more liberal guidelines for reimbursing telehealth, though the guidelines for reimbursement vary from state to state and company to company (a good resource is www.telehealthlawcenter.org). However, these restrictions undermine the development of telehealth and e-health technologies and implementation of such technologies in the field by limiting financial incentives for their use. Since 2005, the Medicare Telehealth Enhancement Act (in 2009 bill #H.R. 2068; see http://www.govtrack.us/congress/bill.xpd?bill=h111-2068; 111th Congress, 2009) has been introduced to allow Medicare to reimburse for telehealth services in nonrural areas, expand eligible healthcare providers to include all Medicare providers, expand the technologies to be reimbursed for delivery of treatment, and refinance grant programs to fund infrastructure, training, licensing, and equipment needed to develop telehealth programs in underserved areas. However, this bill has not been passed to date.

The most significant barrier is the lack of dissemination, training, and education about e-health and telehealth in clinical practice. Whitfield and Williams (2004) surveyed the British Association for Behavioral and Cognitive Psychotherapies members' use of CCBT with patients, knowledge of CCBT availability, and beliefs about efficacy. They found that only 2.4% incorporated CCBT in their practice. The most frequently endorsed barrier to use was lack of knowledge about the interventions available or their efficacy. This is saddled on other well-documented barriers to dissemination of evidence-based therapies in general, such as skepticism in practicing professionals about the scalability and generalizability of randomized clinical trials and lack of training with empirically supported treatments in general (see Becker, Stice, Shaw, & Woda, 2009; Shafran et al., 2009; Weissman et al., 2006). Clearly, if practitioners in the field do not know about e-health technologies and are not aware of potential for stepped-care approaches to treatment to extend their practice while providing affordable mental healthcare, then these technologies will not be used.

Another important concern for dissemination and utilization is the actual reach of these technologies. While these technologies, especially telehealth, have the potential to reach virtually anyone in the United States, there are concerns, particularly for e-health, that access and utilization of the delivery medium may be limited by factors such as income and age. The proportion of people who have access to the Internet is large and rapidly expanding. As of December 2009, the Pew Internet and American Life Project estimated that about 74% of the U.S. population had Internet access—a figure that has remained relatively stable since 2006 (http://www.pewinternet.org/Static-Pages/Trend-Data/Whos-Online.aspx). These estimates vary based on ethnicity, age, and income bracket.

In terms of ethnicity, the numbers were 74% for White, non-Hispanic persons; 70% for Black; and 64% for Hispanic. Income also varied, ranging from 60% for the under $30,000 per year bracket up to 94% in the over $75,000 bracket. In terms of age, Internet use ranged from 93% (for ages 18–29) to 81% (ages 30–49) to 70% (ages 50–64) to 38% (over age 65). While concerns about access are an important consideration, there do appear to be shifts that may mitigate some of these disparities over time. First, though overall numbers of those in the United States who have access to the Internet have been fairly stable since 2006, there has been significant growth in the number of Latinos and Blacks who have Internet access (http://www.pewinternet.org/Commentary/2009/ December/ Latinos-Online-20062008.aspx).

The second trend that might mitigate some of these disparities is the aging of the Baby Boomer generation, the leading edge of which is approaching 65 years of age. The aging of this cohort is anticipated to have a profound impact on American society and overall healthcare expenditures (www.gao.gov/new.items/d02544t.pdf). However, Baby Boomers tend to be technically savvy, particularly compared to older generations (http://www.pewinternet.org/Reports/2004/Older-Americans-and-the-Internet/5-Implications-for-the-future/02-Tomorrows-seniors-will-transform-the-wired-senior-stereotype.aspx?r=1). Thus, the percentages of older Americans who use the Internet is projected to grow as Baby Boomers continue to mature, reducing the aged-based digital divide.

Another important issue in utilization of e-health and telehealth is concerns about confidentiality and privacy. Unencrypted Internet connections, wireless devices, work computers, and telephones do not provide adequate security to ensure appropriate levels of confidentiality required for psychotherapy. In dealing with Internet security, there are three main areas of concern for e-health interventions to maintain HIPAA and 21 CFR 11 technical compliance: (a) sign-in, (b) data transfer, and (c) data storage. Use of certificates in authentication and secure sockets layer (SSL) protocols can obviate many of these problems during sign-in and data transfer for Internet-based protocols using private 128-bit encryption keys contained in SSL certificates, and it may provide security solutions for VOIP used for telehealth as well (see Bellazzi et al., 2001).

Data storage is particularly important when sensitive data are stored in a database connected to the Internet. Many database encryption programs are available to meet this need. Security is also an issue for non-Internet-based treatments such as CD-ROM-based or videoconferencing-based interventions. With use of these technologies, confidentiality and privacy issues revolve around where the computer or videoconferencing technology is accessed by the user and who else has access to the computers or rooms where the technology is located. This can be obviated by providers with provision of dedicated computers and dedicated private rooms when feasible.

BIG PICTURE

E-health and telehealth have enormous potential to stretch mental health resources to reach a vast number of people not receiving needed care. Initial empirical support examining efficacy, cost, and best practices for the utilization of both technologies is promising but lacking, despite over a decade of research and many meta-analytic studies demonstrating overall efficacy. Without adequate research demonstrating the utility and promise of these technologies as a means to deliver good care to those in need, it is unlikely that the necessary changes on the state and federal levels to provide financial incentive for the use of these technologies will occur, nor will practitioners adopt minimal contact treatment modalities without assurances that people will get better who use them.

To date, this research shortfall has been mainly due to lack of funding. In terms of funding for research and development of programs that take advantage of these technologies, NIMH is currently the main funding source for non-VA employees. Funding is through the general R01, R03, R34, and STTR grant mechanisms, but e-health and telehealth are not defined research priorities despite IOM recommendations to the Department of Health and Humans Services. As a result there have been few large-scale, well-controlled, randomized clinical trials. Consequently, most of the clinical research done on telehealth and especially e-health interventions in the United States has not moved beyond initial proof-of-concept, pilot stages and has not provided the empirical basis that could lead to large-scale integration of e-health and telehealth into standard practice nationally.

One exception has been the Veterans Administration, which currently provides targeted research dollars for the development and implementation of e-health and telehealth technologies for VA researchers in their solicitation of applications for health services research and development pilot projects program announcement and the targeted solicitation of concept papers to develop full proposal for quality enhancement research initiative (QUERI) center in e-health program announcement. The VA's successful implementation of use of electronic medical records (EMRs) set the stage for the current push for the utilization of EMRs in standard healthcare practice, as exemplified by the Health Information Technology for Economic and Clinical Health Act (HITECH Act), which provides incentives for healthcare providers to adopt EMRs.

Given the current lack of clear legislative agenda, the VA may become the leader in development and implementation of e-health and telehealth, as it did with EMRs, and the results of these efforts will eventually shape policy-making and funding priorities on a national level. However, in order for these resources to become available sooner rather than later, strong advocacy by national professional organizations and government representatives in the current healthcare reform debates is needed, but these voices are currently not present or effective.

Of course, advocating for increases in earmarked research dollars for telehealth and e-health may be putting the cart before the horse as Medicare reimbursement procedures, fuzzy legal boundaries involving licensing and scope of practice, and lack of organizational investment in the integration of the technologies into local healthcare infrastructures undermine the use of any program developed. To date, investments in the integration of these technologies into standard healthcare delivery systems have fallen well short of what is needed to make them viable treatment delivery modalities. On the legislative front, efforts to pass the Medicare Telehealth Enhancement Act (MTEA) have not borne fruit to date, leaving a vacuum that some state legislatures have addressed based on the unique needs of each state (e.g., California, Texas, New Hampshire, Maine); for example, the New Hampshire Telemedicine Act passed in 2009 requires "insurance coverage for telemedicine services if the healthcare service would be covered by the insurer if it were provided through in-person consultation between the patient and provider."

However, even if the MTEA were to be passed tomorrow, it would be just one step in a series of legislation necessary to provide the financial incentive structure necessary for wide-scale implementation of telehealth technologies. Most pressing is the inclusion of e-health because the proposed MTEA does not include provisions for reimbursement for use of e-health technologies such as therapist-supported or -monitored, Internet-delivered, self-management interventions. On the state level, the most pressing legislative issue beyond Medicare is licensing issues. As discussed before, current laws on the use of these technologies are both limiting and inconstant from state to state. Federal efforts to address these barriers include the Health Resources & Services Administration's Licensure Portability Grant Program, which provided $700,000 for two awards in 2009 to support state professional licensing boards' efforts to reduce regulatory barriers to telemedicine alone.

Federal funding does exist to assist healthcare organizations with up-front implementation cost associated with integrating e-health and telehealth into their practices. These programs include congressionally mandated health information technology grants, which awarded approximately $22,936,330 in 2009; telehealth resource center grants, which awarded approximately $975,000 in 2009; and telehealth network grants, which awarded approximately $3,430,000 in 2009. However, when compared to total U.S. healthcare expenditures (about $2.3 trillion in 2008 per the Department of Health and Human Services Centers for Medicare and Medicaid Services), these programs are woefully underfunded.

Addressing efficacy research shortfalls, providing the financial incentive for providers to use these technologies and then assist with the costs of integrating e-health and telehealth into practice, and addressing the licensing barriers for use are all at the heart of what is needed in order for telehealth and e-health to become viable treatment options. All of these issues can be addressed to one degree or another by acknowledging e-health's and telehealth's potential roles as means to stretch healthcare resources and shift healthcare and research priorities and funding both at state and federal levels.

Without an accumulation of large-scale demonstrations that specific e-health and telehealth protocols can be effective treatments for at least low to moderate levels of pathology via completion of well-controlled, adequately powered, randomized clinical trials (e.g., Morland et al., 2010; Taylor et al., 2006) and clear, well-publicized economic analysis of the costs related to their use by larger organizations (such as Kaiser Permanente, the VA, Ontario Ministry of Health, Indian Health Services, etc.; see O'Reilly et al., 2007; Savin et al., 2006; Shore et al., 2007), these issues will not have much impact on the larger healthcare debate in our country. They also will not receive the resources or legislative support necessary to make these technologies a routine part of clinical practice.

However, changes on the government level are not enough; practitioners need to want to pursue these modalities. Clearly, education and dissemination have been a problem (Whitfield & Williams, 2004). This can be addressed via changes in training of specific specialties and/or by provision of continuing education credits that emphasize the stepped-care possibilities and associated reduction in cost while increasing over populations served. But in this case also, support from the organizations and departments responsible is contingent on convincing evidence that encourages use.

In sum, e-health and telehealth have great potential to expand the range and reach of existing healthcare resources when added to traditional face-to-face services. A number of financial and legislative changes need to occur before wide-scale implementation of these modalities is likely to occur. However, the political support required for these to happen is not likely to come together until there are adequate empirical support and clear cost analyses for specific protocols' integration into standard care for the barriers to make more than incremental change in the near future.

Thus, e-health and telehealth are stuck in a place of needing earmarked research dollars to provide the data to support the need for near-term systematic shifts in the utilization of these modalities while not having amassed enough data to become a clear research priority for agencies like NIMH. It is most likely that increased utilization by large organizations, such as the VA, is likely to have an incremental effect on bringing these modalities into mainstream practice and making them research priorities. There are signs that these incremental effects are beginning to cause these shifts to occur (e.g., see the study by Taylor et al., 2006). It is our hope that continued empirical support and dissemination of research results, and current large-scale investment by organizations like the Veterans Administration will provide the basis for its introduction into the current healthcare debate.

REFERENCES

111th Congress, 2009–2010. (2009). Medicare Telehealth Enhancement Act of 2009 (legislation no. H.R. 2068). United States Congress. Retrieved on May 15, 2010, from http://www.govtrack.us/congress/bill.xpd?bill=h111-2068

Aarons, G. A., Wells, R. S., Zagursky, K., Fettes, D. L., & Palinkas, L. A. (2009). Implementing evidence-based practice in community mental health agencies: A multiple stakeholder analysis. *American Journal of Public Health, 99*(11), 2087–2095.

Alleman, J. R. (2002). Online counseling: The Internet and mental health treatment. *Psychotherapy: Theory, Research, Practice, Training, 39*(2), 199–209.

American Psychological Association. (2010). APA: Health-care reform. Retrieved on May 15, 2010, from http://www.apa.org/health-reform/index.html

Andersson, G., & Kaldo, V. (2004). Internet-based cognitive behavioral therapy for tinnitus. *Journal of Clinical Psychology, 60*(2), 171–178.

Antonuccio, D. O., Thomas, M., & Danton, W. G. (1997). A cost-effectiveness analysis of cognitive behavior therapy and fluoxetine (Prozac) in the treatment of depression. *Behavior Therapy, 28*(2), 187–210.

Astin, M. C., & Rothbaum, B. O. (2000). Exposure therapy for the treatment of posttraumatic stress disorder. *National Center for Posttraumatic Stress Disorder: Clinical Quarterly, 9,* 49–51.

Bados, A., Balaguer, G., & Saldaña, C. (2007). The efficacy of cognitive-behavioral therapy and the problem of drop-out. *Journal of Clinical Psychology, 63*(6), 585–592.

Baer, L., Brown-Beasley, M. W., Sorce, J., & Henriques, A. I. (1993). Computer-assisted telephone administration of a structured interview for obsessive-compulsive disorder. *American Journal of Psychiatry, 150*(11), 1737–1738.

Bakke, B., Mitchell, J., Wonderlich, S., & Erickson, R. (2001). Administering cognitive-behavioral therapy for bulimia nervosa via telemedicine in rural settings. *International Journal of Eating Disorders, 30*(4), 454–457.

Barak, A., & Gluck-Ofri, O. (2007). Degree and reciprocity of self-disclosure in online forums. *Cyberpsychology & Behavior, 10*(3), 407–417.

Barak, A., Hen, L., Boniel-Nissim, M., & Shapira, N. (2008). A comprehensive review and a meta-analysis of the effectiveness of Internet-based psychotherapeutic interventions. *Journal of Technology in Human Services, 26*(2), 109–160.

Bastien, C. H., Morin, C. M., Ouellet, M., Blais, F. C., & Bouchard, S. (2004). Cognitive-behavioral therapy for insomnia: Comparison of individual therapy, group therapy, and telephone consultations. *Journal of Consulting and Clinical Psychology, 72*(4), 653–659.

Bauer, S., de Niet, J., Timman, R., & Kordy, H. (2010). Enhancement of care through self-monitoring and tailored feedback via text messaging and their use in the treatment of childhood overweight. *Patient Education and Counseling, 79*(3), 315–319.

Becker, C. B., Stice, E., Shaw, H., & Woda, S. (2009). Use of empirically supported interventions for psychopathology: Can the participatory approach move us beyond the research-to-practice gap? *Behavior Research and Therapy, 47*(4), 265–274.

Becker, C. B., Zayfert, C., & Anderson, E. (2004). A survey of psychologists' attitudes towards and utilization of exposure therapy for PTSD. *Behavior Research and Therapy, 42*(3), 277–292.

Bellazzi, R., Montani, S., Riva, A., & Stefanelli, M. (2001). Web-based telemedicine systems for home-care: Technical issues and experiences. *Computer Methods and Programs in Biomedicine, 64*(3), 175–187.

Bodenheimer, T., Lorig, K., Holman, H., & Grumbach, K. (2002). Patient self-management of chronic disease in primary care. *JAMA, 288*(19), 2469–2475.

Bosmans, J. E., Hermens, M. L. M., de Bruijne, M. C., van Hout, H. P. J., Terluin, B., Bouter, L. M., Stalman, W. A. B., et al. (2008). Cost-effectiveness of usual general practitioner care with or without antidepressant medication for patients with minor or mild-major depression. *Journal of Affective Disorders, 111*(1), 106–112.

Bouchard, S., Paquin, B., Payeur, R., Allard, M., Rivard, V., Fournier, T., Renaud, P., et al. (2004). Delivering cognitive-behavior therapy for panic disorder with agoraphobia in videoconference. *Telemedicine Journal & e-Health, 10*, 13–24.

Bower, P., & Gilbody, S. (2005). Stepped care in psychological therapies: Access, effectiveness and efficiency: Narrative literature review. *British Journal of Psychiatry, 186*, 11–17.

Brown, C., Conner, K. O., Copeland, V. C., Grote, N., Beach, S., Battista, D., & Reynolds, C. F. (2010). Depression stigma, race, and treatment seeking behavior and attitudes. *Journal of Community Psychology, 38*(3), 350–368.

Buhrman, M., Fältenhag, S., Ström, L., & Andersson, G. (2004). Controlled trial of Internet-based treatment with telephone support for chronic back pain. *Pain, 111*(3), 368–377.

Calear, A. L., Christensen, H., Mackinnon, A., Griffiths, K. M., & O'Kearney, R. (2009). The YouthMood project: A cluster randomized controlled trial of an online cognitive behavioral program with adolescents. *Journal of Consulting and Clinical Psychology, 77*(6), 1021–1032.

Carlbring, P., Nilsson-Ihrfelt, E., Waara, J., Kollenstam, C., Buhrman, M., Kaldo, V.,...Andersson, G. (2005). Treatment of panic disorder: Live therapy vs. self-help via the Internet. *Behavior Research and Therapy, 43*(10), 1321–1333.

Carragher, N., Adamson, G., Bunting, B., & McCann, S. (2010). Treatment-seeking behaviors for depression in the general population: Results from the National Epidemiologic Survey on Alcohol and Related Conditions. *Journal of Affective Disorders, 121*(1/2), 59–67.

Carter, J. A., Buckey, J. C., Greenhalgh, L., Holland, A. W., & Hegel, M. T. (2005). An interactive media program for managing psychosocial problems on long-duration spaceflights. *Aviation, Space, and Environmental Medicine, 76*(Supplement 1), B213–B223.

Cavanagh, K., Shapiro, D. A., Van Den Berg, S., Swain, S., Barkham, M., & Proudfoot, J. (2006). The effectiveness of computerized cognitive behavioral therapy in routine care. *British Journal of Clinical Psychology, 45*(4), 499–514.

Celio, A. A., Winzelberg, A. J., Wilfley, D. E., Eppstein-Herald, D., Springer, E. A., Dev, P., & Taylor, C. B. (2000). Reducing risk factors for eating disorders: Comparison of an Internet- and a classroom-delivered psychoeducational program. *Journal of Consulting and Clinical Psychology, 68*(4), 650–657.

Chamberlin, J. (2010). The digital shift: Telepsychology and electronic record-keeping are around the corner. Is your practice ready? *Monitor on Psychology, 41*(5), 46.

Childress, C. A. (2000). Ethical issues in providing online psychotherapeutic interventions. *Journal of Medical Internet Research, 2*(1), e5.

Chiles, J. A., Lambert, M. J., & Hatch, A. L. (1999). The impact of psychological interventions on medical cost offset: A meta-analytic review. *Clinical Psychology: Science and Practice, 6*(2), 204–220.

Christensen, H., Griffiths, K. M., & Jorm, A. F. (2004). Delivering interventions for depression by using the Internet: Randomized controlled trial. *British Medical Journal, 328*(7434), 265.

Christensen, H., Griffiths, K. M., & Korten, A. (2002). Web-based cognitive behavior therapy: Analysis of site usage and changes in depression and anxiety scores. *Journal of Medical Internet Research, 4*(1), e3.

Corrigan, P., McCracken, S., & Blaser, B. (2003). Disseminating evidence-based mental health practices. *Evidence Based Mental Health, 6*(1), 4–5.

Crossley, M., Morgan, D., Lanting, S., Dal Bellow-Haas, V., & Kirk, A. (2008). Interdisciplinary research and interprofessional collaborative care in a memory clinic for rural and northern residents of western Canada: Unique training ground for clinical psychology graduate students. *Australian Psychologist, 43*(4), 231–238.

Cuijpers, P., Donker, T., van Straten, A., Li, J., & Andersson, G. (In press). Is guided self-help as effective as face-to-face psychotherapy for depression and anxiety disorders? A systematic review and meta-analysis of comparative outcome studies. *Psychological Medicine,* Epub ahead of print April 21, 2010, 1–15; retrieved June 2, 2010.

Cuijpers, P., Marks, I. M., van Straten, A., Cavanagh, K., Gega, L., & Andersson, G. (2009). Computer-aided psychotherapy for anxiety disorders: A meta-analytic review. *Cognitive Behavior Therapy, 38*(2), 66–82.

Curran, V. R., Fleet, L., & Kirby, F. (2006). Factors influencing rural health care professionals' access to continuing professional education. *Australian Journal of Rural Health, 14*(2), 51–55.

Darin, E. R., & Kurniawan, S. H. (2000). Increasing the usability of online information for older users: A case study in participatory design. *International Journal of Human–Computer Interaction, 12*(2), 263–276.

Davison, G. C. (2000). Stepped care: Doing more with less? *Journal of Consulting and Clinical Psychology, 68*(4), 580–585.

Day, S., & Schneider, P. L. (2002). Psychotherapy using distance technology: A comparison of face-to-face, video, and audio treatment. *Journal of Counseling Psychology, 49*(4), 499–503.

Demiris, G., Finkelstein, S. M., & Speedie, S. M. (2001). Considerations for the design of a Web-based clinical monitoring and educational system for elderly patients. *Journal of the American Medical Informatics Association, 8*(5), 468–472.

Devineni, T., & Blanchard, E. B. (2005). A randomized controlled trial of an Internet-based treatment for chronic headache. *Behavior Research and Therapy, 43*(3), 277–292.

Dimidjian, S., Hollon, S. D., Dobson, K. S., Schmaling, K. B., Kohlenberg, R. J., Addis, M. E., Gallop, R., et al. (2006). Randomized trial of behavioral activation, cognitive therapy, and antidepressant medication in the acute treatment of adults with major depression. *Journal of Consulting and Clinical Psychology, 74*(4), 658–670.

Dodge, J. A., Janz, N. K., & Clark, N. M. (2002). The evolution of an innovative heart disease management program for older women: Integrating quantitative and qualitative methods in practice. *Health Promotion Practice, 3*(1), 30–42.

Draper, C., Hall, M. R., & O'Donohue, W. T. (2008). Adjunctive e-health. In *Evidence-based adjunctive treatments* (pp. 107–122). San Diego, CA: Academic Press.

Dumesnil, H., & Verger, P. (2009). Public awareness campaigns about depression and suicide: A review. *Psychiatric Services* (Washington, DC), *60*(9), 1203–1213.

Elliott, T. R., Brossart, D., Berry, J. W., & Fine, P. R. (2008). Problem-solving training via videoconferencing for family caregivers of persons with spinal cord injuries: A randomized controlled trial. *Behavior Research and Therapy, 46*(11), 1220–1229.

Espie, C. A. (2009). "Stepped care": A health technology solution for delivering cognitive behavioral therapy as a first line insomnia treatment. *Sleep: Journal of Sleep and Sleep Disorders Research, 32*(12), 1549–1558.

Flagg, B. N. (1990). *Formative evaluation for educational technologies.* New York, NY: Routledge.

Foa, E. B., Keane, T. M., & Friedman, M. J. (2008). *Effective treatments for PTSD: Practice guidelines from the International Society for Traumatic Stress Studies.* New York, NY: Guilford Press.

FDA. (1997). Food and Drug Administration Modernization Act of 1997. Retrieved July 21, 2010, from http://www.fda.gov/RegulatoryInformation/Legislation/%20FederalFoodDrugandCosmeticActFDCAct/SignificantAmendmentstotheFDCAct/FDAMA/FullTextofFDAMAlaw/default.htm

Fox, S. (2006). Summary of findings: Pew Internet & American Life Project. Retrieved April 3, 2010 from http://www.pewinternet.org/Reports/2006/Online-Health-Search-2006.aspx?r=1

Frueh, B. C., Henderson, S., & Myrick, H. (2005). Telehealth service delivery for persons with alcoholism. *Journal of Telemedicine and Telecare, 11*(7), 372–375.

Frueh, B. C., Monnier, J., Grubaugh, A. L., Elhai, J. D., Yim, E., & Knapp, R. (2007). Therapist adherence and competence with manualized cognitive-behavioral therapy for PTSD delivered via videoconferencing technology. *Behavior Modification, 31*(6), 856–866.

Furstenberg, C. T., Carter, J. A., Henderson, J. V., & Ahles, T. A. (2002). Formative evaluation of a multimedia program for patients about the side effects of cancer treatment. *Patient Education and Counseling, 47*(1), 57–62.

Gega, L., Marks, I., & Mataix-Cols, D. (2004). Computer-aided CBT self-help for anxiety and depressive disorders: Experience of a London clinic and future directions. *Journal of Clinical Psychology, 60*(2), 147–157.

Gellatly, J., Bower, P., Hennessy, S., Richards, D., Gilbody, S., & Lovell, K. (2007).What makes self-help interventions effective in the management of depressive symptoms? Meta-analysis and meta-regression. *Psychological Medicine, 37*, 1217–28.

Germain, V., Marchand, A., Bouchard, S., Drouin, M., & Guay, S. (2009). Effectiveness of cognitive behavioral therapy administered by videoconference for posttraumatic stress disorder. *Cognitive Behavior Therapy, 38*(1), 42–53.

Glueckauf, R. L., Ketterson, T. U., Loomis, J. S., & Dages, P. (2004). Online support and education for dementia caregivers: Overview, utilization, and initial program evaluation. *Telemedicine Journal and e-Health, 10*(2), 223–232.

Glueckauf, R. L., Pickett, T. C., Ketterson, T. U., Loomis, J. S., & Rozensky, R. H. (2003). Preparation for the delivery of telehealth services: A self-study framework for expansion of practice. *Professional Psychology: Research and Practice, 34*(2), 159–163.

Godleski, L., Nieves, J. E., Darkins, A., & Lehmann, L. (2008). VA telemental health: Suicide assessment. *Behavioral Sciences & the Law, 26*(3), 271–286.

Green, K. E., & Iverson, K. M. (2009). Computerized cognitive-behavioral therapy in a stepped care model of treatment. *Professional Psychology: Research and Practice, 40*(1), 96–103.

Greenwood, J., & Williams, R. (2008). Continuing professional development for Australian rural psychiatrists by videoconference. *Australasian Psychiatry, 16*(4), 273–276.

Greist, J. H. (1998). The computer as clinician assistant: Assessment made simple. *Psychiatric Services, 49*(4), 467–472.

Greist, J. H., Marks, I. M., Baer, L., Kobak, K. A., Wenzel, K. W., Hirsch, M. J.,...Clary, C. M., (2002). Behavior therapy for obsessive-compulsive disorder guided by a computer or by a clinician compared with relaxation as a control. *Journal of Clinical Psychiatry, 63*(2), 138–145.

Gribble, J. N., Miller, H. G., Cooley, P. C., Catania, J. A., Pollack, L., & Turner, C. F. (2000). The impact of T-ACASI interviewing on reported drug use among men who have sex with men. *Substance Use & Misuse, 35*(6–8), 869–890.

Griffiths, K. M., & Christensen, H. (2007). Internet-based mental health programs: A powerful tool in the rural medical kit. *Australian Journal of Rural Health, 15*(2), 81–87.

Griffiths, K. M., Farrer, L., & Christensen, H. (2010). The efficacy of Internet interventions for depression and anxiety disorders: A review of randomized controlled trials. *Medical Journal of Australia, 192*(11 Suppl), S4–11.

Hare, J., Osmond, A., Yang, Y., Wills, G., Weal, M., De Roure, D.,...Yardley, L. (2009). LifeGuide: A platform for performing Web-based behavioral interventions. In *Proceedings of the WebSci'09: Society,* online, March 18–20, 2009, Athens, Greece. Retrieved July 21, 2010, from http://eprints.ecs.soton.ac.uk/17201/

Hassija, C. M., & Gray, M. J. (2009). Telehealth-based exposure therapy for motor vehicle accident-related posttraumatic stress disorder. *Clinical Case Studies, 8*(1), 84–94.

Hauenstein, E. J., Petterson, S., Rovnyak, V., Merwin, E., Heise, B., & Wagner, D. (2007). Rurality and mental health treatment. *Administration and Policy in Mental Health and Mental Health Services Research, 34*(3), 255–267.

Hayward, L., MacGregor, A. D., Peck, D. F., & Wilkes, P. (2007). The feasibility and effectiveness of computer-guided CBT (fearfighter) in a rural area. *Behavioral and Cognitive Psychotherapy, 35*(4), 409–419.

Heckman, T. G., Anderson, E. S., Sikkema, K. J., Kochman, A., Kalichman, S. C., & Anderson, T. (2004). Emotional distress in nonmetropolitan persons living with HIV disease enrolled in a telephone-delivered, coping improvement group intervention. *Health Psychology, 23*(1), 94–100.

Heckner, C., & Giard, A. (2005). A comparison of on-site and telepsychiatry supervision. *Journal of the American Psychiatric Nurses Association, 11*(1), 35–38.

Hembree, E. A., Foa, E. B., Dorfan, N. M., Street, G. P., Kowalski, J., & Tu, X. (2003). Do patients drop out prematurely from exposure therapy for PTSD? *Journal of Traumatic Stress, 16*(6), 555–562.

Heuzenroeder, L., Donnelly, M., Haby, M. M., Mihalopoulos, C., Rossell, R., Carter, R.,...Vos, T. (2004). Cost-effectiveness of psychological and pharmacological interventions for generalized anxiety disorder and panic disorder. *Australian and New Zealand Journal of Psychiatry, 38*(8), 602–612.

Hildebrand, R., Chow, H., Williams, C., Nelson, M., & Wass, P. (2004). Feasibility of neuropsychological testing of older adults via videoconference: Implications for assessing the capacity for independent living. *Journal of Telemedicine and Telecare, 10*(3), 130–134.

Hilty, D. M., Alverson, D. C., Alpert, J. E., Tong, L., Sagduyu, K., Boland, R. J.,...Yellowlees, P. M. (2006). Virtual reality, telemedicine, web and data processing innovations in medical and psychiatric education and clinical care. *Academic Psychiatry, 30*(6), 528–533.

Himle, J. A., Fischer, D. J., Muroff, J. R., Van Etten, M. L., Lokers, L. M., Abelson, J. L., & Hanna, G. L. (2006). Videoconferencing-based cognitive-behavioral therapy for obsessive-compulsive disorder. *Behavior Research and Therapy, 44*(12), 1821–1829.

Hockey, A. D., Yellowlees, P. M., & Murphy, S. (2004). Evaluation of a pilot second-opinion child telepsychiatry service. *Journal of Telemedicine and Telecare, 10,* 48–50.

Hoge, C. W., Auchterlonie, J. L., & Milliken, C. S. (2006). Mental health problems, use of mental health services, and attrition from military service after returning from deployment to Iraq or Afghanistan. *JAMA, 295*(9), 1023–1032.

Horvath, A. O., & Greenberg, L. S. (1989). Development and validation of the working alliance inventory. *Journal of Counseling Psychology, 36,* 223–233.

Institute of Medicine. (2004). *Quality through collaboration: The future of rural health.* Washington, DC: National Academies Press.

Institute of Medicine. (2008). *Treatment of posttraumatic stress disorder: An assessment of the evidence.* Washington, DC: National Academies Press.

Jackson, H., Judd, F., Komiti, A., Fraser, C., Murray, G., Robins, G.,...Wearing, A. (2007). Mental health problems in rural contexts: What are the barriers to seeking help from professional providers? *Australian Psychologist, 42*(2), 147–160.

Jacobson, N. S., Martell, C. R., & Dimidjian, S. (2001). Behavioral activation treatment for depression: Returning to contextual roots. *Clinical Psychology: Science and Practice, 8*(3), 255–270.

Joinson, A. (1999). Social desirability, anonymity, and Internet-based questionnaires. *Behavior Research Methods, Instruments & Computers, 31*(3), 433–438.

Joinson, A. N. (2001). Self-disclosure in computer-mediated communication: The role of self-awareness and visual anonymity. *European Journal of Social Psychology, 31*(2), 177–192.

Joinson, A. N. (2004). Self-esteem, interpersonal risk, and preference for e-mail to face-to-face communication. *CyberPsychology & Behavior, 7*(4), 472–478.

Kaiser Commission on Key Facts. (2003). The uninsured in rural America. The Henry J. Kaiser Family Foundation. Retrieved on March 15, 2010, from http://www.kff.org/uninsured/upload/The-Uninsured-in-Rural-America-Update-PDF.pdf

Kaltenthaler, E., Brazier, J., De Nigris, E., Tumur, I., Ferriter, M., Beverley, C., Parry, G., et al. (2006). Computerized cognitive behaviour therapy for depression and anxiety update: A systematic review and economic evaluation. *Health Technology Assessment, 10*(33), 1–168.

Katon, W., Von Korff, M., Lin, E., Simon, G., Walker, E., Unutzer, J.,...Ludman, E. (1999). Stepped collaborative care for primary care patients with persistent symptoms of depression—A randomized trial. *Archives of General Psychiatry, 56*, 1109–1115.

Kenardy, J., McCafferty, K., & Rosa, V. (2003). Internet-delivered indicated prevention for anxiety disorders: A randomized controlled trial. *Behavioural and Cognitive Psychotherapy, 31*(3), 279–289.

Kenwright, M., Marks, I., Graham, C., Franses, A., & Mataix-Cols, D. (2005). Brief scheduled phone support from a clinician to enhance computer-aided self-help for obsessive-compulsive disorder: Randomized controlled trial. *Journal of Clinical Psychology, 61*(12), 1499–1508.

Kenwright, M., Marks, I. M., Gega, L., & Mataix-Cols, D. (2004). Computer-aided self-help for phobia/panic via Internet at home: A pilot study. *British Journal of Psychiatry, 184*(5), 448–449.

Kessler, R. C., Bergiund, P. A., Bruce, M. L., Koch, J. R., Laska, E. M., Leaf, P. J.,...Wang, P. S. (2001). The prevalence and correlates of untreated serious mental illness. *Health Services Research, 36*(6), 987–1007.

Kessler, R. C., Zhao, S., Blazer, D. G., & Swartz, M. (1997). Prevalence, correlates, and course of minor depression and major depression in the national comorbidity survey. *Journal of Affective Disorders, 45*(1–2), 19–30.

Knaevelsrud, C., & Maercker, A. (2007). Internet-based treatment for PTSD reduces distress and facilitates the development of a strong therapeutic alliance: A randomized controlled clinical trial. *BMC Psychiatry, 7*(1), 13.

Kohn, R., Saxena, S., Levav, I., & Saraceno, B. (2004). The treatment gap in mental health care. *Bulletin of the World Health Organization, 82*(11), 858–866.

Lange, A., Rietdijk, D., Hudcovicova, M., Schrieken, B., Emmelkamp, P. M., & van de Ven, J. P. (2003). Interapy: A controlled randomized trial of the standardized treatment of posttraumatic stress through the Internet. *Journal of Consulting and Clinical Psychology, 71*(5), 901–909.

Lange, A., Van de Ven, J. P., & Schrieken, B. (2003). Interapy: Treatment of posttraumatic stress via the Internet. *Cognitive Behavior Therapy, 32*(3), 110–124.

Lewis, Y. L., Bredfeldt, R. P., Strode, S. W., & D'Arezzo, K. W. (1998). Changes in residents' attitudes and achievement after distance learning via two-way interactive video. *Family Medicine, 30*(7), 497–500.

Litz, B. T., Engel, C. C., Bryant, R. A., & Papa, A. (2007). A randomized, controlled proof-of-concept trial of an Internet-based, therapist-assisted self-management treatment for posttraumatic stress disorder. *American Journal of Psychiatry, 164*(11), 1676–1684.

Litz, B. T., & Salters-Pedneault, K. (2007). The art of evidence-based treatment of trauma survivors. In S. G. Hofmann & J. Weinberger (Eds.), *The art and science of psychotherapy* (pp. 211–230). New York, NY: Routledge.

Lorig, K. R., & Holman, H. R. (2003). Self-management education: History, definition, outcomes, and mechanisms. *Annals of Behavioral Medicine, 26*(1), 1–7.

Lorig, K., Ritter, P. L., Laurent, D. D., Plant, K., Green, M., Jernigan, V. B. B., & Case, S. (2010). Online diabetes self-management program: A randomized study. *Diabetes Care, 33*(6), 1275–1281.

Lorig, K., Ritter, P. L., Villa, F. J., & Armas, J. (2009). Community-based peer-led diabetes self-management: A randomized trial. *Diabetes Educator, 35*(4), 641–651.

Lorig, K. R., Ritter, P. L., Dost, A., Plant, K., Laurent, D. D., & McNeil, I. (2008). The expert patients program online, a 1-year study of an Internet-based self-management program for people with long-term conditions. *Chronic Illness, 4*(4), 247–256.

Lorig, K. R., Ritter, P. L., Laurent, D. D., & Plant, K. (2006). Internet-based chronic disease self-management: A randomized trial. *Medical Care, 44*(11), 964–971.

Lorig, K. R., Ritter, P. L., Laurent, D. D., & Plant, K. (2008). The Internet-based arthritis self-management program: A one-year randomized trial for patients with arthritis or fibromyalgia. *Arthritis and Rheumatism, 59*(7), 1009–1017.

Lorig, K. R., Ritter, P., Stewart, A. L., Sobel, D. S., William Brown, Jr., B., Bandura, A.,…Holman, H. (2001). Chronic disease self-management program: 2-Year health status and health care utilization outcomes. *Medical Care, 39*(11), 1217–1223.

Lorig, K., Sobel, D. S., Stewart, A. L., Brown, B. W., Bandura, A., Ritter, P.,…Holman, H. R. (1999). Evidence suggesting that a chronic disease self-management program can improve health status while reducing hospitalization: A randomized trial. *Medical Care, 37*(1), 5–14.

Lovell, K., & Richards, D. (2000). Multiple access points and levels of entry (MAPLE): Ensuring choice, accessibility and equity for CBT services. *Behavioral and Cognitive Psychotherapy, 28*(4), 379–391.

Luce, K. H., Winzelberg, A. J., Zabinski, M. F., & Osborne, M. I. (2003). Internet-delivered psychological interventions for body image dissatisfaction and disordered eating. *Psychotherapy: Theory, Research, Practice, Training, 40*(1–2), 148–154.

Magaletta, P. R., Fagan, T. J., & Ax, R. K. (1998). Advancing psychology services through telehealth in the Federal Bureau of Prisons. *Professional Psychology: Research and Practice, 29*(6), 543–548.

Marks, I., Cuijpers, P., Cavanagh, K., van Straten, A., Gega, L., & Andersson, G. (2009). Meta-analysis of computer-aided psychotherapy: Problems and partial solutions. *Cognitive Behavior Therapy, 38*(2), 83–90.

Marks, I. M., Baer, L., Greist, J. H., Park, J., Bachofen, M., Nakagawa, A., Wenzel, K. W., et al. (1998). Home self-assessment of obsessive–compulsive disorder: Use of a manual and a computer-conducted telephone interview: Two UK–US studies. *British Journal of Psychiatry, 172*, 406–412.

Marks, I. M., Cavanagh, K., & Gega, L. (2007). *Hands-on help: Computer-aided psychotherapy.* New York, NY: Psychology Press.

Marks, I., & Cavanagh, K. (2009). Computer-aided psychological treatments: Evolving issues. *Annual Review of Clinical Psychology, 5*, 121–141.

Marks, I. M., Mataix-Cols, D., Kenwright, M., Cameron, R., Hirsch, S., & Gega, L. (2003). Pragmatic evaluation of computer-aided self-help for anxiety and depression. *British Journal of Psychiatry 183*(1), 57–65.

McKay, J. R., Lynch, K. G., Shepard, D. S., Ratichek, S., Morrison, R., Koppenhaver, J., & Pettinati, H. M. (2004). The effectiveness of telephone-based continuing care in the clinical management of alcohol and cocaine use disorders: 12-Month outcomes. *Journal of Consulting and Clinical Psychology, 72*(6), 967–979.

Mermelstein, R., Hedeker, D., & Wong, S. C. (2003). Extended telephone counseling for smoking cessation: Does content matter? *Journal of Consulting and Clinical Psychology, 71*(3), 565–574.

Midkiff, D. M., & Wyatt, W. J. (2008). Ethical issues in the provision of online mental health services (etherapy). *Journal of Technology in Human Services, 26*(2–4), 310–332.

Mojtabai, R. (2005). Trends in contacts with mental health professionals and cost barriers to mental health care among adults with significant psychological distress in the United States: 1997–2002. *American Journal of Public Health, 95*(11), 2009–2014.

Mojtabai, R. (2007). Americans' attitudes toward mental health treatment seeking: 1990–2003. *Psychiatric Services, 58*(5), 642–651.

Morland, L. A., Greene, C. J., Rosen, C. S., Foy, D., Reilly, P., Shore, J.,...Frueh, B. C. (2010). Telemedicine for anger management therapy in a rural population of combat veterans with posttraumatic stress disorder: A randomized noninferiority trial. *Journal of Clinical Psychiatry, 71*(7), 855–863.

Mouton-Odum, S., Keuthen, N. J., Wagener, P. D., Stanley, M. A., & DeBakey, M. E. (2006). StopPulling.com: An interactive, self-help program for trichotillomania. *Cognitive and Behavioral Practice, 13*(3), 215–226.

NCHS Pressroom. (2004). Half of Americans use at least one prescription. Retrieved April 18, 2010, from http://www.cdc.gov/nchs/pressroom/04news/hus04.htm

National Institute of Mental Health. (2008). NIMH. The numbers count: Mental disorders in America. Retrieved April 18, 2010, from http://www.nimh.nih.gov/health/publications/ the-numbers-count-mental-disorders-in-america/index.shtml

Nelson, E., Barnard, M., & Cain, S. (2006). Feasibility of telemedicine intervention for childhood depression. *Counseling & Psychotherapy Research, 6*(3), 191–195.

Newman, M. G. (2000). Recommendations for a cost-offset model of psychotherapy allocation using generalized anxiety disorder as an example. *Journal of Consulting and Clinical Psychology, 68*(4), 549–555.

Newman, M. G., Erickson, T., Przeworski, A., & Dzus, E. (2003). Self-help and minimal-contact therapies for anxiety disorders: Is human contact necessary for therapeutic efficacy? *Journal of Clinical Psychology, 59*(3), 251–274.

Newton, M. S., & Ciliska, D. (2006). Internet-based innovations for the prevention of eating disorders: A systematic review. *Eating Disorders: Journal of Treatment & Prevention, 14*(5), 365–384.

O'Donohue, W. T., Draper, C., (2010). *Stepped care and e-health: Practical applications to behavioral disorders.* New York, NY: Springer Publishing.

Oliveira, J. M., Austin, A. A., Miyamoto, R. E., Kaholokula, J. K., Yano, K. B., & Lunasco, T. (2006). The rural Hawaii behavioral health program: Increasing access to primary care behavioral health for native Hawaiians in rural settings. *Professional Psychology: Research and Practice, 37*(2), 174–182.

O'Reilly, R., Bishop, J., Maddox, K., Hutchinson, L., Fisman, M., & Takhar, J. (2007). Is telepsychiatry equivalent to face-to-face psychiatry? Results from a randomized controlled equivalence trial. *Psychiatric Services, 58*(6), 836.

Papa, A., & Litz, B. T. (in press). Grief. In O'Donohue, W. T., Draper, C. (Eds.), *Stepped care and e-health: Practical applications to behavioral disorders*. New York, NY: Springer.

Pietrzak, R. H., Johnson, D. C., Goldstein, M. B., Malley, J. C., & Southwick, S. M. (2009). Perceived stigma and barriers to mental health care utilization among OEF-OIF veterans. *Psychiatric Services, 60*(8), 1118–1122.

Proudfoot, J., Ryden, C., Everitt, B., Shapiro, D. A., Goldberg, D., Mann, A., Tylee, A., et al. (2004). Clinical efficacy of computerised cognitive-behavioural therapy for anxiety and depression in primary care: Randomized controlled trial. *British Journal of Psychiatry, 185*(1), 46–54.

Raylu, N., Oei, T. P. S., & Loo, J. (2008). The current status and future direction of self-help treatments for problem gamblers. *Clinical Psychology Review, 28*(8), 1372–1385.

Reger, M. A., & Gahm, G. A. (2009). A meta-analysis of the effects of Internet- and computer-based cognitive-behavioral treatments for anxiety. *Journal of Clinical Psychology, 65*(1), 53–75.

Richardson, L. K., Frueh, B. C., Grubaugh, A. L., Egede, L., & Elhai, J. D. (2009). Current directions in videoconferencing tele-mental health research. *Clinical Psychology: Science and Practice, 16*(3), 323–338.

Ritterband, L. M., Gonder-Frederick, L. A., Cox, D. J., Clifton, A. D., West, R. W., & Borowitz, S. M. (2003). Internet interventions: In review, in use, and into the future. *Professional Psychology: Research and Practice, 34*(5), 527–534.

Rosen, C. S., Chow, H. C., Finney, J. F., Greenbaum, M. A., Moos, R. H., Sheikh, J. I., & Yesavage, J. A. (2004). VA practice patterns and practice guidelines for treating posttraumatic stress disorder. *Journal of Traumatic Stress, 17*(3), 213–222.

Ruskin, P. E., Silver-Aylaian, M., Kling, M. A., Reed, S. A., Bradham, D. D., Hebel, J. R., Barrett, D., et al. (2004). Treatment outcomes in depression: Comparison of remote treatment through telepsychiatry to in-person treatment. *American Journal of Psychiatry, 161*(8), 1471.

Savin, D., Garry, M. T., Zuccaro, P., & Novins, D. (2006). Telepsychiatry for treating rural American Indian Youth. *Journal of the American Academy of Child & Adolescent Psychiatry, 45*(4), 484–488.

Schneider, A. J., Mataix-Cols, D., Marks, I. M., & Bachofen, M. (2005). Internet-guided self-help with or without exposure therapy for phobic and panic disorders. *Psychotherapy and Psychosomatics, 74*(3), 154–164.

Shafran, R., Clark, D. M., Fairburn, C. G., Arntz, A., Barlow, D. H., Ehlers, A., Freeston, M., et al. (2009). Mind the gap: Improving the dissemination of CBT. *Behaviour Research and Therapy, 47*(11), 902–909.

Schopp, L. H., Demiris, G., & Glueckauf, R. L. (2006). Rural backwaters or front-runners? Rural telehealth in the vanguard of psychology practice. *Professional Psychology: Research and Practice, 37*(2), 165–173.

Schopp, L., Johnstone, B., & Merrill, D. (2000). Telehealth and neuropsychological assessment: New opportunities for psychologists. *Professional Psychology: Research and Practice, 31*(2), 179–183.

Shore, J. H., Brooks, E., Savin, D. M., Manson, S. M., & Libby, A. M. (2007). An economic evaluation of telehealth data collection with rural populations. *Psychiatric Services, 58*(6), 830–835.

Simpson, S. (2009). Psychotherapy via videoconferencing: A review. *British Journal of Guidance & Counseling, 37*(3), 271–286.

Simpson, S., Bell, L., Britton, P., Mitchell, D., Morrow, E., Johnston, A. L., & Brebner, J. (2006). Does video therapy work? A single case series of bulimic disorders. *European Eating Disorders Review, 14*(4), 226–241.

Spek, V., Cuijpers, P., Nyklíček, I., Riper, H., Keyzer, J., & Pop, V. (2007). Internet-based cognitive behaviour therapy for symptoms of depression and anxiety: A meta-analysis. *Psychological Medicine: A Journal of Research in Psychiatry and the Allied Sciences, 37*(3), 319–328.

Taylor, C. B., Bryson, S., Luce, K. H., Cunning, D., Doyle, A. C., Abascal, L. B., Rockwell, R., et al. (2006). Prevention of eating disorders in at-risk college-age women. *Archives of General Psychiatry, 63*(8), 881.

Tuerk, P. W., Yode, M., Ruggier, K. J., Gro, D. F., & Acierno, R. (2010). A pilot study of prolonged exposure therapy for posttraumatic stress disorder delivered via telehealth technology. *Journal of Traumatic Stress, 23*(1), 116–123.

USDA Economic Research Service (November 11, 2008). ERS/USDA research emphasis—An enhanced quality of life for rural Americans. Retrieved March 2, 2010, from http://www.ers.usda.gov/Emphases/Rural/.

Vergara Rojas, S., & Gagnon, M. (2008). A systematic review of the key indicators for assessing telehomecare cost-effectiveness. *Telemedicine and e-Health, 14.9*, 896–904.

Vos, T., Corry, J., Haby, M. M., Carter, R., & Andrews, G. (2005). Cost-effectiveness of cognitive-behavioral therapy and drug interventions for major depression. *Australian and New Zealand Journal of Psychiatry, 39*(8), 683–692.

Wagner, B., Knaevelsrud, C., & Maercker, A. (2005). Internet-based treatment for complicated grief: Concepts and case study. *Journal of Loss and Trauma, 10*(5), 409–432.

Wagner, B., Knaevelsrud, C., & Maercker, A. (2006). Internet-based cognitive-behavioral therapy for complicated grief: A randomized controlled trial. *Death Studies, 30*(5), 429–453.

Wagner, B., & Maercker, A. (2007). A 1.5-year follow-up of an Internet-based intervention for complicated grief. *Journal of Traumatic Stress, 20*(4), 625–630.

Walter, D. A., Rosenquist, P. B., & Bawtinhimer, G. (2004). Distance learning technologies in the training of psychiatry residents: A critical assessment. *Academic Psychiatry, 28*(1), 60–65.

Wang, P. S., Berglund, P., Olfson, M., Pincus, H. A., Wells, K. B., & Kessler, R. C. (2005). Failure and delay in initial treatment contact after first onset of mental disorders in the National Comorbidity Survey Replication. *Archives of General Psychiatry, 62*(6), 603–613.

Wang, P. S., Lane, M., Olfson, M., Pincus, H. A., Wells, K. B., & Kessler, R. C. (2005). Twelve-month use of mental health services in the United States: Results from the National Comorbidity Survey Replication. *Archives of General Psychiatry, 62*(6), 629–640.

Weissman, M. M., Verdeli, H., Gameroff, M. J., Bledsoe, S. E., Betts, K., Mufson, L., Fitterling, H., et al. (2006). National survey of psychotherapy training in psychiatry, psychology, and social work. *Archives of General Psychiatry, 63*(8), 925.

Westen, D. (2005). Are research patients and clinical trials representative of clinical practice? In J. C. Norcross, L. Beutler, & R. F. Levant (Eds.), *Evidence-based practices in mental health: Debate and dialogue on the fundamental questions* (pp. 161–189). Washington, DC: American Psychological Association.

Wheeler, J. R. (2003). Can a disease self-management program reduce health care costs? The case of older women with heart disease. *Medical Care, 41*(6), 706.

Whitfield, G., Hinshelwood, R., Pashely, A., Campsie, L., & Williams, C. (2006). The impact of a novel computerized CBT CD ROM (overcoming depression) offered to patients referred to clinical psychology. *Behavioral and Cognitive Psychotherapy, 34*(1), 1–11.

Whitfield, G., & Williams, C. (2004). If the evidence is so good— Why doesn't anyone use them? A national survey of the use of computerized cognitive behavior therapy. *Behavioral and Cognitive Psychotherapy, 32*(1), 57–65.

Williams, C., & Martinez, R. (2008). Increasing access to CBT: Stepped care and CBT self-help models in practice. *Behavioral and Cognitive Psychotherapy, 36*(6). Developments in the theory and practice of cognitive and behavioral therapies, 675–683.

Wood, J. A. V., Miller, T. W., & Hargrove, D. S. (2005). Clinical supervision in rural settings: A telehealth model. *Professional Psychology: Research and Practice, 36*(2), 173–179.

Wright, K. M., Cabrera, O. A., Bliese, P. D., Adler, A. B., Hoge, C. W., & Castro. C. A. (2009). Stigma and barriers to care in soldiers postcombat. *Psychological Services, 6*(2), 108–116.

Young, K. S. (2005). An empirical examination of client attitudes towards online counseling. *CyberPsychology & Behavior, 8*(2), 172–177.

Zoellner, L. A., Feeny, N. C., Cochran, B., & Pruitt, L. (2003). Treatment choice for PTSD. *Behavior Research and Therapy, 41*(8), 879–886.

Six

Can Prescribing Psychologists Assist in Providing More Cost-Effective, Quality Mental Healthcare?

MORGAN T. SAMMONS

INTRODUCTION

Although in 2008 U.S. total expenditures for healthcare declined for the first time in 48 years, the American populace spent approximately $2.3 trillion in pursuit of better health—or over $7,000 per person. Measured as a percentage of the total gross domestic product, we spent 16.2% of our GDP on healthcare, an amount that almost doubles that of most other industrialized nations (CMS, 2009). While it is tempting to believe that this amount has brought us better or even more healthcare, this assumption is erroneous. The quality of healthcare rendered to Americans continues to lag behind that provided in other nations, and larger numbers of our population are going without needed healthcare services. What we do tend to pay for, unfortunately, is the cost of expensive medical technologies and procedures (few of which have been demonstrated to result in overall improvements in patient outcome or well-being), higher fees for certain medical specialties, and higher administrative costs to managed healthcare organizations.

As costs for overall healthcare provision have risen, costs of providing mental healthcare have kept pace. Mental disorders are now among the five most costly health conditions for both children and adults (Agency for Healthcare Research and Quality, 2009a).

For children, mental healthcare emerges as the most expensive sector of health expenditures, with a total expenditure of $8.9 billion in 2006 (an average of $1,931 per child), outranking asthma ($8.0 billion), trauma-related disorders ($6.1 billion), acute bronchitis ($3.1 billion), and infectious diseases ($2.9 billion). Similarly, for adults, mental disorders ranked among the five most costly conditions in 2006, joining heart conditions, cancer, trauma-related disorders, and asthma (Agency for Healthcare Research and Quality, 2009b). Of these five conditions, relative increases in expenditures for the period 1996–2006 were highest for trauma and mental disorders. The number of people incurring costs for mental disorders almost doubled in this decade, from 19.3 million to 36.2 individuals, resulting in an increase in expenditures from $35.2 billion (annualized dollars) to $57.5 billion in 2006.

We also possess compelling evidence that while our expenditures for mental healthcare have increased dramatically, patient outcomes, particularly for mental disorders, have remained frustratingly poor. This seems particularly the case for common mental disorders treated by nonspecialists in primary care settings.

Data presented by Schwenk et al. (2004) provide an illustration. These researchers examined the results of a naturalistic survey of 1,000 depressed patients treated in primary care and their physicians. Most of these patients (approximately 60%) suffered from depression that was at least of moderate severity. Almost all received a medication for their depression, and almost universally, this was the only intervention offered these patients. Most patients experienced a modest improvement in their depressive symptoms, but even 3–5 years later, many remained symptomatic. Many had stopped their medication due to side effects or an absence of notable improvement.

It is also apparent that among those seeking treatment for the most common mental disorder, depression, current trends are away from the provision of psychotherapy and focus much more on provision of pharmacological interventions. Given the limitations of pharmacological interventions for depression, this trend suggests that the needs of increasing numbers of patients treated for depression are not being met.

In line with the epidemiological data reported before, Olfson and Marcus (2009), using data abstracted from the Medical

Expenditure Panel Survey, reported in 2003 that 20% of the U.S. population had sought mental health treatment, compared with 12% approximately a decade previously. During this time, the rate of use of antidepressants almost doubled, from 13 million patients to 23 million patients annually. Of patients seeking treatment for depression, increasing numbers were offered pharmacotherapy rather than psychotherapy, and fewer than 20% of all those patients getting an antidepressant were also afforded psychotherapy, as compared with 30% a decade earlier (among patients receiving psychotherapy, the number of sessions remained essentially constant, averaging eight visits). Alarmingly, but not unsurprisingly, Olfson and Marcus (2009) reported significantly increased use of antipsychotics in patients with depressive spectrum diagnoses.

Trends in psychotropic drug use among children and adolescents are even more dramatic. Antidepressants were prescribed in 5.5% of all U.S. outpatient office visits for adolescents in 1999–2001. This represented an astonishing 206.1% growth in such prescriptions since 1994 (Thomas, Conrad, Casler, & Goodman, 2006). Due to the well-demonstrated and occasionally severe unwanted effects associated with their use, including the incidence of suicidal ideation (particularly in children and adolescents; Olfson, Marcus, & Shaffer, 2006), it seems unquestionable that the administration of antidepressants to this population in the current primary care environment, with stove-piped care and little coordination of services between prescribers and other members of the treatment team, is suboptimal.

Data exist for other common mental disorders and behavioral problems. Domestic violence perpetrated against women, for example, is one of the most pernicious public health issues of our time. The primary care system not only is the venue in which most abused women seek services, but also represents the most likely place where a comprehensive treatment protocol could be implemented. Yet data suggest that simply implementing screening for domestic violence in primary care, with follow-up using treatment as usual models (provision of referral information to external domestic abuse agencies), does not result in differences in outcome between women offered screening and those who were not (MacMillan et al., 2009).

Other recognized unmet practice needs include pediatric behavioral health disorders. While the vast majority of these are treated in the primary care rather than the specialty mental health area, most pediatricians have more familiarity with diagnoses such as attention deficit hyperactivity disorder than with other commonly occurring problems, such as conduct disorder (Williams, Klinepeter, Palmes, Pulley, & Foy, 2004).

The management of mental disorders, then, is demonstrably suboptimal in that setting where most patients seek such services: the primary care arena. Current primary care delivery systems are lacking in numerous respects and do not foster the type of collaborative environment that is necessary for integrating treatment of mental disorders. Using an ethnographic data collection method, Chesluk and Holmboe (2010) observed that current systems are more organized around meeting the needs of physician practitioners (which they do poorly) than in providing a platform for integrated care:

> Physicians' hectic routine forces them to work in a manner that inhibits reflection and collaboration...Professional and administrative staff cannot step in to collaborate with physicians the way they do with each other...To the extent that the entire practice team does come together, it is around physicians and facilitating their schedules, rather than around patients and their experiences. (p. 878)

Better integration of mental health services, via proposals such as "medical home" models, presents opportunities to address a fundamental failing in current stove-piped systems of care: that preventable medical conditions are the leading cause of premature death among people with severe and persistent mental disorders (Alakeson, Frank, & Katz, 2010). Alakeson and colleagues (2010) noted that at present only two fully integrated federally qualified healthcare centers exist: the Cherokee Health System in Tennessee and the Crider Center in Missouri. While the data on integrating behavioral health into primary care are promising, acknowledged gaps exist in our understanding of the efficacy of such integration, particularly in areas like substance abuse. It is nevertheless apparent that the vast majority of patients with mental disorders seek treatment in primary care and that the services currently offered are suboptimal (Annapolis Coalition, 2007; Butler et al., 2008).

Some authors (like me) have argued that integrating specifically trained psychologists into the primary care setting—particularly those who possess the ability to integrate a regimen of psychotherapy with psychotropic drugs—is likely to result in more comprehensive care that leads to enhanced patient outcomes. But if this supposition is true, three issues must be successfully addressed:

- Mental disorders can be successfully treated in primary care versus specialty mental health settings.
- In most cases, a combination of medication and psychotherapy represents the optimum treatment strategy for common mental disorders.
- Psychologists can be suitably trained to prescribe safely and effectively.

CAN MENTAL DISORDERS BE SUCCESSFULLY TREATED IN NONSPECIALTY HEALTHCARE SETTINGS?

In answering this question, it is important to understand that the past decade has seen a dramatic shift not only in the number of individuals seeking mental healthcare but also in the setting in which they receive such care. Using the epidemiological catchment area updated survey, Mauer and Druss (2009) found that 50% of all mental healthcare is received in primary care settings. These researchers also reported that over the past 20 years, the proportion of individuals receiving mental healthcare increased from 12 to 20% of the health-seeking population. Those seeking care in medical settings only, as opposed to specialty mental health settings, increased by 154%. The number treated in community health centers for either mental health or substance abuse issues increased from 210,000 annually two decades ago to 800,000 annually in the first decade of the twenty-first century.

DOES THE COMBINATION OF MEDICATION AND PSYCHOTHERAPY YIELD ENHANCED OUTCOMES FOR PATIENTS WITH COMMON MENTAL DISORDERS?

Numerous studies have demonstrated the superiority of combined interventions for depression, bipolar disorder, and psychotic spectrum disorders. While it seems true for the treatment of depression that placebo is equivalent to pharmacological intervention for at least mild to moderate forms of the disorder, rates of medication-specific response increase substantially in the case of severe depression (Fournier et al., 2010). Regarding combined treatments for unipolar depression, a meta-analysis of 15 years of data demonstrated that combined treatments confer specific benefits and enhance probability of response over monotherapies (Hollon et al., 2005).

Similar results can be found for anxiety spectrum disorders like social anxiety disorder (Blanco et al., 2010). For bipolar disorder, one of the most disabling and refractory of mental disorders, the addition of a psychosocial component to a medication regimen resulted in a shorter time to recovery and significantly more patients in the combined treatment arm were rated as clinically well (Miklowitz et al., 2007). Results supporting the use of combined treatments have also been reported in adolescent depression (TADS Team, 2007) and other disorders such as insomnia (Morin, Vallières, Guay, Ivers, & Savard, 2009).

Results of these studies are buttressed by a more informal yet credible study performed by the Consumer's Union, the author of the mass-market periodical *Consumer Reports*. Similarly to a study performed by this group in 1995 indicating that consumers of psychotherapy reported benefits from it (*Consumer Reports*, 1995), this more recent study indicated that consumers who sought treatment for anxiety or depression benefited most from and preferred a combination of medication and psychotherapy (*Consumer Reports*, 2010). These results are consistent with reports in the scientific literature; moreover, they provide an insight into individual preferences that academic studies tend to neglect.

These findings notwithstanding, a current of thought remains among psychologists and other nonphysician mental health providers that psychotherapy may provide a superior intervention to pharmacotherapy for many common mental disorders (e.g., Jensen et al., 2007; Kennard, Silva, Vitiello, Curry, & Kratochvil, 2009). As McGrath and Sammons (submitted) note, it is therefore at least theoretically possible to support an argument that psychologists should eschew training in psychopharmacology because the market for psychotherapy services will continue to grow and the profession would be better served if psychology redoubled its efforts to provide effective, evidence-based behavioral treatments.

Unfortunately, it is likely that this argument will be proven to be more meretricious than meritorious, for several reasons. First, the majority of patients seeking treatment for most medical disorders receive medication but not psychotherapy. This is due to a number of factors, including that standards of practice in primary care focus on pharmacological interventions and also the very real barriers in reimbursement and referral policies that impede access to psychotherapy services due to reimbursement. But another salient factor is patient choice. Some patients simply prefer the ease of pharmacological interventions over the more time-intensive process of psychotherapy. While it can be argued that pharmacological cures are not permanent, it can also be argued with equal ease that numbers of patients who report lasting benefit from psychotherapy are in the minority.

It is unfortunately true that while psychotherapy "beats" pharmacotherapy in a number of head-to head experimental paradigms, the total number of patients who improve after receiving either intervention remains suboptimal (Rush, 2007). Even using well-designed, carefully employed interventions, response rates to either condition are likely to be relatively low (e.g., DeRubeis et al., 2005). Finally, well-designed comparative effectiveness studies indicate that for a number of conditions—from less disabling conditions such as insomnia and mild or moderate depression to psychotic spectrum conditions like schizophrenia or severe affective disorders like bipolar disorder—combined treatment with medication and psychotherapy results in better outcome for larger numbers of patients. Thus, insistence on a "psychotherapy only" professional focus is likely misguided.

Treatment as usual in primary care can be improved by basic provider education and the enhancement of care via placement of trained providers in primary care clinics. Wells et al. (2005) found that the addition of a psychotherapy quality improvement model in outpatient clinics treating milder forms of depression resulted in a reduction in medication use and an increase in psychotherapy utilization. At a follow-up approaching 5 years, patients in clinics exposed to either a medication or a psychotherapy quality improvement intervention were less likely to have unmet treatment needs, and the chance of an unmet treatment need was significantly less in those patients attending a clinic receiving a psychotherapy quality improvement intervention. These patients were also less likely to have had a primary care visit for depression in the 6 months prior to exit from the study.

Primary care patients with serious and persistent mental illness did similarly better when exposed to an enhanced care model utilizing care managers to provide advocacy, education, communication with providers, and patient support (Druss et al., 2010). At 12-month follow-up, patients receiving enhanced care showed significantly improved mental-health-related quality of life as opposed to those in the treatment-as-usual condition. Interestingly, this study also examined physical outcomes; it found that at 12 months, there were improvements, albeit nonsignificant, on certain physiological measures, including cardiovascular health. This suggested the possibility that longer term exposure to the enhanced care model might result in improvements in physical as well as mental health.

Integration of behavioral interventions with primary care services will significantly improve not only outcomes but also the ability of patients, particularly those in vulnerable or underserved groups, to access such care. Laraque and Sia (2010) presented a current example of an abused preschooler with significant mental health needs who was able to get a broad range of services utilizing an integrated family medical home primary care model. As these authors observed, the Patient Protection and Affordable Care Act (PPACA), recently signed into law by President Obama, will provide many more opportunities for similarly integrating behavioral health and primary medical services.

In particular, the PPACA will require funding of mental health and substance abuse screening, brief intervention, and referral and recovery services in primary care, funded over 5 years with $30 million beginning in 2011. Eligible participants will include those primary care entities that attempt to integrate behavioral health into primary care services, establish relationships with behavioral healthcare providers, and can demonstrate a need to integrate behavioral healthcare (Sundararaman, R., 2009).

OBJECTIONS TO PSYCHOLOGISTS' PRESCRIBING PSYCHOTROPICS

Although most objections to the addition of psychotropic medications to the armamentarium of clinical psychologists come from the medical and, in particular, the psychiatric professions, psychology as a profession is rather unique in that there is a small but vocal minority within the profession who ardently oppose the acquisition of prescriptive authority. Most surveys of psychologists indicate that approximately 75% of those polled from specialties across the discipline endorse prescriptive authority; approximately

25% are opposed. These numbers have remained rather static for much of the past two decades (Sammons, Gorny, Allen, & Zinner, 2000).

Those opposed present a variety of reasons for their opposition, ranging from the risible (e.g., that psychologists are not intellectually equipped to prescribe drugs) to the moral or philosophical (that psychotherapy presents a superior mechanism for dealing with individual distress). More reasonable arguments, however, tend toward three themes: that the training of psychologists is insufficient to allow them to prescribe, that (generally, but not always by extension) psychologists will therefore represent a hazard to the health-seeking public, and that because there are defined limits to the use of psychotropic agents, psychologists should eschew their use.

Many of these arguments are immediately dismissible, but several deserve some attention. Of course, psychology as a profession would be remiss if we did not satisfactorily address the issue of patient safety. Will the well-being of patients who receive psychotropic medication from psychologists be affirmatively harmed?

In the past, we had scant data to answer this question. The 10 graduates of the psychopharmacology demonstration project were deemed by both the American College of Neuropsychopharmacology (ACNP; the external advisory board that had been contracted to review the Department of Defense's psychopharmacology demonstration project) and the General Accounting Office (later the Government Accountability Office; GAO) to be practicing safely and effectively (see Sammons, 2010, for a review of these documents and the psychopharmacology demonstration project). But beyond this, few data existed, and the experiences of 10 prescribers could not be generalized to represent the practice of a profession.

At this point, however, approximately 100 prescribing psychologists are utilizing those skills within the Department of Defense, other federal agencies, and the two states in which psychologists have been granted legislative authority to prescribe (New Mexico and Louisiana). To date, there has been no evidence of any of these providers harming patients by deviating from the standard of care in the utilization of psychotropics, although these psychologists practice in a number of jurisdictions and healthcare systems, so there is not a central database that accrues data to determine whether their practice as a group differs from that of other healthcare providers. In the absence of a central database for prescribing psychologists, we must at this point rely on either individual reports of substandard practice collected via routine quality assurance measures (to the best of this author's knowledge, there have been none) or the safety record of other nonphysician healthcare providers, who have conclusively demonstrated (see following discussion) that their practice regarding psychotropics is as safe and effective as that of physician providers.

It must be understood that the patient safety argument has traditionally been employed by the medical profession when any other healthcare profession has attempted to expand its scope of practice into areas that were previously the exclusive purview of medicine. Expansion of the scope of practice of nurse anesthetists, advance practice nurses in other fields of healthcare, physician assistants, optometrists, podiatrists, dentists, physical therapists, chiropractors, and others have all been opposed by various physician specialties with the argument that, absent training that replicated that of physicians, patient safety would suffer. This argument has been definitively repudiated (see DeLeon, Kenkel, Oliviera-Berry, & Sammons, in press; Fox et al., 2009; Sammons, 2003).

The expansion of the scope of practice of many nonphysician healthcare provider groups over the past two decades has been exponential. Advanced practice nurses can now prescribe medications in all 50 of the United States as well as in the District of Columbia. They have completely independent prescriptive authority in 14 states and, with some degree of physician involvement, more limited prescriptive authority in 33 (Phillips, 2007). There are now approximately 168,000 advance nurse practitioners in the United States (Phillips, 2006). The care provided by nurse practitioners has been deemed equivalent to that provided by physicians (Naylor & Kurtzman, 2010). Programs for nurse practitioners expanded 61% between 1995 and 2006, even though many applicants were turned away due to a lack of instructors. Substitution of nurse practitioners for physicians for patient visits has been demonstrated to provide immediate cost savings.

If the numbers of nurse practitioners are combined with those of physician assistants, who increasingly provide care with limited physician oversight, a sea change in the composition of primary care providers is evident. The number of physician assistants in the workforce doubled between 1997 and 2007. Of the 68,000 physician assistants practicing in 2007, approximately 37% worked in primary care settings, although increasing numbers provided services in specialty settings such as dermatology, surgical specialties, and emergency medicine (Morgan & Hooker, 2010). In 2008, physician assistants wrote a total of 332,000,000 prescriptions in the United States, and they practice with generally minimal oversight from physicians (American Academy of Physician Assistants, 2010). These providers outnumber general and family physicians and general pediatricians (U.S. Department of Health and Human Services, cited in Fox et al., 2010).

If patient safety had been harmed or patient care otherwise suffered as a result of the expansion of the scope of practice of nurses, PAs, optometrists, and other nonphysician groups, the continued expansion of their scopes of practice would definitely not have occurred. Simply put, there is no evidence that patient safety suffers when nonphysician groups acquire skills previously monopolized by medicine, and there is compelling evidence that nonphysician healthcare providers reduce costs while providing high-quality care (Lenz, Mundinger, Kane, Hopkins, & Lin, 2004; Speer & Bess, 2003).

At the same time, we must take care to heed the cautions by those who argue against a headlong embrace of pharmacological interventions. Antidepressants in many instances are of relatively modest benefit over placebo, at least as they are widely employed (e.g., as stand-alone interventions with no other intervention); because it principally reflects industry-sponsored drug trials, the literature supporting their use in many instances is suspect at best (Greenberg, 2010; Healy, 2004). Those supporting the use of psychotropics by psychologists, however, have always argued that psychologists, who bring an orientation to the understanding of mental disorders that is not exclusively rooted in a neurobiological heuristic and are highly adept in the deployment of psychotherapeutic and other behavioral approaches, will utilize these agents in a fundamentally different fashion (Sammons, 2003; Sammons & Newman, 2010).

Although there remain few systematically collected data to support this hypothesis, the practice of the growing number of prescribing psychologists and my experience as a prescribing psychologist seem to bear such claims out. Prescribing psychologists report that they do use medication in conjunction with psychotherapy and rather than as stand-alone interventions and that a significant portion of their practice involves either simplifying medication regimens or stopping the use of psychotropics altogether.

PREPARING PSYCHOLOGISTS FOR PRACTICE IN THE PRIMARY CARE ENVIRONMENT

Psychologists must become more conversant with the clinical management of the general medical patient if the profession is to be a competitive presence in the healthcare marketplace. In 1998, I made the argument that more specific, clinically appropriate education in certain components of clinical medicine was essential to train psychologists who could be competitive in the healthcare marketplace:

> The key issue is that educators continue to fail to produce psychologists who can function as true scientist-practitioners in today's health care marketplace. Significant curricular changes must take place if this glaring deficiency is to be rectified... Psychologists in training must no longer be allowed to discuss knowledge of Axis III conditions as being outside the scope of knowledge of psychology. Physiological and pathophysiological processes are intimately linked to a broad spectrum of mental disorders, and woe betide the practitioner who cannot adequately assess such conditions in order to provide appropriate, multimodal intervention. Psychologists who are ignorant of basic physiological processes are marginalized as members of multidisciplinary treatment teams in health care settings... Employers in the not too distant future will ask why they should hire a psychologist, whose training has left her or him bereft of core skills necessary to work in health care settings, when another practitioner (say, a nurse with some training in behavioral interventions) can function effectively in both roles. (Sammons, 1998, p. 38)

Such arguments are not dissimilar to others made in support of curricular changes that would allow psychologists to become more competitive in the primary healthcare setting. Cummings, O'Donohue, and Cummings (2009) noted that the training of psychologists continues to be inadequate in the application of psychological interventions in fast-paced, nonspecialty mental healthcare settings and that recognition of medical conditions, in addition to training in health economics and practice management, are vital educational prerequisites to the effective and competitive providers in the primary care arena.

The potential results of making these curricular changes are anything but theoretical. Cummings et al. (2009) reported that the presence of appropriately trained behavioral healthcare specialists in the primary care environment resulted in a dramatic increase in the number of completed referrals to mental health (in most healthcare settings, a very small percentage—an estimated 10%—of referrals written for specialty mental health are ever completed by the patient). It also resulted in more efficient utilization of physician time, a reduction in overall medical costs, and greater adherence to recommended medical regimens.

Another compelling argument for the inclusion of psychologists trained in psychopharmacology in the primary care environment rests in the undeniable shortage of providers with specialty training in psychopharmacology. A restriction on the supply of mental health providers with broad clinical skills, including psychopharmacology, is undoubtedly a factor in both limiting access to services and keeping the cost of those services relatively high. In particular, a shortage of providers skilled in the use of psychotropic medications can be implicated in both poorer outcomes and less cost-effective care, and this observation is as applicable in the primary care environment as it is in specialty mental health.

It has long been apparent that the numbers of psychiatrists treating adults and treating children have been insufficient to meet demand. There are currently fewer than 7,000 child psychiatrists practicing in the United States, and it has been estimated that approximately 30,000 of such specialists would be necessary to meet demand. The number of child psychiatry residencies continues to dwindle, and over 30% of them are now filled by international medical graduates. Similar projections are also true for psychiatrists treating adults; although the decline in medical students entering psychiatric residencies has stabilized, demand continues to outpace supply (American Academy of Child and Adolescent Psychiatry, 2009).

Changes in practice are dependent on changes in training. If we presume that the integration of psychologists—in this instance, those with prescriptive authority—into the primary care setting is a goal worthy of achievement, we must then begin by restructuring the graduate curriculum for clinical psychologists. An in-depth analysis of what curricular changes will be required is beyond the scope of this chapter. The following list provides at least the basis for further discussion:

> Courses in clinical psychopharmacology should be standard, not elective, offerings in the curriculum.
> Courses in neurosciences, including psychophysiology, neuroanatomy, and neuropsychology, should address

not only the assessment but also the clinical management of neurological disorders.

Courses in biological bases of behavior should be expanded to include a review of physical symptoms or correlates of commonly presenting physical illnesses, as well as an introduction to common Axis III complaints that the primary care psychologist is likely to encounter in routine practice.

Elective course work in physical assessment should be made available to interested students.

For prescribing psychologists, the pathway to practice is lengthy and opportunities are limited. Prescribing psychologists must first obtain licensure as a doctoral-level psychologist. They must then pursue a curriculum in clinical psychopharmacology that averages at least 450 didactic contact hours, followed by an extensive supervised practicum. In those jurisdictions enabling psychologists to prescribe, passage of a national examination, similar to the psychopharmacology examination for psychologists offered by the American Psychological Association, is required. To expedite this process, it is suggested that psychologists be able to integrate some of the current postdoctoral didactic material into the graduate curriculum. Additional postdoctoral clinical training sites, such as might be obtained by collaboration with schools of nursing, should be sought in order to enlarge the number of potential sites. Finally, psychologists interested in pursuing prescriptive authority may wish to consider postdoctoral curricula in advanced practice nursing or in similar fields.

The Annapolis Coalition (2007), a broadly based policy group of healthcare policy makers brought together by the Substance Abuse and Mental Health Services Administration (SAMHSA), outlined a number of challenges that are in many respects ascribable not only to fragmented systems of healthcare delivery but also to the inability of mental health specialists to provide services appropriately in places where most patients seek them: the primary care clinic. This group noted many challenges facing behavioral healthcare providers, among them

inadequate workforce and treatment capacity
changing profiles of individuals seeking services including increased comorbidity of mental health, medical, and substance abuse problems

rapidly evolving patterns of licit and illicit drug use
a shift in financing to public systems accompanied by declines in private coverage and restrictive managed care policies and practices

It is eminently clear that the inclusion of psychologists trained in the appropriate use of psychotropics in primary care settings would, if present in sufficient numbers, make considerable progress toward addressing some of these identified deficits.

As Collins, Hewson, Munger, and Wade (2010) stated,

> Integrating mental health services into a primary care setting offers a promising, viable, and efficient way of ensuring that people have access to needed mental health services. Additionally, mental health care delivered in an integrated setting can help to minimize stigma and discrimination, while increasing opportunities to improve overall health outcomes. Successful integration requires the support of a strengthened primary care delivery system as well as a long-term commitment from policymakers at the federal, state, and private levels. (p. 3)

To this list of involved parties we must also add professional associations, such as the American Psychological Association, and training programs that prepare psychologists for clinical practice. Without the leadership of these entities, we will continue to graduate psychologists who have neither the intervention skills nor the appropriate fund of knowledge to practice in that setting where most patients with mental health needs seek services: the primary care environment. To neglect this vital area of practice is a disservice to both our patients and our profession.

REFERENCES

Agency for Healthcare Research and Quality. (2009a). *Issue brief #242: The five most costly children's conditions, 2006. Estimates for the U.S. civilian noninstitutionalized children aged 0–17*. Rockville, MD: Author.

Agency for Healthcare Research and Quality. (2009b). *Statistical brief #248: The five most costly conditions, 1996 and 2006: Estimates for the U.S. civilian noninstitutionalized population*. Rockville, MD: Author.

Alakeson, V., Frank, R. G., & Katz, R. E. (2010). Specialty care medical homes for people with severe, persistent mental disorders. *Health Affairs, 29,* 867–873.

American Academy of Child and Adolescent Psychiatry. (2009). AACAP workforce fact sheet. Online access verified June 20, 2010, at ww.aacap.org/cs/root/legislative_action/aacap_workforce_fact_sheet

American Academy of Physician Assistants. (2010). Our practice areas. Retrieved June, 20, 2010, from http://www.aapa.org/about-pas/our-practice-areas

Annapolis Coalition. (2007). *An action plan for behavioral workforce development.* Rockville, MD: Substance Abuse and Mental Health Services Administration.

Blanco, C., Heimberg, R. G., Schneier, F. R., Fresco, D. M., et al. (2010). A placebo controlled trial of phenelzine, cognitive behavioral group therapy, and their combination for social anxiety disorder. *Archives of General Psychiatry, 67,* 286–295.

Butler, M., Kane, R. L., McAlpine, D., Kathol, R. G., Fu, S. S., Hagedorn, H., & Wilt, T. J. (2008). Integration of mental health/substance abuse and primary care. AHRQ publication no. 09-E003. Rockville, MD: Agency for Healthcare Research and Quality.

CMS (Centers for Medicare and Medicaid Services). (2009). Centers for Medicare and Medicaid Services, Office of the Actuary, National Health Statistics Group, retrieved June 16, 2010, at http://www.cms.gov/NationalHealthExpendData/downloads/highlights.pdf

Chesluk, B. J., & Holmboe, E. S. (2010). How teams work—or don't—in primary care: A field study on internal medicine practices. *Health Affairs, 29,* 874–879.

Collins, C., Hewson, D. L., Munger, R., & Wade, T. (2010). *Evolving models of behavioral health integration in primary care.* New York, NY: Milbank Memorial Fund.

Consumer Reports. (1995). Mental health: Does therapy help? *November,* 734–739.

Consumer Reports. (2010). Depression and anxiety. Readers reveal the therapists and drugs that helped. *July,* 28–31.

Cummings, N. T., O'Donohue, W., & Cummings, J. (2009). Financial dimension of integrated behavioral/primary care. *Journal of Clinical Psychology in Medical Settings, 16,* 31–29.

DeLeon, P. H., Sammons, M. T., & Fox, R. (2000). Prescription privileges. In A. E. Kazdin (Ed.), *Encyclopedia of psychology* (Vol. 6, pp. 285–287). Washington, DC: American Psychological Association and Oxford University Press.

DeLeon, P. H., Kenkel, M. B., Oliveira-Berry, J., & Sammons, M. T. (submitted). Emerging policy issues for psychology: A key to the future of the profession.

DeRubeis, R. J., Hollon, S. D., Amsterdam, J. D., Shelton, R. C., Young, P. R., et al. (2005). Cognitive therapy versus medications in the treatment of moderate to severe depression. *Archives of General Psychiatry, 62,* 409–416.

Druss, B., von Esenwein, S., Compton, M., Rask, K., Zhao, L., & Parker, R. (2010). A randomized trial of medical care management for community mental health settings: The primary care access referral and evaluation (PCARE) study. *American Journal of Psychiatry, 167,* 151–159.

Fournier, J. C., DeRubeis, R. J., Hollon, S. J., Dimidjian, S., Amsterdam, J. D., et al. (2010). Antidepressant drug effects and depression severity: A patient level analysis. *Journal of the American Medical Association, 303,* 47–53.

Fox, R. E., DeLeon, P. H., Newman, R., Sammons, M. T., Dunivin, D., & Baker, D. C. (2009). Prescriptive authority and psychology: A status report. *American Psychologist, 64,* 257–268.

Greenberg, R. P. (2010). Prescriptive authority in the face of research revelations. *American Psychologist, 65,* 136–137.

Healy, D. (2004). *Let them eat Prozac: The unhealthy relationship between the pharmaceutical industry and depression.* New York, NY: New York University Press.

Hollon, S. D., Jarrett, R. B., Nieremberg, A. A., Thase, M. E., Trivedi, M., & Rush, A. J. (2005). Psychotherapy and medication in the treatment of adult and geriatric depression: Which monotherapy or combined treatment? *Journal of Clinical Psychiatry, 66,* 455–468.

Jensen, P. S., Arnold, L. E., Swanson, J., Vitiello, B., Abikoff, H. B., et al. (2007). Follow-up of the NIMH MTA study at 36 months after randomization. *Journal of the American Academy of Child and Adolescent Psychiatry, 46,* 989–1002.

Kennard, B. D., Silva, S., Vitiello, B., Curry, J., & Kratochvil, C. (2009). Readmission and residual symptoms after acute treatment of adolescents with major depressive disorder. *Journal of the American Academy of Child and Adolescent Psychiatry, 48,* 186–195.

Laraque, D., & Sia, C. C. J. (2010). Health care reform and the opportunity to implement a family-centered medical home for children. *Journal of the American Medical Association, 303,* 2407–2408.

Lenz, E. R., Mundinger, M. O., Kane, R. L., Hopkins, S. C., & Lin, S. X. (2004). Primary care outcomes in patients treated by nurse practitioners or physicians: Two-year follow-up. *Medical Care Research and Review, 61,* 332–351.

MacMillan, H. L., Wathen, C. N., Jamieson, E., Boyle, M. H., Shannon, H. S., et al. (2009). Screening for intimate partner violence in health care settings: A randomized trial. *Journal of the American Medical Association, 302,* 493–501.

Mauer, B. J., & Druss, B. G. (2009). Mind and body reunited: Improving care at the behavioral and primary healthcare interface. *Journal of Behavioral Health Services and Research,* published online April 2, 2009.

Miklowitz, D. J., Otto, M. W., Frank, E., Reilly-Harrington, N. A., Kogan, J. N., et al. (2007). Intensive psychosocial intervention enhances functioning in patients with bipolar depression: Results from a 9-month randomized controlled trial. *American Journal of Psychiatry, 164,* 1340–1347.

McGrath, R. E., & Sammons, M. T. (Submitted). Prescribing and primary care psychology: Complementary paths for professional psychology.

Morgan, P. A., & Hooker, R. S. (2010). Choice of specialties among physician assistants in the United States. *Health Affairs, 29,* 897–892.

Morin, C. M., Vallières, A., Guay, B., Ivers, H., & Savard, J. (2009). Cognitive behavioral therapy singly and combined with Rx for persistent insomnia. *Journal of the American Medical Association, 301,* 2005–2015.

Naylor, M. D., & Kurtzman, E. T. (2010). The role of nurse practitioners in reinventing primary care. *Health Affairs, 29,* 893–899.

Newman, R., Phelps, R., Sammons, M. T., Dunivin, D., & Cullen, E. (2000). Evaluation of the psychopharmacology demonstration project: A retrospective analysis. *Professional Psychology: Research and Practice, 31*(6), 598–603.

Olfson, M., & Marcus, S. (2009). National patterns in antidepressant medication treatment. *Archives of General Psychiatry, 66,* 848–856.

Olfson, M., Marcus, S. C., & Shaffer, D. (2006). Antidepressant drug therapy and suicide in severely depressed children and adults: A case-control study. *Archives of General Psychiatry, 63,* 865–872.

Phillips, S. J. (2006). 18th Annual legislative update. *Nurse Practitioner, 31,* 6–38.

Phillips, S. J. (2007). 19th Annual legislative update. *Nurse Practitioner, 32,* 14–42.

Rush, A. J. (2007). STAR*D: What have we learned? *American Journal of Psychiatry, 164,* 201–204.

Sammons, M. T. (1998). The case for prescription privileges for psychologists. An overview. In S. C. Hayes and E. M. Heiby (Eds.), *Prescriptive privileges for psychologists: A critical appraisal* (pp. 11–46). Reno, NV: Context Press.

Sammons, M. T. (2002). Enhancing rural mental health care delivery: The role of prescription privileges. In B. Hudnall-Stamm (Ed.), *Behavioral health care in rural and frontier areas: An interdisciplinary perspective* (pp. 121–132). Washington, DC: American Psychological Association.

Sammons, M. T. (2003). Some paradoxes and pragmatics surrounding the prescriptive authority movement. In M. T. Sammons, R. U. Paige, & R. F. Levant, (Eds.). *The evolution of prescribing psychology: A history and guide.* Washington, DC: American Psychological Association.

Sammons, M. T. (2010). The psychopharmacology demonstration project: What did it teach us, and where are we now? In R. E. McGrath & B. E. Moore (Eds.), *Pharmacotherapy for psychologists* (pp. 49–68). Washington, DC: American Psychological Association.

Sammons, M. T., Gorny, S., Allen, R., & Zinner, E. (2000). Prescriptive authority for psychologists: A consensus of support. *Professional Psychology: Research and Practice, 31,* 604–609.

Sammons, M. T., & Levant, R. (1999). Combining pharmacological and psychological treatment strategies for mental disorders. *Journal of Clinical Psychology in Medical Settings, 6,* 1–10.

Sammons, M. T., & Newman, R. (2010). Effects of an uncertain literature on all facets of clinical decision making. *American Psychologist, 65,* 137–138.

Schwenk, T. L., Evans, D. L., Laden, S. K., and Lewis, L. (2004). Treatment outcome and physician-patient communication in primary care patients with chronic, recurrent depression. *American Journal of Psychiatry, 161,* 1892–901.

Speer, A., & Bess, D. (2003). Evaluation of compensation of nonphysician providers. *American Journal of Health-System Pharmacy, 60,* 78–80.

Sundararaman, R. (2009). Behavioral Health Care in Health Care Reform Legislation. Washington, DC: Congressional Research Service.

TADS Team. (2007). The TADS study: Long-term effectiveness and safety outcomes. *Archives of General Psychiatry, 64,* 1132–1143.

Thomas, C. P., Conrad, P., Casler, R., & Goodman, E. (2006). Trends in the use of psychotropic medications among adolescents, 1994–2001. *Psychiatric Services, 57,* 63–69.

Wells, K., Sherbourne, C., Duan, N., Unützer, J., Miranda, J., Schoenbaum, M.,...Rubenstein, L. (2005). Quality improvement for depression in primary care: Do patients with subthreshold depression benefit in the long run? *American Journal of Psychiatry, 162,* 1149–1157.

Williams, J., Klinepeter, K., Palmes, G., Pulley, A., & Foy, J. M. (2004). Diagnosis and treatment of behavioral health disorders in pediatric practice. *Pediatrics, 114,* 601–606.

Seven

Diagnostic System Innovations

THOMAS A. WIDIGER

INTRODUCTION

The *Diagnostic and Statistical Manual of Mental Disorders* (DSM) is the classification of psychopathology developed under the authority of the American Psychiatric Association (APA). The current version of this nomenclature is DSM-IV-TR (APA, 2000). Work is now proceeding on the next edition, DSM-5 (Regier, Narrow, Kuhl, & Kupfer, 2010). DSM-5 is expected to be published in 2013.

The primary purpose of an official diagnostic nomenclature is to provide a common language of communication (Kendell, 1975; Sartorius et al., 1993). A common language is necessary if there is to be any meaningful communication among clinicians, researchers, and various public healthcare agencies. However, as an official diagnostic nomenclature, the DSM-IV-TR is an exceedingly powerful document, impacting many important social, scientific, forensic, clinical, and other professional decisions (Schwartz & Wiggins, 2002). Persons think in terms of their language, and the predominant language of psychopathology is DSM-IV-TR.

"DSM-IV is a categorical classification that divides mental disorders into types based on criterion sets with defining features" (APA, 2000, p. xxxi). The categorical model of classification is consistent with a medical tradition in which it is believed (and often confirmed in other areas of medicine) that individual disorders have specific etiologies, pathologies, and treatments (Guze, 1978; Guze & Helzer, 1987; Zachar & Kendler, 2007). Following this lead, clinicians diagnose and conceptualize the conditions presented in DSM-IV-TR as disorders that are qualitatively distinct from normal functioning and from one another.

However, a long-standing question within psychiatry has been whether mental disorders are, in fact, discrete clinical conditions or, instead, arbitrary distinctions along continuous dimensions of functioning (Kendell, 1975). The significance of this question is escalating with the growing recognition of the limitations of the categorical model (Widiger & Clark, 2000; Widiger & Samuel, 2005). As expressed by the vice chair of DSM-5:

> The failure of DSM-III criteria to specifically define individuals with only one disorder served as an alert that the strict neo-Kraepelinian categorical approach to mental disorder diagnoses advocated by Robins and Guze (1970), Spitzer, Endicott, & Robins (1975), and others could have some serious problems. (Regier, 2008, p. xxi)

As expressed by Drs. Kupfer, First, and Regier (two of whom are the chair and vice chair of DSM-5):

> In the more than 30 years since the introduction of the Feighner criteria by Robins and Guze, which eventually led to DSM-III, the goal of validating these syndromes and discovering common etiologies has remained elusive. Despite many proposed candidates, not one laboratory marker has been found to be specific in identifying any of the DSM-defined syndromes. Epidemiologic and clinical studies have shown extremely high rates of comorbidities among the disorders, undermining the hypothesis that the syndromes represent distinct etiologies. Furthermore, epidemiologic studies have shown a high degree of short-term diagnostic instability for many disorders. With regard to treatment, lack of treatment specificity is the rule rather than the exception. (Kupfer, First, & Regier, 2002, p. xviii)

The Robins and Guze (1970) paradigm for the validation of categorical diagnosis has been widely influential within psychiatry (Klerman, 1983; Kupfer et al., 2002). In 1989, Robins and Barrett (1989) edited a text in honor of this classic paper. Kendell (1989) provided the final word in his closing chapter. His conclusions, however, were curiously negative: "Ninety years have now elapsed since Kraepelin first provided the framework of a plausible classification of mental disorders. Why then, with so many potential validators available, have we made so little progress since that time?" (Kendell, 1989, p. 313). He answered his rhetorical question in the next paragraph:

"One important possibility is that the discrete clusters of psychiatric symptoms we are trying to delineate do not actually exist but are as much a mirage as discrete personality types" (p. 313).

Most (if not all) mental disorders appear to be the result of a complex interaction of an array of interacting biological vulnerabilities and dispositions with a number of significant environmental, psychosocial events that often exert their effects over a progressively developing period of time (Rutter, 2003). The symptoms and pathologies of mental disorders appear to be highly responsive to a wide variety of neurobiological, interpersonal, cognitive, and other mediating and moderating variables that help to develop, shape, and form a particular individual's psychopathology profile. This complex etiological history and individual psychopathology profile are unlikely to be well described by single diagnostic categories that attempt to make distinctions at nonexistent discrete joints along the continuous distributions (Widiger & Samuel, 2005). The publication of DSM-III provided a significant, major advance in the diagnosis and classification of psychopathology (Klerman, 1983). As Craddock and Owen (2002) suggest, perhaps it is time to move on.

The psychiatric diagnostic system is currently failing in many ways, including in an absence of a provision of reliably distinct boundaries, an absence of a credible rationale for diagnostic thresholds, an inadequate coverage of existing clinical populations, and the absence of specific etiologies and treatments (Kupfer et al., 2002; Regier et al., 1989; Widiger & Trull, 2007). Discussed herein will be, in particular, the difficulties with diagnostic co-occurrence and arbitrary diagnostic thresholds. This will be followed by a description of a dimensional classification that could serve as a model for the rest of the diagnostic manual. The chapter will conclude with a brief discussion of the forthcoming DSM-5 and recommendations for the future.

EXCESSIVE DIAGNOSTIC CO-OCCURRENCE

One of the more problematic findings for the validity of the DSM-IV-TR categorical model of classification has been the excessive comorbidity among diagnoses (Krueger & Markon, 2006; Maser & Patterson, 2002; Widiger & Clark, 2000). The term "comorbidity" refers to the co-occurrence of distinct disorders, each presumably with its own etiology, pathology, and treatment implications. However, as recognized years ago, "the greatest challenge that the extensive comorbidity data pose to the current nosological system concerns the validity of the diagnostic categories themselves—Do these disorders constitute distinct clinical entities?" (Mineka, Watson, & Clark, 1998, p. 380). Concurrent diagnostic comorbidity is the norm rather than the exception, with the rate dramatically increasing if one considers lifetime comorbidity (Brown, Campbell, Lehman, Grisham, & Mancill, 2001; Kessler et al., 1994).

The widely cited National Institute of Mental Health's epidemiologic catchment area (ECA) program provided one of the most extensive studies of the epidemiology of mental disorders across rural and urban America. Its most revealing finding was the substantial degree of diagnostic comorbidity (Regier et al., 1998), despite being confined to just a small proportion of all of the disorders included within the diagnostic manual. The ECA findings led in turn to the National Comorbidity Survey (NCS), which focused on the comorbidity of substance use with other disorders (Kessler et al., 1994). The NCS reported that "the vast majority of lifetime disorders in the NCS (79%) were comorbid disorders" (Kessler et al., 1994, p. 11)—a finding again understated by the fact that only a minority of the disorders included in DSM-IV were surveyed. The NCS was followed by the National Epidemiologic Survey on Alcohol and Related Conditions (NESARC), which again reported the occurrence of a "pervasive" diagnostic comorbidity (Grant et al., 2004, p. 361).

DSM-IV-TR provides diagnostic criterion sets to help guide clinicians toward a single, correct diagnosis and an additional supplementary section devoted to differential diagnosis that indicates "how to differentiate [the] disorder from other disorders that have similar presenting characteristics" (APA, 2000, p. 10). The intention of the diagnostic manual is to help the clinician determine which particular mental disorder is present, the selection of which would presumably indicate the presence of a specific pathology that will explain the occurrence of the symptoms and suggest a specific treatment that will ameliorate the patient's suffering (Frances, First, & Pincus, 1995; Kendell, 1975). Considerable effort is spent by the authors of each edition of the diagnostic manual to further buttress each disorder's criterion set, trying to shore up discriminant validity and distinctiveness, following the rubric of Robins and Guze (1970) that the validity of a diagnosis rests in large part on its "delimitation from other disorders...These criteria should...permit exclusion of borderline cases and doubtful cases (an undiagnosed group) so that the index group may be as homogeneous as possible" (p. 108).

However, it is evident from the extensive comorbidity reported by the ECA, NCS, and NESARC that the effort to construct a manual that will direct clinicians to a single diagnosis has not succeeded. Indeed, as suggested more recently by Kendell and Jablensky (2003), "If no detectable discontinuities in symptoms are found in large tracts of the territory of psychiatric disorder, it is likely that, sooner or later, our existing typology will be abandoned and replaced by a dimensional classification" (p. 8).

In some instances, the presence of multiple diagnoses suggests distinct yet comorbid psychopathologies; however, in most instances, the presence of co-occurring diagnoses suggests instead common, shared pathologies (Widiger & Clark, 2000). Psychosocial and pharmacologic interventions, with few exceptions, target and have effects upon a number of different disorders rather than being specific to individual diagnostic categories (Parker, 2000). Underlying the problematic diagnostic co-occurrence across the substance, mood, anxiety, and other mental disorders appear to be (in part) common domains of functioning that correspond closely to broad dimensions of general personality functioning, identified as neuroticism (or negative affectivity), positive affectivity (extraversion), disinhibition (or low constraint, conscientiousness), and antagonism (Krueger & Tackett, 2003).

Krueger and his colleagues have been particularly productive in replicating within a variety of populations the two dimensions of internalization and externalization identified by Achenbach and Edelbrock (1978) many years ago within childhood psychopathology (Goldberg, Krueger, Andrews, & Hobbs, 2009). These broad domains of functioning are governed in large part by fundamental temperaments (McCrae & Costa, 2003) that provide neurobiological dispositions toward the development of a number of DSM-IV-TR mental disorders (Krueger & Tackett, 2003):

> Comorbidity may be trying to show us that many current treatments are not so much treatments for transient "state" mental disorders of affect and anxiety as they are treatments for core processes, such as negative affectivity, that span normal and abnormal variation as well as undergird multiple mental disorders. (Krueger, 2002, p. 44)

However, it is not yet clear how the APA diagnostic manual could in fact be reorganized with respect to internalization and externalization. Public healthcare, insurance, and other agencies communicate information concerning psychopathology using the DSM-IV-TR alphabetical and numerical coding system, developed originally by the World Health Organization (WHO) for the international classification of diseases (ICD-10; WHO, 1992). Mental disorders are within the section of the ICD identified by the letter "F," followed by a numerical code to indicate which specific disorder is present. Acute stress disorder, for example, has the code of F308.3, and major depressive disorder, recurrent, has the code of F296.3. This alphanumerical coding system is effective for a universal, cross-language communication of the diagnostic categories, but it would be difficult to record at the same time within the existing system broad dimensions that cut across the existing diagnostic categories (Frances et al., 1995).

ARBITRARY DIAGNOSTIC THRESHOLDS

Each revision to the APA diagnostic manual generates substantial confusion in that seemingly minor changes to diagnostic criterion sets often result in unexpected and quite substantial shifts in prevalence rates that profoundly complicate scientific theory and public healthcare decisions (Narrow, Rae, Robins, & Regier, 2002). According to Regier et al. (1998), "We are...in need of clear information on the prevalence rates of psychiatric disorders for public policy and constituent groups who support and ultimately benefit from our research activities" (p. 114). Regier and Narrow (2000) state that "a major goal of the next generation of psychiatric epidemiology will be to establish a more precise and clinically relevant baseline than was accomplished by the ECA program and the NCS" (p. 28).

Establishing a single, fixed diagnostic threshold that would lead to consistent prevalence estimates is exceedingly difficult in the absence of any clear, distinct boundary between normal and abnormal functioning. There is currently no consistently applied or well understood threshold for the presence of any single DSM-IV-TR mental disorder. None of the thresholds for a DSM-IV-TR mental disorder were set at a distinct point of demarcation. All of the diagnostic thresholds are largely arbitrary, set at that point at which it seems reasonable to conclude that a respective disorder is present. There is no gold standard to guide these decisions or no objective laboratory measure that can objectively confirm the presence versus absence of a respective disorder (Epstein, Isenberg, Stern, & Silbersweig, 2002). As a result, the thresholds vary considerably across revisions to the diagnostic manual as the authors of these criterion sets tinker with their number and content in an effort to improve differential diagnosis.

The most popular diagnosis in many clinical settings is the wastebasket category of "not otherwise specified" (NOS). NOS is used when a clinician has determined that a mental disorder is present but the person fails to meet the diagnostic criteria for one of the existing diagnostic categories (APA, 2000). The fact that NOS is used so frequently suggests that the existing diagnostic categories lack clinical utility (Mullins-Sweatt & Widiger, 2009). A substantial number of persons are seeking treatment for conditions that fail to meet diagnostic criteria for a particular DSM-IV-TR anxiety, mood, eating, personality, or other form of psychopathology (e.g., Magruder & Calderone, 2000; Shisslak, Crago, & Estes, 1995; Stein, Walker, Hazen, & Forde, 1997).

Consider, for example, subthreshold depression (Pincus, McQueen, & Elinson, 2003). "The majority of cases of clinical depression go unrecognized and untreated" (Munoz, Hollon, McGrath, Rehm, & VandenBos, 1994, p. 42). Persons with subthreshold levels of depression exhibit high rates of healthcare utilization and require substantial medical care costs (Johnson, Weissman, & Klerman, 1992). Nearly half of all pharmacologic interventions for depression are prescribed by primary care physicians, with many of these patients failing to meet diagnostic criteria for any existing mood disorder diagnosis (Merikangas, Ernst, Maier, Hoyer, & Angst, 1996).

Even the namesake for the neo-Kraepelinian movement that led to DSM-III appears to have known that it does not really work. Kraepelin (1917) acknowledged that "wherever we try to mark out the frontier between mental health and disease, we find a neutral territory, in which the imperceptible change from the realm of normal life to that of obvious derangement takes place" (p. 295). A simple inspection of the diagnostic criteria for major depressive disorder would not lend confidence to a conceptualization of this disorder as a condition qualitatively distinct from normal depression or sadness (Andrews et al., 2008). The diagnostic criteria include depressed mood, loss of interest or pleasure, weight loss (or gain), insomnia (or hypersomnia), psychomotor retardation (or agitation), loss of energy, feelings of worthlessness, and/or diminished capacity to make decisions.

Each of these diagnostic criteria is readily placed along a continuum of severity that would shade imperceptibly into what would be considered a normal sadness or depression. DSM-IV-TR, therefore, includes specific thresholds for each diagnostic criterion, but the words that are inserted are simply demarcating arbitrary levels of severity (e.g., "nearly every day," "markedly diminished," and at least a "2 week" period; APA, 2000). The diagnosis requires five of these nine criteria, with no apparent rationale for this threshold other than it would appear to be severe enough to be defensible to be titled as a "major" depressive episode, as distinguished from a "minor" depressive episode, which is then distinguished from "normal" sadness (APA, 2000).

Depression does appear to shade imperceptibly into "normal" sadness (Andrews et al., 2008). Ustun and Sartorius (1995) conducted a study of 5,000 primary care attendees in 14 countries and reported a linear relationship between disability and number of depressive symptoms. Kessler, Zhao, Blazer, and Swartz (1997) examined the distribution of minor and major symptoms of depression using data from the National Comorbidity Survey. They examined the relationship of these symptoms with parental history of mental disorder, number and duration of depressive episodes, and comorbidity with other forms of psychopathology. Relationship increased with increasing number of symptoms, with no clear, distinct break in relationships. Sakashita, Slade, and Andrews (2007) examined the relationship between the number of symptoms of depression and four measures of impairment using data from the Australian National Survey of Mental Health and Well-Being; they found that the relationship was again simply linear, with no clear or natural discontinuity to support the selection of any particular cutoff point.

A dimensional model would recognize the existence of this continuity, provide a means for tracking subthreshold conditions, and facilitate the development of more precise, consistent, and uniform points of demarcation along the continuum for different social, clinical decisions. The existing diagnostic categories are frustrating and troublesome to clinicians in part because the existing diagnostic thresholds do not have a clear meaning or functional relevance to their clinical decisions (Mullins-Sweatt & Widiger, 2009). The current diagnostic thresholds are not set at a point that is optimal for any one particular social or clinical decision, and yet they are used to inform a wide variety of public healthcare concerns. As a result, the thresholds are largely ineffective for each one of them.

Kraemer, Noda, and O'Hara (2004) argue that, in the mental health profession, "a categorical diagnosis is necessary" (p. 21). Kraemer and colleagues state that "clinicians who must decide whether to treat or not treat a patient, to hospitalize or not, to treat a patient with a drug or with psychotherapy, or what type, must inevitably use a categorical approach to diagnosis" (p. 12). While seemingly compelling, this is not an accurate characterization of actual clinical practice.

In many common clinical situations, the decision is not actually categorical. Clinicians and social agencies make decisions with respect to frequency of therapy sessions, degree of medication dosage, and even degrees of hospitalization (e.g., day hospital, partial hospitalization, residential program, or traditional hospitalization). Even more importantly, it is evident that the many different important social, clinical decisions will not be well informed by the same diagnostic threshold (e.g., pharmacotherapy, hospitalization, psychotherapy, disability, and insurance coverage). A dimensional model would increase the credibility of mental disorder classification by providing the means with which to identify more explicitly and reliably precise points along respective continua that would be optimal for these different decisions, rather than assuming that a single diagnostic threshold, which is itself largely arbitrary, is optimal for all of the different decisions that must be made.

INTELLECTUAL DISABILITY

Many persons write as if a shift to a dimensional classification represents a new, fundamental change to the diagnostic manual (e.g., Regier, 2008; Rounsaville et al., 2002). For much of the manual, such a shift would certainly represent a fundamental change in how mental disorders are conceptualized and classified (Guze, 1978; Guze & Helzer, 1987; Robins & Guze, 1970). Nevertheless, there is a clear precedent for a dimensional classification of psychopathology already included within DSM-IV-TR: the diagnosis of mental retardation (APA, 2000).

In DSM-IV-TR, mental retardation is diagnosed along a continuum of intellectual and social functioning—more specifically, "significantly subaverage intellectual functioning: an IQ [intelligence quotient] of approximately 70 or below" (APA,

2000, p. 49), along with related deficits or impairments in adaptive functioning. An IQ of 70 does not carve nature at a discrete joint or identify the presence of a qualitatively distinct condition, disease, or disorder. On the contrary, it is a quantitative cutoff point along a continuum of functioning. An IQ of 70 is simply two standard deviations below the mean of an appropriate assessment instrument (American Association of Mental Retardation [AAMR], 2002).

Intelligence involves the ability to reason, plan, solve problems, think abstractly, comprehend complex ideas, learn quickly, and learn from experience (AAMR, 2002). It is distributed as a hierarchical, multifactorial continuous variable because most persons' level of intelligence, including most of those with mental retardation, is the result of a complex interaction of multiple genetic, fetal, and infant development, and environmental influences (Deary, Spinath, & Bates, 2006). There are no discrete breaks in its distribution that would provide an absolute distinction between normal and abnormal intelligence. The point of demarcation for the diagnosis of an intellectual disability (the more current term for the disorder) is an arbitrary, quantitative distinction along the normally distributed levels of hierarchically and multifactorially defined intelligence. This point of demarcation is arbitrary in the sense that it does not carve nature at a discrete joint, but it was not, of course, randomly or mindlessly chosen. It is a defensible selection that was informed by the impairments in functioning commonly associated with an IQ of 70 or below (AAMR, 2002).

In addition, the disorder of mental retardation is not diagnosed simply by the presence of an IQ of 70 or below. It must be accompanied by a documented impairment to functioning. "Mental retardation is a disability characterized by significant limitation in both intellectual functioning and in adaptive behavior as expressed in conceptual, social, and practical adaptive skills" (AAMR, 2002, p. 23). Persons with IQ scores lower than 70 who can function effectively would not be diagnosed. The diagnosis is understood in the context of the social, practical requirements of everyday functioning that must be met by the person (Luckasson & Reeve, 2002). The purpose of the diagnosis is not to suggest that a specific pathology is present, but rather to identify persons who, on the basis of their intellectual disability, would be eligible for public healthcare services and benefits to help them overcome or compensate for their relatively lower level of intelligence.

Many instances of intellectual disability are due in large part to specific etiologies, such as tuberous sclerosis, microcephaly, von Recklinghausen's disease, trisomy 21, mosaicism, Prader–Willi syndrome, and many, many more (Kendell & Jablensky, 2003). Nevertheless, the disorders that result from these specific etiologies are generally understood as medical conditions, an associated feature of which is also an intellectual disability that would be diagnosed concurrently and independently as mental retardation. The intellectual disability diagnosed as a mental disorder within DSM-IV-TR is itself a multifactorially determined and heterogeneous dimensional construct falling along the broad continuum of intellectual functioning. "The causes of intellectual disabilities are typically complex interactions of biological, behavioral/psychological, and sociocultural factors" (Naglieri, Salter, & Rojahn, 2008, p. 409). An important postnatal cause for intellectual disability is "simply" psychosocial deprivation, resulting from poverty, chaotic living environment, and/or child abuse or neglect. As expressed in DSM-IV-TR, "In approximately 30–40% of individuals seen in clinical settings, no clear etiology for the mental retardation can be determined despite extensive evaluation efforts" (APA, 2000, p. 45).

In sum, in the classification of intellectual disability (mental retardation), one diagnoses a multifactorial disorder on the basis of a normative cutoff point and level of impairment without any implication of there being a qualitative distinction. Intellectual disability may serve as an effective model for the classification of the rest of the diagnostic manual, including mood, psychotic, personality, anxiety, and other mental disorders.

DSM-5 AND DIMENSIONAL CLASSIFICATION

The first paragraph of the introduction to DSM-IV-TR states that "our highest priority has been to provide a helpful guide to clinical practice" (APA, 2000, p. xxiii). First (2005) argued in his rejoinder to proposals for shifting the diagnostic manual into a dimension model, that "the most important obstacle standing in the way of its implementation in DSM-V (and beyond) is questions about clinical utility" (p. 561). Nevertheless, one must question whether the existing diagnostic manual in fact has appreciable clinical utility (Mullins-Sweatt & Widiger, 2009). "Apologists for categorical diagnoses argue that the system has clinical utility, being easy to use and valuable in formulating cases and planning treatment [but] there is little evidence for these assertions" (Livesley, 2001, p. 278). First (2005) suggested in one context that "the current categorical system of DSM has clinical utility with regard to the treatment of individuals" (p. 562), but within another context stated that "with regard to treatment, lack of treatment specificity is the rule rather than the exception" (Kupfer et al., 2002, p. xviii).

The heterogeneity of diagnostic membership, the lack of precision in description, the excessive diagnostic co-occurrence, the failure to lead to a specific diagnosis, the reliance on the "not otherwise specified" wastebasket diagnosis, and the unstable and arbitrary diagnostic boundaries of the DSM-IV-TR diagnostic categories are matters of clinical utility that are a source of considerable frustration for clinicians and public healthcare agencies (Mullins-Sweatt & Widiger, 2009).

In 1999, a DSM-5 research planning conference was held under joint sponsorship of the APA and the National Institute of Mental Health (NIMH); the purpose was to set research priorities that would optimally inform future classifications. An impetus for this effort was the frustration with the existing nomenclature (Kupfer et al., 2002). At this conference, DSM-5 research planning work groups were formed to develop white papers that would set a research agenda for DSM-5. The nomenclature work group, charged with addressing fundamental assumptions of the diagnostic system, concluded that it would be "important that consideration be given to advantages and disadvantages of basing part or all of DSM-V on dimensions rather than categories" (Rounsaville et al., 2002, p. 12).

The white papers developed by the DSM-5 research planning work groups were followed by a series of international conferences whose purpose was to further enrich the empirical database in preparation for the eventual development of DSM-5 (a description of this conference series can be found at www.dsm5.org). The first conference was devoted to shifting personality disorders to a dimensional model of classification (Widiger, Simonsen, Krueger, Livesley, & Verheul, 2005). The final conference was devoted to dimensional approaches across the diagnostic manual, including substance use disorders, major depressive disorder, psychoses, anxiety disorders, and developmental psychopathology, as well as the personality disorders (Helzer, Kraemer, et al., 2008).

Work on DSM-5 is now well underway, and it is evident that a primary goal is to shift the manual toward a dimensional classification (Helzer, Wittchen, Krueger, & Kraemer, 2008; Regier et al., 2010). This effort is a clear recognition of the failure of the categorical system. Nevertheless, it also appears to be the case that the shifts likely to be taken in DSM-5 will be neither fundamental nor significant. The effort is likely to fall considerably short of a true paradigm shift. Current proposals appear, for the most part, to be quite tentative, if not timid. "What is being proposed for DSM-V is not to substitute dimensional scales for categorical diagnoses, but to add a dimensional option to the usual categorical diagnoses for DSM-V[sic]" (Kraemer, 2008, p. 9).

As acknowledged by Helzer, Kraemer, and Krueger (2006), "Our proposal not only preserves categorical definitions but also does not alter the process by which these definitions would be developed. Those charged with developing criteria for specific mental disorders would operate just as their predecessors have" (p. 1675). In other words, work groups will continue to develop diagnostic criteria to describe prototypic cases in a manner that will maximize homogeneity and differential diagnosis (Robins & Guze, 1970; Spitzer, Williams, & Skodol, 1980), thereby continuing to fail to describe typical cases adequately and again leaving many patients to receive the diagnosis of NOS.

Dimensional proposals for DSM-5 have been posted on the official APA Web site (www.dsm5.org). However, all of the proposals are only to develop "supplementary dimensional approaches to the categorical definitions that would also relate back to the categorical definitions" (Helzer, Wittchen, et al., 2008, p. 116). These dimensions will only serve as ancillary descriptions that will lack any official representation within a patient's medical record (i.e., they will have no official alphanumerical code and may then not even be communicated to any public healthcare agency). In sum, "what is being proposed for DSM-V is not to substitute dimensional scales for categorical diagnoses, but to add a dimensional option to the usual categorical diagnoses for DSM-V" (Kraemer, 2008, p. 9). In the end, DSM-5 will remain a categorical diagnostic system.

DSM-III is often said to have provided a significant paradigm shift in how psychopathology is diagnosed (Kendell & Jablensky, 2003; Klerman, 1983; Regier, 2008). Much of the credit for the innovative nature and success of DSM-III is due to the foresight, resolve, and perhaps even courage of its chair, Dr. Robert Spitzer. The primary authors of DSM-5 fully recognize the failure of the categorical model of classification (Kupfer et al., 2002; Regier, 2008; Regier et al., 2010). They have the empirical support and the opportunity to lead the field of psychiatry to a comparably bold new future in diagnosis and classification, but it does not appear that this will in fact occur.

RECOMMENDATIONS FOR THE FUTURE

Three recommendations follow from this discussion; these include implementing a true paradigm shift in the conceptualization and classification of mental disorders, separating the assessment of disorder from the impairment it causes, and collaborating with public healthcare agencies to establish diagnostic thresholds that have a specific meaning and function for each particular social, clinical decision. Each of these recommendations will be discussed briefly in turn.

Implement a True Paradigm Shift

It is apparent to the chair and vice chair of DSM-5 that the diagnosis of psychopathology should shift from a categorical to a dimensional classification (Kupfer et al., 2002; Regier, 2008; Regier et al., 2010). Yet, DSM-5 will remain a categorical model of classification. What is needed instead is a true paradigm shift in the classification of psychopathology from diagnostic categories to a dimensional classification.

This shift must include the provision of the dimensional classification with official diagnostic coding so that it will in fact be used in clinical practice and will be used for official communications among various public healthcare agencies. Relegating the dimensional classification to an ancillary, supplementary option will mean that it will carry no official recognition within a patient's medical record. Clinicians and public healthcare agencies will continue to use primarily if not solely the categorical diagnoses. For the dimensional classifications created by each DSM-5 work group to have any real impact, they need to be part of the official medical record of each respective patient. This shift would require a major change in the ICD-10 and DSM-IV-TR alphanumerical coding system, but it would be a shame for a bureaucratic coding tradition to prevent a shift in classification that would dramatically improve the validity and clinical utility of psychiatric diagnosis.

Separate the Assessment of Disorder From Impairment

The classification of each mental disorder should include separate scales for the assessment of the presence of the disorder and for level of impairment (Sartorius, 2009). Not all persons sharing the same disorder will have the same level of impairment. The inclusion of separate scales is also consistent with the current interest within psychiatry to separate the diagnosis of disorder from the assessment of disability in the theory that some persons with a disorder may not in fact be suffering from any significant impairment (Lehman, Alexopolous, Goldman, Jeste, & Ustun, 2002).

The presence of a clinically significant impairment, however, may also remain a fundamental and necessary component for determining at what point a mental disorder is said to be present (Widiger & Clark, 2000). In any case, the presence of a separate scale for level of impairment will allow for a more uniform, meaningful, and consistent threshold across all disorders (and revisions to the diagnostic manual) for determining when a disorder is considered to be present, rather than leaving it up to the subjective interests and whims of each separate work group.

Establish Different Thresholds for Different Social, Clinical Needs

The third recommendation is to work closely with different public healthcare agencies to establish additional thresholds (also likely based on level of impairment) that are optimally suitable for their particular needs and concerns. The presence of a mental disorder does not necessarily suggest the need for insurance coverage, hospitalization, disability, or mitigation of criminal responsibility. Given that there is no qualitative point of demarcation for an absolute judgment for the presence of a mental disorder, points of demarcation should instead be based on pragmatic implications and be optimally suitable for different social, clinical decisions. The development of different cutoff points for different social, clinical decisions will require a willingness to collaborate closely with different agencies and associations; in the end, this collaboration will result in a diagnostic system that has much better credibility, meaning, and value for everyone concerned.

REFERENCES

Achenbach, T. M., & Edelbrock, C. S. (1978). The classification of child psychopathology: A review and analysis of empirical efforts. *Psychological Bulletin, 85,* 1275–1301.

AAMR (American Association on Mental Retardation). (2002). *Mental retardation: Definition, classification, and systems of support* (10th ed.). Washington, DC: Author.

APA (American Psychiatric Association). (2000). *Diagnostic and statistical manual of mental disorders. Text Revision* (4th ed., rev. ed.). Washington, DC: Author.

Andrews, G., Brugha, T., Thase, M., Duffy, F. F., Rucci, P., & Slade, T. (2008). Dimensionality and the category of major depressive episode. In J. E. Helzer, H. C. Kraemer, R. F. Krueger, H-U. Wittchen, P. J. Sirovatka, & D. A. Regier (Eds.), *Dimensional approaches to diagnostic classification. Refining the research agenda for DSM-V* (pp. 35–51). Washington, DC: American Psychiatric Association.

Brown, T. A., Campbell, L. A., Lehman, C. L., Grisham, J. R., & Mancill, R. B. (2001). Current and lifetime comorbidity of the DSM-IV anxiety and mood disorders in a large clinical sample. *Journal of Abnormal Psychology, 110,* 585–599.

Craddock, N., & Owen, M. J. (2005). The beginning of the end for the Kraepelinian dichotomy. *British Journal of Psychiatry, 186,* 364–366.

Deary, I. J., Spinath, F. M., & Bates, T. C. (2006). Genetics of intelligence. *European Journal of Human Genetics, 14,* 690–700.

Epstein, J., Isenberg, N., Stern, E., & Silbersweig, D. (2002). Toward a neuroanatomical understanding of psychiatric illness: The role of functional imaging. In J. E. Helzer & J. J. Hudziak (Eds.), *Defining psychopathology in the 21st century* (pp. 57–69). Washington, DC: American Psychiatric Press.

First, M. B. (2005). Clinical utility: A prerequisite for the adoption of a dimensional approach in DSM. *Journal of Abnormal Psychology, 114,* 560–564.

Frances, A. J., First, M. B., & Pincus, H. A. (1995). *DSM-IV guidebook.* Washington, DC: American Psychiatric Press.

Goldberg, D. P., Krueger, R. F., Andrews, G., & Hobbs, M. J. (2009). Emotional disorders: Cluster 4 of the proposed meta-structure for DSM-V and ICD-11. *Psychological Medicine, 39,* 2043–2059.

Grant, B. F., Stinson, F. S., Dawson, D. A., Chou, S. P., Ruan, W. J., & Pickering, R. P. (2004). Co-occurrence of 12-month alcohol and drug use disorders and personality disorders in the United States: Results from the National Epidemiologic Survey on Alcohol and Related Conditions. *Archives of General Psychiatry, 61,* 361–368.

Guze, S. B. (1978). Nature of psychiatric illness: Why psychiatry is a branch of medicine. *Comprehensive Psychiatry, 19,* 295–307.

Guze, S. B., & Helzer, J. E. (1987). The medical model and psychiatric disorders. In R. Michels & J. Cavenar (Eds.), *Psychiatry* (Vol. 1, chap. 51, pp. 1–8). Philadelphia, PA: J. B. Lippincott.

Helzer, J. E., Kraemer, H. C., & Krueger, R. F. (2006). The feasibility and need for dimensional psychiatric diagnoses. *Psychological Medicine, 36,* 1671–1680.

Helzer, J. E., Kraemer, H. C., Krueger, R. F., Wittchen, H-U., Sirovatka, P. J., & Regier, D. A. (Eds.). (2008). *Dimensional approaches in diagnostic classification.* Washington, DC: American Psychiatric Association.

Helzer, J. E., Wittchen, H-U., Krueger, R. F., & Kraemer, H. C. (2008). Dimensional options for DSM-V: The way forward. In J. E. Helzer, H. C. Kraemer, R. F. Krueger, H-U. Wittchen, P. J. Sirovatka, & D. A. Regier (Eds.), *Dimensional approaches to diagnostic classification. Refining the research agenda for DSM-V* (pp. 115–127). Washington, DC: American Psychiatric Association.

Johnson, J., Weissman, M. M., & Klerman, G. L. (1992). Service utilization and social morbidity associated with depressive symptoms in the community. *Journal of the American Medical Association, 267,* 1478–1483.

Kendell, R. E. (1975). *The role of diagnosis in psychiatry.* Oxford, England: Blackwell Scientific Publications.

Kendell, R. E. (1989). Clinical validity. In L. N. Robins & J. E. Barrett (Eds.), *The validity of psychiatric diagnosis* (pp. 305–321). New York, NY: Raven Press.

Kendell, R. E., & Jablensky, A. (2003). Distinguishing between the validity and utility of psychiatric diagnosis. *American Journal of Psychiatry, 160,* 4–12.

Kessler, R. C., McGonagle, K. A., Zhao, S., Nelson, C. B., Hughes, M., Eshleman, S.,...Kendler, K. S. (1994). Lifetime and 12-month prevalence of DSM-III-R psychiatric disorders in the United States: Results from the national comorbidity survey. *Archives of General Psychiatry, 51,* 8–19.

Kessler, R. C., Zhao, S., Blazer, D. G., & Swartz, M. (1997). Prevalence, correlates, and course of minor depression and major depression in the national comorbidity survey. *Journal of Affective Disorders, 45,* 19–30.

Klerman, G. L. (1983). The significance of DSM-III in American psychiatry. In. R. L. Spitzer, J. B. W. Williams, & A. E. Skodol (Eds.), *International perspectives on DSM-III* (pp. 3–26). Washington, DC: American Psychiatric Press.

Kraemer, H. C. (2008). DSM categories and dimensions in clinical and research contexts. In J. E. Helzer, H. C. Kraemer, R. F. Krueger, H-U. Wittchen, P. J. Sirovatka, & D. A. Regier (Eds.), *Dimensional approaches to diagnostic classification. Refining the research agenda for DSM-V* (pp. 5–17). Washington, DC: American Psychiatric Association.

Kraemer, H. C., Noda, A., & O'Hara, R. (2004). Categorical versus dimensional approaches to diagnosis: Methodological challenges. *Journal of Psychiatric Research, 38,* 17–25.

Kraepelin, E. (1917). *Lectures on clinical psychiatry* (3rd ed.). New York, NY: William Wood.

Krueger, R. F. (2002). Psychometric perspectives on comorbidity. In J. E. Helzer & J. J. Hudziak (Eds.), *Defining psychopathology in the 21st century. DSM-V and beyond* (pp. 41–54). Washington, DC: American Psychiatric Publishing.

Krueger, R. F., & Markon, K. E. (2006). Reinterpreting comorbidity: A model-based approach to understanding and classifying psychopathology. *Annual Review of Clinical Psychology, 2,* 111–133.

Krueger, R. F., & Tackett, J. L. (2003). Personality and psychopathology: Working toward the bigger picture. *Journal of Personality Disorders, 17,* 109–1128.

Kupfer, D. J., First, M. B., & Regier, D. A. (Eds.). (2002). Introduction. In D. J. Kupfer, M. B. First, & D. A. Regier (Eds.), *A research agenda for DSM-V* (pp. xv–xxiii). Washington, DC: American Psychiatric Association.

Lehman, A. F., Alexopolous, G. S., Goldman, H., Jeste, D., & Ustun, B. (2002). Mental disorder and disability: Time to reevaulate the relationship? In D. J. Kupfer, M. B. First, & D. A. Regier (Eds.), *A research agenda for DSM-V* (pp. 201–218). Washington, DC: American Psychiatric Association.

Livesley, W. J. (2001). Commentary on reconceptualizing personality disorder categories using trait dimensions. *Journal of Personality, 69,* 277–286.

Luckasson, R., & Reeve, A. (2001). Naming, defining, and classifying in mental retardation. *Mental Retardation, 39,* 47–52.

Magruder, K. M., & Calderone, G. E. (2000). Public health consequences of different thresholds for the diagnosis of mental disorders. *Comprehensive Psychiatry, 41,* 14–18.

Maser, J. D., & Patterson, T. (2002). Spectrum and nosology: implications for DSM-V. *Psychiatric Clinics of North America, 25,* 855–885.

McCrae, R. R., & Costa, P. T. (2003). *Personality in adulthood: A five-factor theory perspective.* New York: NY: Guilford.

Merikangas, K. R., Ernst, C., Maier, W., Hoyer, E. B., & Angst, J. (1996). In T. A. Widiger, A. J. Frances, H. A. Pincus, R. Ross, M. B. First, & W. W. Davis (Eds.), *DSM-IV sourcebook* (Vol. 2, pp. 97–110). Washington, DC: American Psychiatric Association.

Mineka, S., Watson, D., & Clark, L. A. (1998). Comorbidity of anxiety and unipolar mood disorders. *Annual Review of Psychology, 49,* 377–412.

Mullins-Sweatt, S. N., & Widiger, T. A. (2009). Clinical utility and DSM-V. *Psychological Assessment, 21,* 302–312.

Munoz, R. F., Hollon, S. D., McGrath, E., Rehm, L. P., & VandenBos, G. P. (1994). On the AHCPR depression in primary care guidelines. *American Psychologist, 49,* 42–61.

Naglieri, J., Salter, C., & Rojahn, J. (2008). Cognitive disorders of childhood. Specific learning and intellectual disabilities. In J. E. Maddux & B. A. Winstead (Eds.), *Psychopathology. Foundations for a contemporary understanding* (2nd ed., pp. 401–416). Mahwah, NJ: Lawrence Erlbaum Associates.

Narrow, W. E., Rae, D. S., Robins, L. N., & Regier, D. A. (2002). Revised prevalence estimates of mental disorders in the United States. Using a clinical significance criterion to reconcile 2 surveys' estimates. *Archives of General Psychiatry, 59,* 115–123.

Parker, G. (2000). Classifying depression: Should paradigms lost be regained? *Archives of General Psychiatry, 157,* 1195–1203.

Pincus, H. A., McQueen, L. E., & Elinson, L. (2003). Subthreshold mental disorders: Nosological and research recommendations. In K. A. Phillips, M. B. First, & H. A. Pincus (Eds.), *Advancing DSM. Dilemmas in psychiatric diagnosis* (pp. 129–144). Washington, DC: American Psychiatric Association.

Regier, D. A. (2008). Forward: Dimensional approaches to psychiatric classification. In J. E. Helzer, H. C. Kraemer, R. F. Krueger, H-U. Wittchen, P. J. Sirovatka, & D. A. Regier (Eds.), *Dimensional approaches to diagnostic classification. Refining the research agenda for DSM-V.* Washington, DC: American Psychiatric Association.

Regier, D. A., Kaelber, C. T., Rae, D. S., Farmer, M. E., Knauper, B., Kessler, R. C., & Norquist, G. S. (1998). Limitations of diagnostic criteria and assessment instruments for mental disorders. Implications for research and policy. *Archives of General Psychiatry, 55,* 109–115.

Regier, D. A., & Narrow, W. E. (2002). Defining clinically significant psychopathology with epidemiologic data. In J. E. Helzier & J. J. Hudziak (Eds.), *Defining psychopathology in the 21st century. DSM-V and beyond* (pp. 19–30). Washington, DC: American Psychiatric Publishing.

Regier, D. A., Narrow, W. E., Kuhl, E. A., & Kupfer, D. J. (2010). The conceptual development of DSM-V. *American Journal of Psychiatry, 166,* 645–655.

Robins, E., & Guze, S. B. (1970). Establishment of diagnostic validity in psychiatric illness: Its application to schizophrenia. *American Journal of Psychiatry, 126,* 107–111.

Robins, L. N., & Barrett, J. E. (Eds.). (1989). *The validity of psychiatric diagnosis.* New York, NY: Raven Press.

Rounsaville, B. J., Alarcon, R. D., Andrews, G., Jackson, J. S., Kendell, R. E., & Kendler, K. (2002). Basic nomenclature issues for DSM-V. In D. J. Kupfer, M. B. First, & D. E. Regier (Eds.), *A research agenda for DSM-V* (pp. 1–29). Washington, DC: American Psychiatric Association.

Rutter, M. (2003, October). *Pathways of genetic influences on psychopathology.* Zubin award address at the 18th Annual Meeting of the Society for Research in Psychopathology, Toronto, Ontario.

Sakashita, C., Slade, T., & Andrews, G. (2007). An empirical analysis of two assumptions in the diagnosis of DSM-IV major depressive episode. *Australian and New Zealand Journal of Psychiatry, 41,* 17–23.

Sartorius, N. (2009). Disability and mental illness are different entities and should be assessed separately. *World Psychiatry, 8,* 86.

Sartorius, N., Kaelber, C. T., Cooper, J. E., Roper, M., Rae, D. S., Gulbinat, W.,...Regier, D. A. (1993). Progress toward achieving a common language in psychiatry. *Archives of General Psychiatry, 50,* 115–124.

Schwartz, M. A., & Wiggins, O. P. (2002). The hegemony of the DSMs. In J. Sadler (Ed.), *Descriptions and prescriptions: Values, mental disorders, and the DSM* (pp. 199–209). Baltimore, MD: Johns Hopkins University Press.

Shisslak, C. M., Crago, M., & Estes, L. S. (1995). The spectrum of eating disturbances. *International Journal of Eating Disorders, 18,* 209–219.

Spitzer, R. L., Endicott, J., & Robins, E. (1975). Clinical criteria for psychiatric diagnosis and DSM-III. *American Journal of Psychiatry, 132,* 1187–1192.

Spitzer, R. L., Williams, J. B. W., & Skodol, A. E. (1980). DSM-III: The major achievements and an overview. *American Journal of Psychiatry, 137,* 151–164.

Stein, M. B., Walker, J. R., Hazen, A. L., & Forde, D. R. (1997). Full and partial posttraumatic stress disorder: Findings from a community survey. *American Journal of Psychiatry, 154,* 1114–1119.

Ustun, T. B., & Sartorius, N. (Eds.). (1995). *Mental illness in general health care: An international study.* London: John Wiley & Sons.

Widiger, T. A., & Clark, L. A. (2000). Toward DSM-V and the classification of psychopathology. *Psychological Bulletin, 126,* 946–963.

Widiger, T. A., & Samuel, D. B. (2005). Diagnostic categories or dimensions: A question for DSM-V. *Journal of Abnormal Psychology, 114,* 494–504.

Widiger, T. A., Simonsen, E., Krueger, R. F., Livesley, W. J., & Verheul, R. (2005). Personality disorder research agenda for the DSM-V. *Journal of Personality Disorders, 19,* 317–340.

Widiger, T. A., & Trull, T. J. (2007). Plate tectonics in the classification of personality disorder: Shifting to a dimensional model. *American Psychologist, 62,* 71–83.

WHO (World Health Organization). (1992). *The ICD-10 classification of mental and behavioral disorders. Clinical descriptions and diagnostic guidelines.* Geneva, Switzerland: Author.

Zachar, P., & Kendler, K. S. (2007). Psychiatric disorders: A conceptual taxonomy. *American Journal of Psychiatry, 164,* 557–565.

Eight

Evidence-Based Treatment

E. DAVID KLONSKY

INTRODUCTION

Recent years have witnessed an increased emphasis on the importance of evidence in behavioral healthcare practice (APA, 2006; Bieschke, Fouad, Collins, & Halonen, 2004; Fisher & O'Donohue, 2009). However, the integration of science and clinical practice has not gone smoothly (e.g., Boisvert & Faust, 2006; Norcross, Klonsky, & Tropiano, 2008). This chapter addresses the integration of scientific evidence into practice, including the importance of basing practice on scientific evidence, differing perspectives on the definition and quantification of "evidence," reasons for the apparent gap between science and practice, and suggestions for bridging this gap and improving mental healthcare for the twenty-first century. Although parts of the chapter focus on issues within the field of psychology, all issues discussed are highly relevant to behavioral healthcare broadly defined.

EARLY EMPHASIS ON INTEGRATING PSYCHOLOGICAL SCIENCE AND PRACTICE

Given the recent emphasis on evidence-based care in psychology (e.g., APA, 2006) and medicine more broadly (e.g., Sackett, Rosenberg, Gray, Haynes, & Richardson, 1996), it may come as a surprise to some that the integration of science and practice has been a central issue in psychology for more than 60 years (Reisman, 1976). The stresses of World War II, unprecedented in scope, led to a substantial increase in individuals seeking psychotherapy, especially among soldiers returning from combat. This steady demand that remained after the war's end, combined with a relative shortage of treatment professionals to meet this demand, led to a reformulation of the field's structure, identity, and approach to training (for a synopsis, see Peterson and Park, 2005).

The American Psychological Association (APA) explored how to standardize the training of those studying to become clinical psychologists and issued the Shakow report on graduate training in clinical psychology in 1947. In 1949, the U.S. government created the National Institute of Mental Health (NIMH) to support research into psychological and behavioral disorders and interventions. These developments paved the way for creation of the scientist–practitioner model of clinical psychology training, also known as the "Boulder model" (Peterson & Park, 2005; Reisman, 1976).

The scientist–practitioner model resulted from the Boulder Conference on Graduate Education in Clinical Psychology, a 14-day meeting in Boulder, Colorado, funded by NIMH and sponsored by APA. The Boulder model has three overarching emphases:

- Practitioners of psychology not only must consume and apply psychological science in their practice, but also must know how to produce science themselves.
- Given this emphasis, clinical psychology training programs must have intensive research requirements, including a dissertation, and result in a doctoral (PhD) degree.
- Graduate training will include an integration of research training, academic course work, and clinical training.

Thus, the Boulder conference provided a foundation for producing generations of psychologists whose delivery of treatments and other clinical services would be closely tied to the scientific evidence. Although the Boulder model is not without its critics (e.g., Frank, 1984; Snyder & Elliott, 2005), it has remained the dominant paradigm for ensuring that psychological clinical practice is based on psychological clinical science.

WHY SCIENCE IS IMPORTANT FOR PRACTICE

To many, it goes without saying that science should be thoroughly integrated into mental health practice. Historically, however, clinical expertise and judgment have routinely proceeded without being checked by scientific investigation. Even today, many mental and behavioral healthcare professionals value clinical experience and expertise more than scientific evidence when making diagnostic or therapeutic decisions (Stewart & Chambless, 2007), a tendency with very real and detrimental consequences for patient care.

Clinical Expertise Unchecked by Science Is Dangerous

Paul Meehl addresses this issue in his seminal article, "Credentialed Persons, Credentialed Knowledge" (Meehl, 1997). Smart, well-meaning, highly trained healthcare professionals have a long tradition of developing, utilizing, and disseminating diagnostic and therapeutic procedures without scientific investigation. For example, beginning in the 1600s, surgeons debated for centuries regarding the merits of debridement for wounds contaminated by gunpowder or metal (i.e., surgically removing tissue contaminated by foreign particles). Some believed wounds should be closed despite the presence of such foreign particles, whereas others felt it was best to cut away contaminated flesh before closing the wound. Opposition to wound debridement persisted into the 1940s, until careful scientific investigation clearly supported the superiority of the approach.

This is not an isolated example. As Meehl notes, medical historians conclude that almost every medical practice utilized before 1890 was useless or harmful. Examples of such standard practices included bleeding, purging, and blistering—none of which was useful and the first two of which were harmful. Lest we think that we in modern times are immune to such misjudgments, recall that prestigious institutions of higher learning and advanced degrees existed then just as they do today. Further, there is no reason to believe that our brains or capacity for reason have greatly improved over the past hundred or couple of hundred years; evolution simply does not work that fast! Thus, we must be ever vigilant about our potential for fallacious reasoning and beliefs (for thorough coverage of the limits of human reasoning, see Gilovich, 1993).

As Meehl argues, possession of a respected credential, such as a doctorate degree or license to practice, does not credential one's knowledge or professional opinion. Like the historical examples cited by Meehl, modern psychological and behavioral healthcare providers are also capable of developing, utilizing, and disseminating ineffective or harmful treatments. For example, several psychological treatments that probably cause harm are in use today, such as critical incident stress debriefing (may increase symptoms of posttraumatic stress disorder), facilitated communication (may lead to false accusations of child abuse), and recovered memory techniques (may lead to false memories of trauma) (for a review, see Lilienfeld, 2007).

Moreover, one of the most popular methods for assessing psychopathology and personality, the Rorschach inkblot test, may overdiagnose psychopathology and fail to meet established standards for reliability and validity (Lilienfeld, Wood, & Garb, 2000). Only through scientific investigation can mental healthcare professionals—even those who are eminently reasonable, intelligent, and well intentioned—confidently distinguish among effective, ineffective, and harmful treatments.

Biases and Heuristics

Howard Garb (1996, 1997, 1998, 2005) further elaborates on the limitations of judgments made in mental health contexts. Specifically, Garb describes a series of biases and cognitive heuristics that can lead highly trained and conscientious practitioners to make inaccurate decisions regarding diagnoses and clinical care. Biases can involve gender, race, and social class. For example, contrary to data from structured interviews, clinicians were more likely to diagnose schizophrenia in African Americans as compared to Caucasians (Pavkov, Lewis, & Lyons, 1989; Simon, Fleiss, Gurland, Stiller, & Sharpe, 1973). In another study, clinicians were biased to see minorities as being at greater risk for rehospitalization than Caucasians. However, at follow-up, rehospitalization rates were equivalent for minorities and Caucasians (Stack, Lannon, & Miley, 1983).

Similarly, when hypothetical case histories that are identical except for the manipulation of gender are viewed, clinicians diagnose histrionic personality disorder more often in women and antisocial personality disorder more often in men (Ford & Widiger, 1989). To be sure, gender might represent diagnostically useful information; but gender should not supersede the presence or absence of defining diagnostic features. There is also evidence that clinicians overpredict violence in men and underpredict violence in women, as compared to actual violent outcomes (McNiel & Binder, 1995).

Cognitive heuristics refers to simple, time-saving "mental shortcuts" that help people make efficient decisions and judgments (Garb, 1996, 1998). In everyday life, these heuristics serve us well. For example, the representativeness heuristic refers to the tendency to judge the category of membership of people or objects based on how closely they match the "typical" or "average" member of that category. If while driving we hear a siren and notice a large red truck behind us with flashing lights, we quickly determine we should pull over to let the fire engine pass. We do not need to read the writing on the side of the vehicle to make this judgment; rather, the sight and sound of the vehicle resembles, or is representative of, our typical conception of a fire engine.

For simple, everyday situations, such as identifying a fire engine, the representativeness heuristic works efficiently. However, this and other heuristics can lead us astray when we are making complex judgments, such as those routinely required in clinical contexts. For example, in the study by Ford and Widiger (1989) described before, the gender-biased diagnoses may have occurred because the typical or representative antisocial patient was considered to be male and the typical histrionic patient to be female. Importantly, there is evidence that the representative heuristic continues to affect diagnostic judgments even when clinicians are instructed to adhere strictly to diagnostic criteria (Garb, 1996).

Another relevant heuristic is the availability heuristic. This occurs when judgments regarding an event are influenced by how easy it is to think of an example of the event. For example, people often associate mental illness with danger and violence because they can easily recall mentally ill violent criminals such as Ted Bundy or John Hinckley (Turk et al., 1988). Similarly, clinicians who regularly treat patients with certain diagnoses can be inclined to see new patients as disproportionately likely to have that diagnosis. For example, a clinician who primarily treats depressed individuals can be more likely to diagnose depression in subthreshold cases or when another distress-oriented diagnosis may be more suitable.

A third heuristic, the anchoring-and-adjustment heuristic, can also harm clinical judgment. This refers to the tendency to begin with a first impression and then insufficiently adjust that impression based on subsequent information. In everyday life, this heuristic may explain the saying that it is important to make good first impressions. Because people give greater weight to initial information, it can take a lot to undo a bad first impression. In clinical settings, there is evidence that during diagnostic interviews, clinicians overvalue initial information and undervalue subsequent information (Turk et al., 1988). This tendency could significantly harm case conceptualization and treatment planning if it goes unchecked.

The biases and heuristics discussed here are not a comprehensive list. For more thorough coverage, see Garb (1998,

2005) and Turk et al. (1988). Yet, even this limited discussion of biases and heuristics suggests the dangers of clinical expertise and judgments unchecked by scientific evidence. The effects of heuristics and biases are powerful and pervasive, yet largely outside our awareness. As will be discussed in further detail later, scientific evidence and objective data collection can help protect us from misjudgments. We must take great care to evaluate (and reevaluate) our judgments critically as a matter of routine. The accuracy of critical decisions regarding diagnosis and treatment is at stake.

Clinical Versus Statistical Prediction

There are convincing arguments regarding the limitations of clinical expertise and the importance of basing practice on science whenever possible. However, in the spirit of the scientific method, it is useful to compare accuracy of judgments based on science versus clinical expertise directly. Paul Meehl, and later William Grove and others, addressed this question across a wide variety of judgments (Grove, 2005; Grove & Meehl, 1996; Grove, Zald, Lebow, Snitz, & Nelson, 2000; Meehl, 1954).

An example serves to describe the issue. Let us suppose that a therapist wishes to select the best treatment for a given client. Such a decision is based on several factors, including presenting problem, diagnostic features, demographic and cultural characteristics of the client, and many other variables. Using statistical prediction to select a treatment refers to utilizing a model statistically optimized based on data obtained from a large sample of similar patients. Using clinical prediction refers to any other method, such as a clinician using her or his best judgment about treatment selection, taking into account all the relevant information. The statistical versus clinical prediction issue applies to a wide range of areas, including those that are health related (such as predicting psychotherapy outcome, recidivism risk, heart disease) and non-health-related areas (such as job performance, graduate school success, and lie detection). Strikingly, in approximately 90% of studies, statistical predictions were comparable or superior to clinical predictions.

Some argue that experts are especially adept at identifying instances when the typical method of statistical prediction may not apply. Meehl refers to this as the "broken leg" phenomenon. We may have an established set of variables that predict whether Joe will go to the movies on a given evening, but if he breaks his leg, it may be best no longer to rely on the statistical mode. However, there is a marked tendency for experts to see "broken legs"—to find a reason to rely on clinical judgment rather than statistical prediction methods—when it is not appropriate. On average, when statistical and clinical predictions disagree, the statistical prediction is correct five out of six times (Meehl, 1954). Included in the data supporting these findings are numerous studies conducted in psychological and behavioral healthcare contexts (Grove et al., 2000). Those interested in a comprehensive review of this literature are referred to Grove (2005).

The "McFall Manifesto"

Among the most passionate and articulate arguments for a scientific approach to psychological practice is Richard McFall's "Manifesto for a Science of Clinical Psychology" (1991). McFall recognizes that the scientific method is the gold standard in healthcare for determining which interventions are effective, and he suggests (convincingly) that "scientific clinical psychology is the only legitimate and acceptable form of clinical psychology." Given the pitfalls of intuition and judgment discussed by Meehl, Garb, Grove, and others, it is clear that behavioral healthcare must be based on science to the greatest extent possible.

INTEGRATING SCIENCE INTO PRACTICE

What does it mean to incorporate science into practice? I suggest that there are two primary ways of integrating science into psychological and behavioral practice. One is to be as familiar as possible with the empirical literature and strive continually to utilize empirically supported procedures as much as possible. A second is to utilize a scientific approach to the implementation of diagnostic and therapeutic procedures. The former has received considerably more attention than the latter, but the approaches are compatible rather than mutually exclusive. This section first discusses the two approaches one at a time; it ends with a discussion of how they can and should be utilized together.

Basing Clinical Care on Scientific Evidence

The first approach to incorporating science into practice has received more attention. This approach involves ensuring a close tie between clinical care and the latest scientific evidence. For example, if a patient has disorder "A" and well-designed and controlled research shows that treatment "X" works best for disorder "A," then the patient should be treated with treatment "X" and not any other treatment. This premise that clinical care should be based on scientific evidence may seem simple and obvious. However, defining evidence is difficult, and perspectives vary widely on exactly what constitutes "evidence."

A seminal definition of evidence for psychological treatments was offered in the mid-1990s. A task force of the Society of Clinical Psychology (Division 12, American Psychological Association) published specific criteria for determining whether a given treatment for a given disorder was "well established" or "probably efficacious" (Chambless & Hollon, 1998). In order to be considered "well established," a treatment must meet one of the following conditions:

- At least two good group design studies, conducted by different investigators, demonstrate efficacy in one or more of the following ways: (a) superior to pill or psychological placebo or to another treatment, or (b) equivalent to an already established treatment.
- A large series of single-case design studies demonstrate efficacy. These studies must have (a) used good experimental designs, or (b) compared the intervention to another effective form of treatment.

Key elements in these criteria include replication, careful controls, and experimental design. As in other healthcare fields, careful control and experimental designs are the only ways to establish a causal relationship between a particular treatment and clinical improvements observed as a result of the treatment. Replication is the only way to ensure that results are not due to chance or idiosyncrasies of a particular study. To be sure, the criteria developed by the Society of Clinical Psychology are not the only means of quantifying research evidence. Discussion of varying approaches is beyond the scope of this chapter, but for those interested, other approaches of note can be found in Nathan and Gorman (2002), Roth and Fonagy (2004), and Weisz (2004).

Some argue that treatments meeting strict criteria for efficacy are not applicable to real-world clinical contexts. For example, it has been argued that research samples are selected for having one clear clinical disorder, whereas clinical patients often present with multiple disorders. Moreover, research-administered treatments follow strict manuals, whereas treatment in clinical contexts often requires flexibility and adaptation (for a discussion, see Addis, Wade, & Hatgis, 1999). Finally, providers in research contexts may receive specialized and ongoing training not available to providers in busy and demanding clinical contexts. For all these reasons, it is important to address the following question directly: Are treatments supported in research contexts more effective compared to usual treatment, and do they remain so in real-world clinical contexts?

Fortunately, a growing body of research addresses this question. John Weisz and colleagues (Weisz, Jensen-Doss, & Hawley, 2006) conducted a meta-analysis of findings from 32 randomized controlled trials comparing research-supported treatments to treatment as usual. They found that treatments with research support outperformed usual care, both immediately after treatment and at follow-up. The pattern of findings did not vary by severity of clinical problems or by ethnicity of the patients. Their findings do not directly address the issue of whether research-supported treatments perform just as well in clinical contexts, but they do provide evidence that research-supported treatments outperform care typically given in clinical contexts.

Perhaps the best evidence to date that research-supported treatments work in "real-world" clinical settings comes from Hunsley and Lee (2007), who noted that efficacy studies examine treatments in carefully controlled research settings, whereas effectiveness studies examine treatments in less controlled, more realistic clinical settings. Therefore, they were interested in treatments that had first been proven efficacious in research contexts and that were later examined in effectiveness studies. Would such treatments perform as well in clinical contexts as they had in their original research trials?

Hunsley and Lee (2007) examined findings from 35 effectiveness studies examining treatments that had previously been supported in research contexts; 21 of the studies focused on adult treatments, and 14 on child and adolescent treatments. A clear pattern emerged. Whether the outcome variable utilized was treatment completion or clinical improvement, the treatments performed just as well in the effectiveness studies as they had done in the original efficacy studies. These findings provide encouraging evidence that patients benefit when efficacious treatments are transported to the clinical contexts.

Bringing a Scientific Mentality Into the Clinic

The second approach to incorporating science into practice involves bringing a scientific mentality into the clinic.

Judgments such as diagnoses and treatment selection can be treated as hypotheses with the potential to be refuted. Typically, before making a diagnosis and choosing an appropriate course of treatment, a clinician obtains lots of relevant information through both structured and unstructured techniques. Judgments about diagnosis and treatment are then made on the basis of this information. However, it is often the case that additional information is no longer obtained in a systematic fashion. The diagnosis is made, treatment begins, and only if things appear to be going wrong after an extended period of time might the clinician revisit the original judgments.

In contrast, a scientific approach treats such initial judgments as hypotheses to be tested. For example, after making decisions regarding diagnosis and treatment, a psychologist can make specific predictions about what should happen after a given number of sessions. Perhaps after six sessions, certain symptoms are expected to decrease, or certain behaviors expected to change, or certain thoughts expected to be replaced by other thoughts. Whatever the expectation regarding improvement is, the psychologist could utilize standardized and valid measures of these symptoms pretreatment, with a plan to re-administer the measures after a given number of sessions or a set period of time. The follow-up data can then be evaluated against the change predicted to occur; if notable discrepancies occur, this would suggest a need to revisit the original case conceptualization and course of treatment.

Thus, the scientific method of *hypothesis formation followed by testable predictions based on the hypothesis, followed by objective data collection, followed by revisions to the hypothesis based on new data, and so on (process continues to repeat)* can be applied not only by scientists in research contexts, but also by behavioral and psychological healthcare providers in the clinic. Kazdin (2008) provides a compelling argument for this type of approach to psychological practice.

Integrating Both Scientific Evidence and a Scientific Mentality Into Clinical Practice

The two approaches described previously—incorporating scientific evidence into practice and incorporating a scientific mentality into practice—are complementary rather than mutually exclusive. They can and should be used together. This can be accomplished through five steps of evidence-based practice articulated in Strauss, Richardson, Glasziou, and Haynes

(2005) and later addressed by Spring (2007). The steps are easily remembered as the five "*As*":

1. Ask the clinical question (e.g., Which treatment approach would be most appropriate and effective for the client's diagnosis?).
2. Acquire the evidence (e.g., be or become familiar with the latest empirical literature relevant to the case).
3. Appraise the evidence (e.g., determine the implications of the empirical literature for the case and clinical question).
4. Apply the results (e.g., implement the optimal treatment).
5. Assess the outcome (e.g., obtain follow-up data from the patient to determine if the treatment and expected outcome are proceeding as expected).

Spring (2007) emphasizes that in Step 1 (asking the clinical questions), it is important to formulate focused, easily answered questions (e.g., Would interpersonal or cognitive-behavioral therapy be better for a client with generalized anxiety?), rather than broader questions (e.g., What are the effective treatments for generalized anxiety?) that would yield too many research citations to be reviewed in the time realistically available to a busy clinician.

There have also been other attempts to describe scientific psychological practice. The definition of scientific psychological practice was addressed in detail by a 2002 work group (Bieschke et al., 2004). A diversity of almost two dozen psychology organizations sponsored the Competencies Conference: Future Directions in Education and Credentialing in Professional Psychology. The conference was composed of different work groups, one of which, the scientific foundation and research competencies work group, identified features of what they termed the scientifically minded psychologist. After 3 days of discussion and debate, the work group identified consensus components that define a scientific approach to current scientific knowledge:

appropriately apply current scientific knowledge
contribute to knowledge
critically evaluate one's own interventions and their outcomes
practice vigilance about how sociocultural variables influence scientific practice

subject work routinely to the scrutiny of colleagues, stakeholders, and the public

Notably, this description includes elements of integrating scientific evidence into practice (e.g., accessing and applying scientific knowledge) as well as bringing a scientific mentality into practice (e.g., critically evaluating one's own interventions and outcomes). Consistent with the intent of the Boulder model, it is indeed possible to be both scientist and practitioner.

EVIDENCE-BASED PRACTICE

As the field increasingly has recognized the importance of basing healthcare practice on evidence, the concept of evidence-based practice (EBP) has become more influential than ever. EBP was initially advanced in medicine (Sackett et al., 1996). Approximately 10 years later, a presidential task force of the American Psychological Association offered a similar definition of EBP (APA, 2006). According to the task force report, EBP consists of three components: best available research evidence, clinical expertise, and patient characteristics.

Best Available Research Evidence

According to the task force report (APA, 2006), best research evidence refers to "scientific results related to intervention strategies, assessment, clinical problems, and patient populations in laboratory and field settings as well as to clinically relevant results of basic research in psychology and related fields" (p. 274). The report endorses multiple types of research evidence. Although some sources of research evidence are more authoritative than others, it is important to recognize that what constitutes "best evidence" depends in part upon the question of interest (Spring, 2007). For example, questions about diagnostic interviews require psychometric investigations, whereas questions about prognosis are best suited to longitudinal designs.

Nevertheless, in regard to intervention research, the task force report identifies randomized controlled trials and other logically equivalent experimental designs as conveying more authoritative information about efficacy than systematized clinical observation, which in turn is considered more authoritative than clinical opinion or consensus. The report also distinguishes between efficacy (scientific evaluation of whether a treatment works) and clinical utility (applicability, feasibility, and usefulness of the treatment in real-world contexts). Whereas the former is best examined in carefully controlled experimental designs, the latter can be examined with uncontrolled pre- and postdesigns in real-world clinical settings. The report also notes the important role of meta-analyses—systematic efforts to quantify results across studies—for synthesizing large bodies of research on a given intervention, procedure, outcome, or variable of interest.

Clinical Expertise

According to the task force report (APA, 2006), clinical expertise refers to "competence attained by psychologists through education, training, and experience that results in effective practice" (p. 275). Clinical expertise helps psychologists determine what types of information are important to obtain for a given case, which research literatures are the most relevant, and how to apply the available research evidence to a particular clinical case. Clinical expertise is also required to integrate research evidence with patient characteristics and values and thereby choose the most appropriate course of treatment. Finally, the skill with which a treatment is delivered is an important aspect of clinical expertise. The task force report notes that treatment outcomes are systematically related to characteristics of the treatment provider, not just the type of treatment provided. It is likely that expertise grows with enhanced training and increased experience in implementing treatments.

Perhaps due to the ambiguous nature of the term, clinical expertise is the most controversial of the three components of EBP (Spring, 2007). For example, how, if at all, can clinical expertise be differentiated from an opinion or intuition offered by a licensed and trained healthcare practitioner? Are all opinions and intuitions provided by appropriately trained clinicians to be regarded as evidence derived from clinical expertise? As discussed earlier, credentialed persons do not inevitably produce credentialed or valid opinions (Meehl, 1997). The task force acknowledges that even well-trained experts are susceptible to biases, heuristics, and errors of judgment (e.g., Garb, 1998, 2005) and suggests that an awareness of one's limits and fallibilities is an important component of clinical expertise.

Patient Characteristics

Patient characteristics include patient culture, values, and preferences. Incorporating patient characteristics into healthcare decisions is important for a number of reasons. For example, a treatment may be differentially effective for some ethnicities, genders, ages, or backgrounds. In addition, as described by Spring (2007), there is an increasing desire to involve patients in their care and develop collaborative relationships between the clinician and patient, as opposed to the more traditional paternalistic model in which a provider makes decisions on the patient's behalf.

In many cases, research evidence may support more than one approach to treatment, and the provider can work with the patient to determine the approach best suited for the patient. Often this involves the clinician providing information to the patient, such as the range of treatment approaches available, which options have more or less research evidence, and the potential risks and drawbacks to different treatments, as well as the consequences and expected prognosis should the patient opt out of treatment.

Critiques of the APA Definition of EBP

The APA task force report on EBP is impressive in many respects. The report manages to incorporate perspectives from a diversity of psychologists, is largely consistent with definitions of EBP found in medicine, and establishes the importance of scientific research for clinical practice. At the same time, the APA definition of EBP is not without its critics, and some have offered alternative definitions of "evidence."

Stuart and Lilienfeld (2008) note three limitations of the APA report on EBP. First, they note that the report does not offer specific criteria for identifying treatments with research support. Instead, it lists several types of research evidence and notes that some forms of research evidence are more authoritative than others for determining efficacy of interventions; however, it does not delineate guidelines for operationalizing research evidence. As a result, a given treatment may be judged as having sufficient research support by some providers but not by others.

Second, the task force report focused on determining which treatments are likely to be effective based on research evidence, but not on treatments with the potential to be harmful. As described previously, several treatments in use today have showed iatrogenic effects in controlled studies (Lilienfeld, 2007). Third, the report did not clearly recommend regular objective monitoring of patient progress and outcome. In other words, the report can be viewed as emphasizing the integration of scientific evidence into practice to a greater extent than it does a scientific mentality.

Another critique of the APA report may be the inclusion of clinical expertise and patient characteristics in the definition of evidence. This is not to argue that clinical expertise and patient characteristics are inconsequential; on the contrary, good practice depends on careful consideration of these factors, and increased clinical experience is very likely to increase competence in delivering an evidence-based treatment. At the same time, perhaps it is more accurate to refer to research evidence as evidence and to suggest that this evidence should be integrated with clinical expertise and patient values. Is it useful, or accurate, to include clinical expertise and patient characteristics as forms of evidence? Does referring to clinical expertise as "evidence" encourage some to value clinical expertise over research evidence?

Perhaps for this reason, some definitions of evidence refer to research evidence and only to research evidence. For example, Cochrane (1972) and others (Strand, Phelan, & Donovan, 2003) define best evidence as n-of-1 trials, large randomized controlled trials, or systematic reviews (meta-analyses) of multiple medium- and small-sized randomized controlled trials. From this perspective, clinical expertise and patient characteristics remain critical, but they are to be integrated with best research evidence for making healthcare decisions, rather than regarded themselves as forms of evidence.

THE GAP BETWEEN PSYCHOLOGICAL SCIENCE AND PRACTICE

Despite the Boulder conference of 1949 establishing the science–practitioner model of training, despite the emphasis on research-supported treatments that began more than a decade ago (Chambless & Hollon, 1998), and despite the recent consensus around the importance of evidence-based practice (APA, 2006), the integration of science into practice has not been smooth. As noted by Norcross et al. (2008), the relationship between science and practice has been optimistically described as a "strained alliance" (Goldfried & Wolfe, 1996) and, more pessimistically, described as "parallel lines [that] have only rarely touched" (Parloff, 1980). In short, there is a large gap between the science and practice of psychology.

The gap is evident in several respects. One issue is that clinicians rarely engage in research. The Boulder model recommends that psychologists be trained to conduct research, and a competencies task force (Bieschke et al., 2004) suggests that this ability is important for a scientific approach to psychological practice. Yet, it is often the case that research is left behind once one completes graduate school and enters the professional world of psychological practice. A few studies have surveyed clinicians about reasons for not engaging in research and have yielded converging findings (Haynes, Lemsky, & Sexton-Radek, 1987; Sandberg, Johnson, Robila, & Miller, 2002; Vachon et al., 1995). The most common reason cited for not participating in research is insufficient time, followed by client concerns (e.g., effects on the clinical process). If clinicians are to be active participants in the research process, these and other barriers must be addressed.

Whereas a lack of participation in the research process by practitioners is worthy of concern, it is perhaps more concerning if some practitioners are unaware of or apathetic toward clinically relevant psychological research. Unfortunately, evidence suggests that many psychologists receive limited training in research-supported treatments, are unaware of important research findings, and do not value psychological research. A 1995 study of accredited psychology doctoral programs and internships found that only 20% of doctoral programs included at least minimal coverage of research-supported treatments, and that most internship programs did not require competency in research-supported treatments (Crits-Christoph, Frank, Chambless, Brody, & Karp, 1995).

These discouraging findings might not be surprising because they were published 15 years ago, when the emphasis on research-supported treatments was just beginning. However, only modest progress was made in the subsequent decade. Woody, Weisz, and McLean (2005) found that didactic coverage of research-supported treatments by accredited doctoral and internship programs increased between 1993 and 2003, but that supervised training in these treatments declined on average.

Weissman et al. (2006) surveyed a probability sample of training programs in psychiatry (offering an MD), clinical psychology (offering a PhD), psychology (offering a PsyD), and social work (offering a master's level degree). An overwhelming majority of psychiatry programs required both didactic training and clinical supervision in at least one research-supported treatment. However, this figure was reduced to 66% for clinical psychology PhD programs, 33% for psychology PsyD programs, and 38% for master's level social work programs.

Notably, the PsyD and social work program types produce the greatest number of practitioners, suggesting that many practitioners have earned their terminal graduate degree without ever having been trained in a research-supported treatment.

Perhaps due in part to deficiencies in training, there is also evidence that some psychologists are unaware of and/or do not value psychological research. Boisvert and Faust (2006) surveyed practicing psychologists about a variety of issues related to psychological practice and compared their responses to those given by experts in the relevant research. In general, psychologists exhibited modest knowledge of psychological research. Knowledge of research by practitioners was not predicted by theoretical orientation, percentage of time devoted to conducting therapy, or perceived familiarity with research.

Whereas Boisvert and Faust focused on knowledge of research, a subsequent study by Stewart and Chambless (2007) focused on attitudes toward and application of psychological research in a survey of 491 practicing psychologists. Several findings are noteworthy. First, participants expressed only mild agreement that treatment outcome research has meaning for their practice (mean rating of 3.09 on a 7-point scale, where 1 indicates strongly agree and 7 indicates strongly disagree). Second, participants based their treatment decisions on past clinical experiences (mean = 1.53, sd = .91) to a greater extent than current research on treatment outcome (mean = 2.86, sd = 1.59). Experiences in personal therapy and colleagues' advice were given ratings comparable to that for current research on treatment outcome.

Third, to increase their therapy skills and effectiveness, participants relied more on past experiences with patients than treatment materials informed by psychotherapy outcome research findings. Fourth, in a more encouraging finding regarding the integration of research and practice, the majority of participants chose a research-supported treatment when asked to choose a treatment for a patient with panic disorder, and even more chose a research-supported treatment when presented with a summary of the relevant clinical research.

Results present a mixed picture. On the one hand, practicing psychologists appear to value clinical experience more than clinical research; on the other hand, practicing psychologists do value research and demonstrate a willingness and ability to apply research when it is easily available and perceived as relevant.

BRIDGING THE SCIENCE–PRACTICE GAP

As long as there is a gap between psychological science and practice, genuine evidence-based practice will remain elusive. Several researchers and practitioners have offered perspectives on causes for and solutions to the gap. A selection of these perspectives is reviewed in this section.

Understanding the Gap

A recent survey by Norcross et al. (2008) examined the perspectives of both researchers and practitioners on the research–practice gap. A Delphi poll was utilized to obtain information from 11 leading clinical psychological scientists and 13 independent practitioners regarding "the gap between the science and practice of psychology." A variety of reasons and suggestions for bridging the research–practice gap were offered; here I will summarize a selection. Those interested in a full account are referred to Norcross et al.

Although researchers and practitioners were not in full agreement, an important point of consensus emerged. Specifically, both indicated that the field needed to do a better job making research findings accessible to practitioners. For example, this could be done via a psychologist's version of WebMD, user-friendly publications in practitioner-oriented journals, or continuing education offerings. In addition, researchers felt that training could better teach how to incorporate science into practice, and practitioners felt that research could be made more clinically relevant. These three areas—training, clinical relevance of research, and better dissemination—are discussed next.

Improve Psychology Training

The integration of psychological science and practice is the core feature of the Boulder model—the dominant training paradigm in psychology since 1949. Yet, there is ample evidence that the integration of science into practice is not properly taught. As discussed earlier, many doctoral and internship programs offer minimal or no training in research-supported treatments, a trend that has improved only slightly since the 1990s. Baker, McFall, and Shoham (2009) place much of the blame on inadequate standards for accrediting psychology training programs. They argue that APA guidelines for accreditation cover a broad range of programs using different training philosophies, including the practitioner–scholar model, which was developed in opposition to the stringent research training required by the scientist–practitioner model.

Baker et al. (2009) suggest that as practitioner–scholar programs and less research-oriented scientist–practitioner programs have proliferated, APA accreditation standards have evolved to a point that they no longer emphasize research and no longer benefit research-oriented programs. As a result, the system produces more and more practitioners who have little training in and appreciation for psychological science. In response, Baker et al. suggest the development of a new accreditation body, the Psychological Clinical Science Accreditation System (PCSAS).

This suggestion is controversial, to say the least, because it would potentially offer a viable alternative to the APA accreditation system, which has been the only recognized accreditation system for clinical and counseling psychology programs for several decades. PCSAS was officially launched in 2007, and it is designed to produce well-trained, scientifically minded clinical psychologists. Only time will tell whether this new approach to accreditation will improve training and help decrease the science–practice gap.

Make Psychological Research More Relevant and Accessible

A point of consensus between practitioners and researchers is that research must be better delivered to practitioners if we want science to be better integrated into practice (Norcross et al., 2008). This issue can be broken down into two parts. First, the research itself must be perceived as more clinically relevant. Second, the clinically relevant research must be disseminated to practitioners in ways that are maximally accessible.

Making Research More Clinically Relevant

Kazdin (2008) offers three suggestions for making treatment outcome research more clinically relevant. First, he recommends that researchers study mechanisms of change in therapy. Typically, treatment research focuses on *if* treatments lead to change (outcome research) rather than *how* treatments lead to change (process research). Knowing the processes through which treatments effect change can help therapists optimize the therapies they provide and the manner in which they deliver them. As an example, Kazdin describes how discovering mechanisms of fear conditioning and extinction has helped practitioners improve the delivery of exposure therapy. Process research could lead to immediate therapeutic enhancements and amplified interest by practitioners in treatment research.

Second, Kazdin (2008) recommends that research focus on moderators of therapy outcome. "Moderators" refers to variables that influence (enhance or reduce) the effects of therapy. For example, the effects of a given therapy might vary by gender, ethnicity, comorbidity, intelligence, personality traits, or a range of other factors. Kazdin suggests that careful research on the nature of moderator variables and the extent and circumstances of their influence would have clear clinical relevance. Third and finally, Kazdin argues that qualitative research methods could provide more in-depth and clinically relevant accounts of patients' (and therapists') characteristics and experiences, while maintaining the essential scientific features of replicability and validity (Berg, 2001).

Another important issue regarding the clinical relevance and applicability research is the unit of analysis in treatment outcome studies. Typically, efficacy and effectiveness are evaluated on a treatment-by-treatment basis. That is, studies examine whether a particular treatment for a particular disorder is efficacious and/or effective. A consequence of this approach is that more than 100 different treatments can be viewed as having research support (Beutler, Moleiro, & Talebi, 2002).

On the one hand, the large number of research-supported treatments sounds like good news: More research-supported treatments means that more approaches to intervention are available to patients. On the other hand, it is simply not possible for clinicians to learn hundreds of different treatments. Learning even one of these treatments is time consuming and requires didactic components as well as specialized supervision. Even if doctoral and internship programs could somehow teach most of these treatments, new treatments are being developed and tested all the time. To keep up with developments, practitioners would have to spend countless hours in continuing education. This is not a realistic expectation, given the reality and rigors of psychological practice.

As an alternative, Beutler et al. (2002) suggest that it may be more productive to identify common and differential principles of change. Whereas hundreds of different research-supported treatments have been identified, a smaller set of principles seems to cut across the various treatment approaches. Beutler et al. offer a relatively small set of principles of change organized by clinically relevant domains, such as prognosis, level of care, and therapeutic relationships. For example, a principle regarding the therapeutic relationship is as follows: "Therapeutic change is greatest when the therapist is skillful and provides trust, acceptance, acknowledgment, collaboration, and respect for the patient."

Focusing on principles rather than treatments avoids the need to learn a constantly increasing number of different treatments. In addition, research on a relatively small set of principles could be perceived by practitioners as more clinically useful than research on varied and numerous treatments. Of course, a set of principles would have to be validated through careful research and be acceptable to the broad community of psychologists before it could be considered as a serious alternative to the current approach to treatment outcome studies.

Making Research More Clinically Accessible

Another important strategy for bridging the research–practice gap is making psychological research more accessible for practitioners. This is in large part a practical issue. In short, psychological researchers are relatively good at developing and supporting treatments, but not as good at dissemination (i.e., ensuring that the treatments are widely used by practitioners and widely available to patients). This issue has been highlighted by many psychologists (Baker et al., 2009; Persons, 1997; Sobell, 1996).

One reason for poor dissemination might be the format in which psychological research is typically published. Psychological research is typically distributed in formats optimized for other researchers, such as academic journals. Several psychologists have suggested other media, such as a psychology version of WebMD (an online, user-friendly Web site containing medical information) or practitioner-oriented journals (two nice examples include *Cognitive and Behavioral Practice* and *Journal of Clinical Psychology: In Session*) (Norcross et al., 2008; Persons, 1997; Sobell, 1996). Beutler, Williams, Wakefield, and Entwistle (1995) provide encouraging evidence that practitioners are interested in psychological research and willing to make efforts to seek out research and that practitioner-friendly formats could increase these interests and efforts.

Very little research has examined how format or method of presentation affects interest in and perceived clinical relevance of research findings. A notable exception is Stewart and Chambless (2009), who administered research summaries regarding treatments for bulimia to 742 practitioners in private practice. Practitioners found that the research summaries were more compelling and they were more likely to be interested in gaining training if the summaries were accompanied by case examples. The inclusion of extra statistical information with the research summaries did not increase interest beyond inclusion of case examples. Findings suggest that placing psychological research within clinically relevant contexts, such as case examples, could improve clinical accessibility of the research.

Another strategy for improving dissemination is to foster active collaboration between practitioners and researchers (Goldfried & Wolfe, 1996; Sobell, 1996). In part, clinicians may be reluctant to learn and utilize research-supported treatments because the treatments are developed and tested without their involvement and input. Thus, the research-supported treatments developed may not be theoretically or philosophically palatable to many clinicians; in some cases, they may not be optimally practical for clinical settings. Although a full description is beyond the scope of this chapter, Sobell (1996) provides two examples of how practitioner–researcher partnerships led to the successful integration of science and practice, which in turn benefited large numbers of patients.

RECOMMENDATIONS FOR TWENTY-FIRST CENTURY EVIDENCE-BASED BEHAVIORAL HEALTHCARE

As behavioral healthcare enters the twenty-first century, the integration of science into practice is more an aim than a reality. I therefore conclude with a series of recommendations for improving the integration of science and practice. Granted, many of these recommendations are large in scope, perhaps overly ambitious, and could only be implemented by policy makers with the necessary influence and resources. Nonetheless, I offer them in good faith because I believe they would genuinely advance the field and enhance behavioral healthcare for millions of individuals.

Recommendation 1. Reform Graduate Education and Training

As reported by Weissman et al. (2006), the majority of behavioral healthcare professionals are trained by institutions that lack an emphasis on science and the scientific method. As a result, research-supported treatments and scientifically informed behavioral healthcare are not readily available to the general public. To be sure, substantial and difficult reforms would be required to remedy the situation. At least two points of intervention seem important.

First, education of behavioral healthcare providers should include strong and formal emphasis on the limits of human judgment (Garb 1998, 2005; Turk et al., 1988) and the consequent need for a scientific approach in determining the most effective methods of intervention (Grove, 2005; Meehl, 1954). Unfortunately, this topic is typically given minimal coverage in behavioral healthcare training programs. Second, accreditation requirements should ensure that curricula give substantial coverage to limitations of clinical judgment and how a scientific approach helps safeguard against these limitations. The institution in the best position to facilitate such change is the American Psychological Association, which sets accreditation standards through its Committee on Accreditation (CoA). If the CoA does not act, it is increasingly likely that a competing accreditation body will develop (see Baker et al., 2009).

Recommendation 2. Make Public Education Better

A primary limitation in providing evidence-based care to the public is that laypersons are often not sufficiently informed about the nature and research support of the treatments available to them. Understandably, people expect that a healthcare practitioner who has been licensed and earned an appropriate degree would provide services informed by the latest research. Unfortunately, due to the proliferation of healthcare providers graduating from less scientifically minded programs, this is not the case. However, two positive developments would occur if consumers could better identify evidence-based practice and had access to information about which treatments had the best research support for which disorders and conditions; the first is obvious and the second less so. First, consumers would more often access the most effective interventions and shun those with less research support. Second, economic incentive for providers to value and receive training in research-supported treatments would increase. The more that consumers learn to seek out research-supported treatments, the more providers will ensure that they have the relevant training.

A key recommendation, then, is for behavioral healthcare organizations to educate consumers directly. One important approach is through the Internet. Some useful Web sites have already been developed, such as psychologicaltreatments.org, sponsored by the Society of Clinical Psychology (Division 12 of the American Psychological Association). This site is largely geared toward consumers and provides information about dozens of research-supported treatments. Another important site, http://www.abct.org/SCCAP/, is jointly sponsored by the Society of Clinical Child and Adolescent Psychology and the Association for Behavioral and Cognitive Therapies and describes research-supported treatments for child and adolescent behavioral disorders for behavioral and cognitive therapies.

These Web resources are critical first steps toward educating the public. However, only a small proportion of the general public would know to look for these resources and ultimately find them. Now that these resources are available online, serious consideration should be given to advertising campaigns through billboards, newspapers, and even television to make these resources and their importance widely known.

Recommendation 3. Work With Insurance Companies to Ensure Reimbursement of Research-Supported Treatments

Managed care occupies a central place in healthcare. There are many valid concerns about managed care, including whether healthcare providers or insurance company employees ultimately should decide on appropriate interventions. However, there is also an opportunity to partner with insurance companies. Whereas research-supported treatments are valuable because they provide the most efficient and effective care, they are also valuable economically because, in the long run, they will result in quicker remissions and less relapse, both of which translate into fewer dollars required for additional healthcare. First and foremost, evidence-based care is important to reduce suffering and disabling conditions. However, evidence-based care will also reduce the amount of money spent on healthcare; it is incumbent upon scientifically minded healthcare professionals to help insurance companies realize this and incorporate this knowledge into their reimbursement guidelines.

Recommendation 4. Make Continuing Education Better

Research does not stop and the field does not stop progression once a healthcare professional completes graduate school and starts to practice. However, the demands that a full-time practice places on time and energy make it difficult to keep up as new and better treatments are developed. It is for this reason that licensing guidelines for healthcare professionals require a minimum number of hours of continuing education each year.

Unfortunately, all too often continuing education courses teach approaches with little empirical evidence. An important recommendation, then, is for scientifically minded healthcare organizations not only to offer continuing education courses on research-supported techniques, but also to ensure that such courses are readily accessible, affordable, and attractive to a large audience. As described previously, Stewart and Chambless (2009) provide a glimpse into how research-supported treatments can be made more relevant and interesting for practitioners by providing real-world case examples and applications. Ideally, this important work should be only the beginning of efforts to make such information maximally attractive and useful.

Recommendation 5. Create a Clearer Definition of Evidence-Based Practice

The American Psychological Association is arguably the most influential psychological organization in the world. The APA presidential task force statement on evidence-based practice (APA, 2006) should have considerable influence on the field and help establish the kinds of practice that are and are not evidence based. As discussed earlier, the statement identifies three components: research evidence, clinical expertise, and patient characteristics.

A critical potential problem with the definition is the uncertain definition of clinical expertise and the uncertain relationship between research evidence and clinical expertise. For example, if a practitioner has expertise, as evidenced by a license and the appropriate degree, are we to assume that any and all of his or her clinical judgments and decisions are evidence based? If not, by what criteria and on what basis can we differentiate between services that are and are not evidence based? More importantly, if in a particular case a practitioner with appropriate expertise (i.e., component 2 of the APA definition) decides to shun a treatment with research evidence (component 1 of the APA definition), does this still "count" as evidence-based practice? In short, by the current definition, it could be argued that *any* decision made by a licensed healthcare professional could be viewed as meeting component 2 of the APA definition and thus as constituting evidence-based practice.

This is a serious problem with the APA definition of evidence-based practice. In its current form, the definition places few if any conditions on what can be considered evidence-based practice. As a result, practitioners who are not scientifically inclined, as well as training programs that produce such practitioners, not only can continue to operate, but also can continue to advertise themselves as meeting the highest standard of evidence-based practice. Perhaps the single most important change the APA could undertake is to adopt a stronger and clearer stance on evidence-based practice. Everyone stands to gain if practitioners have no choice but to engage in genuinely evidence-based practice.

Recommendation 6. Improve Dissemination of Research-Supported Treatments

Dissemination, rather than a shortage of clinically relevant research, arguably represents the greatest barrier to the continued growth of EBP. Powerful and effective treatments are being improved and developed all the time. However, once a treatment is validated in a research context, how do we go about training thousands of practitioners to provide the treatment? Practitioners have tremendous demands on their time and energy. Time to learn a new treatment, let alone multiple new treatments, is scarce. The time and expense devoted to developing and validating treatments is wasted if these treatments cannot be disseminated widely.

Publication of this volume is timely. At present, unprecedented resources, including billions of dollars, are being channeled into the dissemination of research-supported treatments (McHugh & Barlow, 2010). Examples of national dissemination initiatives include the Improving Access to Psychological Therapies Program in the United Kingdom and the Veterans Health Administration and National Child Traumatic Stress Network initiatives in the United States. Additional dissemination programs have been developed by individual states (e.g., New York and Hawaii), and for particular treatments (e.g., dialectical behavior therapy).

Importantly, although the proliferation of dissemination programs is a very positive development, the programs have necessarily proceeded with little empirical guidance because research on effective dissemination of psychological treatments is in its infancy. McHugh and Barlow (2010) argue that the same urgency motivating the development of these programs must now motivate research into their effectiveness. If the behavioral healthcare field is to continue moving forward, dissemination efforts must undergo the same rigorous outcome and process research as our treatments.

REFERENCES

Addis, M. E., Wade, W. A., & Hatgis, C. (1999). Barriers to dissemination of evidence-based practices: Addressing practitioners' concerns about manual-based psychotherapies. *Clinical Psychology: Science and Practice, 6,* 430–441.

APA (American Psychological Association) Presidential Task Force on Evidence-Based Practice. (2006). Evidence-based practice in psychology. *American Psychologist, 61,* 271–285.

Baker, T. B., McFall, R. M., & Shoham, V. (2009). Current status and future prospects of clinical psychology: Toward a scientifically principled approach to mental and behavioral health care. *Psychological Science in the Public Interest, 9,* 67–103.

Berg, B. L. (2001). *Qualitative research methods for the social sciences* (4th ed.). Needham Heights, MA: Allyn & Bacon.

Beutler, L. E., Moleiro, C., & Talebi, H. (2002). How practitioners can systematically use empirical evidence in treatment selection. *Journal of Clinical Psychology, 58,* 1199–1212.

Beutler, L. E., Williams, R. E., Wakefield, P. J., & Entwistle, S. R. (1995). Bridging scientist and practitioner perspectives in clinical psychology. *American Psychologist, 50,* 984–994.

Bieschke, K. J., Fouad, N. A., Collins, F. L., & Halonen, J. S. (2004). The scientifically minded psychologist: Science as core competency. *Journal of Clinical Psychology, 60,* 713–723.

Boisvert, C. M., & Faust, D. (2006). Practicing psychologists' knowledge of general psychotherapy research findings: Implications for science–practice relations. *Professional Psychology: Research and Practice, 37,* 708–716.

Chambless, D. L., & Hollon, S. D. (1998). Defining empirically supported therapies. *Journal of Consulting and Clinical Psychology, 66,* 7–18.

Cochrane A. (1972). *Effectiveness and efficiency: Random reflections on health services.* London: Nuffield Provincial Hospitals Trust.

Crits-Christoph, P., Frank, E., Chambless, D. L., Brody, C., & Karp, J. F. (1995). Training in empirically validated treatments: What are clinical psychology students learning? *Professional Psychology: Research and Practice, 26,* 514–522.

Fisher, J. E., & O'Donohue, W. (Eds.). (2009). *Practitioner's guide to evidence based psychotherapy.* New York, NY: Springer.

Ford, M. R., & Widiger, T. A. (1989). Sex bias in the diagnosis of histrionic and antisocial personality disorders. *Journal of Consulting and Clinical Psychology, 57,* 301–305.

Frank, G. (1984). The Boulder model: History, rationale, and critique. *Professional Psychology: Research and Practice, 15,* 417–435.

Garb, H. N. (1996). The representativeness and past-behavior heuristics in clinical judgment. *Professional Psychology: Research and Practice, 27,* 272–277.

Garb, H. N. (1997). Race bias, social class bias, and gender bias in clinical judgment. *Clinical Psychology: Science & Practice, 4,* 99–120.

Garb, H. N. (1998). *Studying the clinician: Judgment research and psychological assessment.* Washington, DC: American Psychological Association.

Garb, H. N. (2005). Clinical judgment and decision making. *Annual Review of Clinical Psychology, 55,* 3.1–3.23.

Gilovich, T. (1991). *How we know what isn't so: The fallibility of human reason in everyday life.* New York, NY: Free Press.

Goldfried, M. R., & Wolfe, B. E. (1996). Psychotherapy practice and research: Repairing a strained alliance. *American Psychologist, 51,* 1007–1016.

Grove, W. M. (2005). Clinical versus statistical prediction: The contribution of Paul E. Meehl. *Journal of Clinical Psychology 61,* 1233–1243.

Grove, W. M., & Meehl, P. E. (1996). Comparative efficiency of informal (subjective, impressionistic) and formal (mechanical, algorithmic) prediction procedures: The clinical-statistical controversy. *Psychology, Public Policy, and Law, 2,* 293–323.

Grove, W. M., Zald, D. H., Lebow, B. S., Snitz, B. E., & Nelson, C. (2000). Clinical versus mechanical prediction: A meta-analysis. *Psychological Assessment, 12,* 19–30.

Haynes, S. N., Lemsky, C., & Sexton-Radek, K. (1987). Why clinicians infrequently do research. *Professional Psychology: Research and Practice, 18,* 515–519.

Hunsley, J., & Lee, C. M. (2007). Research-informed benchmarks for psychological treatments: Efficacy studies, effectiveness studies, and beyond. *Professional Psychology: Research and Practice, 38,* 21–33.

Kazdin, A. E. (2008). Evidence-based treatment and practice: New opportunities to bridge clinical research and practice, enhance the knowledge base, and improve patient care. *American Psychologist, 63,* 146–159.

Lilienfeld, S.O. (2007). Psychological treatments that cause harm. *Perspectives on Psychological Science, 2,* 53–70.

Lilienfeld, S. O., Wood, J. M., & Garb, H. N. (2000). The scientific status of projective techniques. *Psychological Science in the Public Interest, 1,* 27–66.

McFall, R. M. (1991). Manifesto for a science of clinical psychology. *Clinical Psychologist, 44,* 75–88.

McHugh, R. K., & Barlow, D. H. (2010). The dissemination and implementation of evidence-based psychological treatments. *American Psychologist, 65,* 73–84.

McNiel, D. E., & Binder, R. L. (1995). Correlates of accuracy in the assessment of psychiatric inpatients' risk of violence. *American Journal of Psychiatry, 152,* 901–906.

Meehl, P. E. (1954). *Clinical versus statistical prediction: A theoretical analysis and a review of the evidence.* Minneapolis, MN: University of Minnesota Press.

Meehl, P. E. (1997). Credentialed persons, credentialed knowledge. *Clinical Psychology: Science and Practice, 4,* 91–98.

Nathan, P. E., & Gorman, J. M. (Eds). (2002). *Treatments that work* (2nd ed.). New York, NY: Oxford University Press.

Norcross, J. C., Klonsky, E. D., & Tropiano, H. L. (2008). The research–practice gap: Clinical scientists and independent practitioners speak. *Clinical Psychologist, 61*(3), 14–17.

Parloff, M. B. (1980). Psychotherapy and research: An anaclitic depression. *Psychiatry, 43,* 279–293.

Pavkov, T. W., Lewis, D. A., & Lyons, J. A. (1989). Psychiatric diagnoses and racial bias: An empirical investigation. *Professional Psychology: Research and Practice, 20,* 364–368.

Persons, J. B. (1997). Dissemination of effective methods: Behavior therapy's next challenge. *Behavior Therapy, 28,* 465–471.

Peterson, C., & Park, N. (2005). The enduring value of the Boulder model: "Upon this rock we build." *Journal of Clinical Psychology, 61,* 1147–1150.

Reisman, J. M. (1976). *A history of clinical psychology.* New York, NY: Irvington.

Roth, A., & Fonagy, P. (2004). *What works for whom? A critical review of psychotherapy research* (2nd ed.). New York, NY: Guilford Press.

Sackett, D. L., Rosenberg, W. M. C., Gray, J. A. M., Haynes, R. B., & Richardson, W. S. (1996). Evidence-based medicine: What it is and what it isn't. *British Medical Journal, 312,* 71–72.

Sandberg, J. G., Johnson, L. N., Robila, M., & Miller, R. B. (2002). Clinician identified barriers to clinical research. *Journal of Marital and Family Therapy, 28,* 61–67.

Simon, R. J., Fleiss, J. L., Gurland, B. J., Stiller, P. R., & Sharpe, L. (1973). Depression and schizophrenia in hospitalized black and white mental patients. *Archives of General Psychiatry, 28,* 509–512.

Snyder, C. R., & Elliott, T. R. (2005). Twenty-first century graduate education in clinical psychology: A four level matrix model. *Journal of Clinical Psychology, 61,* 1033–1054.

Sobell, L. C. (1996). Bridging the gap between scientists and practitioners: The challenge before us. *Behavior Therapy, 27,* 297–320.

Spring, B. (2007). Evidence-based practice in clinical psychology: What it is, why it matters; what you need to know. *Journal of Clinical Psychology, 63,* 611–631.

Stack, L. C., Lannon, P. B., & Miley, A. D. (1983). Accuracy of clinicians' expectancies for psychiatric rehospitalization. *American Journal of Community Psychology, 11,* 99–113.

Stewart, R. E., & Chambless, D. L. (2007). Does psychotherapy research inform treatment decisions in private practice? *Journal of Clinical Psychology, 63,* 267–281.

Stewart, R. E., & Chambless, D. L. (2009). Interesting practitioners in training in empirically supported treatments: Research reviews versus case studies. *Journal of Clinical Psychology, 66,* 73–95.

Strand, M., Phelan, K. J., & Donovan, E. F. (2003). Promoting the uptake and use of evidence: An overview of the problem. *Clinics in Perinatology, 30,* 389–402.

Strauss, S. E., Richardson, W. S., Glasziou, P., & Haynes, B. (2005). *Evidence-based medicine: How to practice and teach EBM* (3rd ed.). New York, NY: Elsevier.

Stuart, R. B., & Lilienfeld, S. O. (2007). The evidence missing from evidence-based practice. *American Psychologist, 62,* 615–616.

Turk, D. C., Salovey, P., & Prentice, D. A. (1988). Psychotherapy: An information processing perspective. In D. C. Turk & P. Salovey (Eds.), *Reasoning, inference, and judgment in clinical psychology* (pp. 1–14). New York, NY: Free Press.

Vachon, D. O., Susman, M., Wynne, M. E., et al. (1995). Reasons therapists give for refusing to participate in psychotherapy process research. *Journal of Counseling Psychology, 42,* 380–382.

Weissman, M. M., Verdeli, H., Gameroff, M. J., Bledsoe, S. E., Betts, K., Mufson, L., et al. (2006). National survey of psychotherapy training programs in psychiatry, psychology, and social work. *Archives of General Psychiatry, 63,* 925–934.

Weisz, J. R. (2004). *Psychotherapy for children and adolescents: Evidence-based treatments and case examples.* Cambridge, UK: Cambridge University Press.

Weisz, J. R., Jensen-Doss, A., & Hawley, K. M. (2006). Evidence-based youth psychotherapies versus usual clinical care: A meta-analysis of direct comparisons. *American Psychologist, 61,* 671–689.

Woody, S. R., Weisz, J., & McLean, C. (2005). Empirically supported treatments: 10 years later. *Clinical Psychologist, 58*(4), 5–11.

Nine

The Quality Improvement Agenda in Behavioral Healthcare Reform
Using Science to Reduce Error

WILLIAM O'DONOHUE, RACHEL AMMIRATI,
AND SCOTT O. LILIENFELD

INTRODUCTION

Every field is built on a set of metaprinciples. These principles comprise the paradigm of a given field and serve as a set of disciplinary commitments that guide members' behavior (Kuhn, 1977). Medicine, for example, is driven by the Hippocratic ethic of "first do no harm," as well as a commitment to engage in practices that are informed by science. Increasingly, quality improvement programs (American Psychological Association, 2009; Deming, 1982, 1986) that incorporate guiding principles associated with business and economics have also begun to shape medicine (Berwick, 2004; Institute of Medicine, 2001).

The essence of quality improvement (QI) is relatively straightforward: a focus on identifying and reducing widespread errors as a vehicle for enhancing the effectiveness and efficiency of a process, service, or product. In this sense, as we will discover, quality improvement mirrors the scientific process in its emphasis on continually rooting out mistakes. In this chapter, we provide readers with a bird's-eye view of the current problems in the behavioral healthcare system and a broad vision of how a QI perspective can alleviate these problems.

THE OVERARCHING PROBLEM

The major problem in behavioral healthcare is its continued lack of a clear set of sound animating principles. Although debates about the importance of practice that is informed by science as opposed to other modes of knowledge generation persist (Westen, Novotny, & Thompson-Brenner, 2004), crucial questions remain unanswered. For example, what factors must we consider when evaluating the effectiveness of a treatment? Are practitioners using treatments that are ineffective or harmful to clients? Is there a legitimate form of "professional knowledge" (as alluded to in the APA's ethical code)—such as intuition or subjective experience—that is distinct from scientific knowledge?

Over the past two decades, there has been an increasing consensus that evidence-based practice is essential to behavioral healthcare (Chambless et al., 1996; Chambless & Ollendick, 2001; Fisher & O'Donohue, 2005; see Chapter 8 in this volume). However, few have acknowledged the potential benefits of adopting what we will argue should be a fundamental tenet of the paradigm guiding our field: a QI philosophy. As the American Psychological Association (2009) recently noted, fields that embrace the QI perspective "systematically collect information from providers or patients with the intention of drawing conclusions about the quality of care provided and improving provider performance, treatment outcome, or efficiency" (p. 551).

Therefore, we believe that a major shift in focus of this kind will serve not only to increase the quality of services we deliver to the beneficiaries of our treatments, but also to better position us to address other key behavioral healthcare problems. We argue that a systematic adoption of a QI orientation is critical if we hope to transform our broken healthcare system into a far more efficient, effective, safe, and accessible one.

AMERICA'S HEALTHCARE CRISIS

There should be little dispute about one point: There is a healthcare crisis in the United States (O'Donohue & Rummel, 2010). We believe that the major dimensions of this crisis include the following:

- *Healthcare is growing increasingly expensive.* In the United States in 1960, healthcare costs were about 5% of gross domestic product (GDP; O'Donohue & Rummel, 2010). Currently, healthcare costs are approximately 17% of GDP and the proportion of the GDP devoted to healthcare is accelerating. Although there are many drivers of healthcare costs, some of the most critical include (a) paying for technological improvements (e.g., more informative but higher cost MRIs as an improvement over lower cost x-rays), (b) increase in the longevity (and hence increased healthcare usage) of patients' lives, and (c) increase in the incidence of costly chronic diseases, such as diabetes, arthritis, and chronic obstructive pulmonary disease (CDC, 2009), as well as attendant problems, such as treatment noncompliance and unhealthy lifestyles (CDC, 2009; O'Donohue, Moore, & Scott, 2007).
- *Problems with access to healthcare.* General access to healthcare is problematic for the poor, minorities, rural communities, and the uninsured (Andrulis, 1998; Ayanian, Weissman, Schneider, Ginsburg, & Zaslavsky, 2000; Balluz, Okoro, & Strine, 2004). Access to quality healthcare is even more difficult (Saha, Arbelaez, & Cooper, 2003). Further, in regard to behavioral healthcare in particular, we tend to neglect the fact that the provision of mental health services primarily in the context of freestanding mental health clinics may restrict access to treatment. After all, the primary care clinic has been called the de facto mental health treatment system in the United States because it is where most depressed mood, anxiety, and increasingly even psychotic disorders are treated (Cummings, O'Donohue, & Ferguson, 2003).
- *Safety in healthcare is problematic.* Medical errors result in tens of thousands of patient deaths each year and even more cases of increased morbidity. In the Institute of Medicine's (2001) influential "Crossing the Quality Chasm" report, the authors estimated that about 90,000 Americans die each year due to medical errors. In regard to behavioral healthcare in particular, it has been difficult to define an error, given the lack of consensus about what constitutes proper assessment and treatment. However, it is clear that behavioral healthcare errors are widespread (Lilienfeld, 2007). Errors include

missed or erroneous diagnoses, problematic assessment results due to the inadequate quality of tests used, and treatments delivered that have little or no demonstrated efficacy or safety data. As a field, we have made little progress in defining and detecting these errors and modifying processes so that they are minimized.

- *Failure to be patient centric.* Behavioral healthcare is rarely designed with significant consumer input. As a field, we know little or nothing about what patients prefer and rarely empower them to make informed decisions about their behavioral healthcare. We are trained in graduate school in the ethic of utilizing the least onerous interventions, but generally rely on 1-hour weekly outpatient individual therapy for the vast majority of our patients (O'Donohue & Cummings, 2008; O'Donohue & Draper, in press). Further, when we focus on improvements, we often focus only on those that we as professionals care about, such as producing more data from randomized controlled trials. Although such trials are important, they are not the be all and end all because they do not answer all legitimate questions. Our field often fails to consider issues about which patients may care, such as improved access to practitioners when they have questions, lower cost treatment options, and less time-consuming interventions.

- *Failure to use information technologies such as electronic health records.* Electronic health record systems can give providers fast access to complete information about a specific patient. Yet, data suggest that behavioral healthcare providers may be reticent to adopt this kind of technology (see Chapter 5 in this volume). Most practitioners simply ask about when and where the patient has received records in the past, which typically results in an incomplete and flawed file. Further, the process of obtaining records via fax or mail can sometimes take months. Still, this system has been in place for the past half century and almost nothing has been done to change it. This is especially troubling given the range of pertinent and impressive technological advances that have emerged in recent years.

- *Failure to be as effective as possible.* As we will soon demonstrate, evidence-based treatments that have been

shown to be the safest and most effective are not used nearly enough by behavioral healthcare providers (see the following section). Instead, clinicians often rely on intuition or personal opinion when choosing treatments and tend not to consider whether data exist that bear on their effectiveness and safety. The use of invalid assessment devices and questionable treatments is ultimately wasteful and contributes to what economists call "the lemon problem." In essence, the existence of lemons in a market depresses the price of a good or service. For example, a consumer may be willing to pay $3 for a gallon of milk. Although the consumer would like the milk to be cheaper (as is the case with all goods), his purchase shows that he is willing to pay the current price. Part of the reason the consumer thinks that this is a fair price is that because virtually all of the milk is of adequate quality (e.g., it is not spoiled or bad tasting, etc.). However, if we imagine that the consumer discovered that half of the milk he purchased was rancid after he purchased it, what would he be willing to pay now? With "lemons" in the market, the consumer might believe that $1.50 seems to be a better price because it results in his risk washing out (i.e., it still takes $3 on average to get a good gallon of milk). Thus, in addition to providing our patients with potentially ineffective or harmful treatments, our use of the equivalent of rancid milk in behavioral healthcare may also depress the value of our services.
- *Too little emphasis on prevention.* The healthcare system is not designed to treat what it can treat most effectively. Instead, it is designed to respond to acute illnesses and to deal with problems that have already emerged. However, President Obama, among others, has stressed that we need to transform the present illness care system into a healthcare system. The key insight is that we all want health, not just an amelioration of illness.

A CLOSER LOOK AT THE BEHAVIORAL HEALTHCARE CRISIS IN PARTICULAR

We have already begun to outline some of the problems that are particularly pressing in the domain of behavioral healthcare. Perhaps most notable of all is the continued disregard for the role of science in mental health practice. As we will demonstrate in the following section, studies that bear on this issue provide ample reason for concern, as well as some grounds for cautious optimism.

Concerns about the gap between science and practice in behavioral healthcare are far from new (e.g., Heppner, Carter, Claiborn, & Brooks, 1992; Shapiro & Wiggins, 1994). Yet, despite compelling calls to action (Baker, McFall, & Shoham, 2009; McFall, 2006), resistance to science persists (see Bloom & Weisberg, 2007, for a discussion of resistance to scientific findings from a developmental perspective). Clearly, all is not well in the field of mental health practice (Lilienfeld, Lynn, & Lohr, 2003). Some authors have compared the treatment choices that many clinical psychologists make to those a child might make in a candy store (Mischel, 2009), and others have raised issues concerning the continued use of potentially harmful psychotherapies (Lilienfeld, 2007). Although impressive advances in our understanding of the relative efficacy of various treatments for debilitating mental health problems continue to be made (Baker et al., 2009; Barlow, 2004), clinical psychology and related fields often seem to be content to stick with the sweet stuff that tastes good, even if it is not good for us.

Despite evidence suggesting at least some improvements in regard to the integration of science and practice in behavioral healthcare (Goodheart, Kazdin, & Sternberg, 2006), there is still a long way to go. This sobering view is borne out by numerous surveys of the treatment practices of mental health providers and of graduate training programs, a sampling of which we review here.

Practitioners and the Use of ESTs and Problematic Treatments

The neglect of empirically supported treatments (ESTs—interventions found to be effective in independently replicated controlled studies) among practitioners has recently been highlighted elsewhere (Baker et al., 2009). Nevertheless, additional surveys over the past few years provide evidence for continued concerns.

One study of college counseling centers found that although 60% of clinicians reported moderate to strong support for the importance of having access to scholarly resources, 25% indicated that they did not use research articles to guide their clinical work (Cooper, Benton, Benton, & Phillips, 2008). Another survey of licensed clinical social workers (LCSWs; Pignotti & Thyer, 2009) revealed similarly mixed findings, suggesting that although most reported using some form of EST in their practice, approximately 75% still continued to use what the authors called "novel unsupported treatments," or treatments for which there is no or questionable empirical support. These treatments included critical incident stress debriefing, which has been found to be ineffective and perhaps harmful in controlled studies (Lilienfeld, 2007), imago relationship therapy, Jungian sandtray therapy, age regression for sexual abuse, past lives therapy, neurolinguistic programming, and psychosynthesis.

Recent surveys of practitioners working with specific populations provide further evidence for the need for quality improvement. One survey of mental health practitioners from both the United States and United Kingdom (Kuller, Ott, Goisman, Wainwright, & Rabin, 2010) suggested that even though the majority of respondents reported using an EST to treat schizophrenia (in this case, cognitive-behavioral therapy [CBT]), approximately 26% of U.S. clinicians (versus approximately 15% of UK clinicians) reported using either humanistic or existential treatments, neither of which is an EST for schizophrenia.

Another survey of practitioners working for the military or VA system found that 90% of clinicians treating posttraumatic stress disorder (PTSD) did not use any of the ESTs (e.g., exposure and response prevention) recommended by the U.S. government (Russell & Silver, 2007). These data dovetail with those of Becker, Zayfert, and Anderson (2004), who found that only half of licensed and provisionally licensed psychotherapists who treat patients with PTSD use imaginal exposure, which is the most scientifically established treatment for this condition. Moreover, fewer than 30% of these psychologists have been trained in exposure techniques (Becker et al., 2004). Even among clinicians who report generally using ESTs, data suggest that many may not be adhering to standardized guidelines (Sheehan, Walrath, & Holden, 2007).

On a somewhat more positive note, a recent survey of practitioners from 15 states revealed that when asked to rate how often they used evidence-based practices on a 4-point scale ranging from 1 = never/almost never to 4 = always/almost always (Nelson & Steele, 2007), most indicated that they did so either sometimes or often (M = 2.62, SD = .86). Nevertheless, it is not clear whether these clinicians actually used practices that are demonstrably evidence based.

Further cause for concern comes from surveys that ask consumers about the treatments they have tried or are using. A sample of parents of children with autism reported that 36% had tried music therapy to treat their children and that 21% were currently using it (Goin-Kochel, Myers, & Mackintosh, 2007). Nevertheless, there is no evidence that music therapy is efficacious for the core symptoms of autism. Large-scale U.S. survey data from individuals with depression and panic attacks similarly suggest that the majority do not receive scientifically supported therapies (Kessler et al., 2001); most receive such unvalidated treatments as herbal remedies, homeopathy, aromatherapy, yoga, hypnosis, biofeedback, and energy therapies.

Training and Education Issues

The continued lack of consistent EST use by practitioners probably stems partly from deficiencies in training and education. Starting more than a decade ago, Crits-Christoph, Frank, Chambless, Brody, and Karp (1995) found that more than 20% of programs did not include training in more than three fourths of ESTs. Horan and Blanchard (2001) similarly found that most internships provided training in fewer than half of 72 ESTs surveyed, and a survey of APA-accredited clinical internship sites suggested that only 28% of sites provided more than 15 hours of training in ESTs (Hays et al., 2002). The variability in EST training was especially pronounced at university counseling centers, and among the major obstacles to training in ESTs cited by training directors were their lack of flexibility in the number of allowable sessions (16.6%) and their ostensible failure to address clients' genuine presenting problems (12.3%).

Have things improved in recent years? It is not clear. Karekla, Lundgren, and Forsyth (2004) found that 31.8% of students in APA-accredited doctoral clinical, counseling, and school psychology programs reported having never taken any course in ESTs, and 51% reported no coursework in EST training manuals. Moreover, in an extensive national survey of psychology, psychiatry, and social work training programs, Weissman et al. (2006) found that large percentages did not require training in evidence-based therapies, which overlapped with but were not identical to ESTs. Among PhD programs, for example, 90 and 97% offered training in behavioral and cognitive-behavioral therapy, respectively, but only 34 and 53%, respectively, required such training.

The corresponding figures for social work programs were markedly lower at 64% and 66%, respectively, and 13% and 21%, respectively. Among the major obstacles to EST training cited were lack of trainee interest (25.9% in PhD programs), an absence of qualified faculty to teach ESTs (11.4% in PhD programs), and the claim that ESTs can be difficult to teach (9.7% in PhD programs).

In addition, when Hunt and Wisocki (2008) surveyed the directors of 165 clinical psychology training programs and related councils, they found that 18% of respondents reported agreeing only "a little" with the statement, "In supervising the clinical work of students, supervisors should require students to refer to the scientific literature in designing treatment programs and in using clinical interventions" (p. 93). One respondent strongly disagreed with this statement! Only 50% of respondents strongly agreed that "systematic assessment of a client's functioning is essential to every therapy," and 61% strongly agreed that "students should be taught clinical methods whose efficacy has been empirically validated" (p. 93). Recent reports of the status of social work training programs have also been less than encouraging, as evidenced by Bledsoe and colleagues' (2007) finding that 62% of such programs that participated in a national survey did not require education or supervision in any EST.

Finally, at least some recent data may offer a silver lining. One study of graduate programs for clinical child psychologists revealed that 93% required that their students be trained, at some level, in evidence-based treatments (Pidano, Kurowski, & McEvoy, 2010). Nevertheless, another recent survey suggested that "students do not appear to view research to be as useful when planning treatments compared to supervisors' input and client-specific evidence" (Luebbe, Radcliffe, Callands, Green, & Thorn, 2007, p. 653). Thus, even if graduate students are being exposed to and trained in ESTs, the negative attitudes of some of their supervisors toward ESTs (e.g., Hunt & Wisocki, 2008) may exert more influence.

Thus, a key problem that we must face in behavioral healthcare is that a significant proportion of clinicians use therapies that (1) lack clear evidence for their effectiveness, (2) are less effective than other available therapies, and (3) may be harmful. Nevertheless, we believe that the adoption of a QI approach to behavioral healthcare may help us to resolve these issues.

THE CURRENT FLAWED APPROACH TO QUALITY: THE SEARCH-AND-PUNISH MISSION FOR "BAD APPLES"

The behavioral healthcare field has tended to rely on what Donald Berwick (2004), who recently became the administrator of the Centers for Medicare and Medicaid Services, calls the "bad apples approach" to identifying defects in quality (p. 42). Specifically, the field emphasizes ethical complaints and audit problems in some accreditation reviews and often relies on whistleblowers to detect and respond to (typically by punishing) individuals thought to be responsible for quality defects.

A number of problems are associated with the bad apples approach. The first is that a defect is often defined only as something fairly egregious, such as having sex with a patient. Other problematic practices, such as giving a patient a Rorschach inkblot or Thematic Apperception Test (TAT) when not supported by research evidence (Lilienfeld et al., 2003), rarely meet the threshold of the typical definition of a defect. As a consequence, we overlook many important defects.

Second, because our system relies primarily on punishment, practitioners have an incentive to hide or deny defects, making it difficult for us to learn about our problems to prevent them from recurring. One of the precepts of QI is that "every defect is a treasure" in that it provides an opportunity to learn about a problem in the system and to change the system so that this defect does not occur again (see Schulz, 2010, for a similar perspective).

Third, the bad apples approach treats defects as static entities and fails to be innovative because it holds practitioners to existing standards rather than encouraging them to ask the question of whether what exists is an old paradigm that needs to be transformed.

Fourth, and finally, this approach to QI is inadequate because it is person- rather than process-centered. It seeks to ask, "Who is a bad apple?" rather than the more informative question, "What problems in the process produced this problematic result?" Deming (1982, 1986) is known to have said that "people blaming approaches" rarely works because they breed distrust, rationalization, and escape and avoidance behaviors. They also overlook the key point that all of us are fallible and prone to error. Thus, Berwick (2004), has more appropriately suggested that the "bad apples" approach to enhancing the quality of a service be replaced by continual QI.

THE QUALITY ROAD MAP

The adoption of a systematic QI program can be a transformative process. It transformed Japan from a producer of relatively low-quality trinkets to one of the top three economies in the world, and Ford Motor Company ("Quality is Job 1") from a company on the brink of bankruptcy to one of international importance (Saunders & Saunders, 1994). Systematic QI has also been recently adopted by China and South Korea, two of the most powerful emerging economies in the world. Although these models of change cannot be directly superimposed on the field of behavioral healthcare, they provide broad examples of how to improve a similarly broken system that provides services (i.e., treatments) to consumers (i.e., patients).

Behavioral healthcare is currently mired in the bad apple approach to quality. To move our field beyond this problematic approach, we propose a number of reforms. Reforms 2 through 8 are nested within the first reform, which is broader than the others.

Reform 1

The first reform we propose is that the more static bad apple approach to ensuring quality in behavioral healthcare be replaced by the more dynamic QI approach. This radical reform will necessitate many changes in our system, including changes to our ethical codes (e.g., mandating that all delivered services must take place in the context of a systematic QI program), models of accreditation, training models, and methods of service delivery. To enact this reform, we will need systematic training in QI technologies (e.g., QI systems of assessment; see Saunders & Saunders, 1994, for a brief description of one such assessment system) in our graduate and continuing education programs, as well as training in basic business skills. Like previously mentioned companies that have successfully used QI programs, we will need to commit ourselves explicitly to excellence and reducing errors.

Reform 2

The second reform we propose is that all behavioral healthcare organizations become learning organizations. This reform involves continually questioning current processes to attempt to improve them, and it utilizes concepts from Deming's QI cycle (Deming, 1986). Specifically, the following steps should be followed:

1. *Identify:* determine what we want to improve.
2. *Analyze:* attempt to understand the processes that are producing the problem.
3. *Test:* implement the change and measure results.
4. *Act:* decide on changes to improve the process.

This QI cycle transforms a static organization into a dynamic learning organization, and it can operate on a variety of processes in the organization at all times. Specifically, the QI cycle should be applied to processes involving safety, access, price, effectiveness, and diagnosis, as well as others. Once we identify meaningful quality indicators such as safety, price, effectiveness, and consumer satisfaction, we can measure, benchmark, and improve them.

It is important to note how similar this QI cycle is to the scientific process. The prominent philosopher of science, Sir Karl Popper (1957), argued that the function of science is to root out errors in our belief systems, and that this goal is accomplished most effectively and efficiently when we advance bold conjectures (i.e., "risky predictions") in an attempt to identify error. Scientists can then collect data to determine if these bold conjectures are false or in need of revision. Deming's (1950) cycle is essentially the same. Unfortunately, though, most who have stridently embraced the scientific process in the field of behavioral healthcare have failed to propose simultaneously that we also adopt a QI perspective (see McFall, 1991, for an important exception).

Some have suggested that the QI approach, although very similar to the scientific process, may have decided advantages over the relatively basic recommendation that practitioners should use evidence-based treatment. Specifically, although evidence-based treatment is certainly superior to treatment that is not based on evidence, it tends to be associated with a rather static, one-dimensional view of quality. In essence, practitioners who use treatments based on scientific evidence believe that it is the scientific evidence that gives rise to the quality of their service. However, this way of thinking engenders a dichotomous way of thinking about quality (i.e., one either does or does not implement treatments based on scientific evidence), rather than fostering a more dimensional and dynamic conceptualization of quality.

Because the QI approach emphasizes error elimination and self-correction, it has the potential to be much richer than the static EST approach. It suggests that opportunities for QI can be found in more than the kind of therapy delivered (e.g., cognitive-behavioral versus psychodynamic) and gives rise to a number of important questions that we can continually ask ourselves, including:

How do we continually drive down prices?
How do we continually improve access?
How do we periodically find out what our patients want (e.g., e-mail access to us for quick questions)?

Further, the QI perspective also forces us to adopt a more quantitative approach to improving the quality of our services and to ask ourselves the following:

What are the benchmarks—such as therapy effect sizes, drop-out rates, and relapse rates—in my organization compared with those in published studies?
How can therapy be altered to improve these benchmarks?

Finally, QI also requires that we continually ask ourselves vital yet basic questions, such as the following:

Is this even the right kind of approach?
What changes might be necessary to improve patient satisfaction (e.g., using effective prevention so that the need for treatment is greatly reduced or even eliminated)?

In line with reform 2, Berwick (2004) provided the following list of key objectives for healthcare organizations that adopt a QI approach:

- *Name the problem(s).* We can use consumer input for this objective, although we are already aware of some of the problems (i.e., use of invalid assessment devices, use of harmful or understudied therapies, poor prescription practices, access problems, lack of affordability, and lack of continuity of care).
- *Identify and build on successes.* What are the best practices? Where are the centers of excellence? What can we learn from them? We do not have to reinvent the wheel, but we must learn from our colleagues, including those who use QI approaches in physical medicine and more distant industries.

- *Take leaps of faith.* We must attempt bold solutions. Many of our problems are too big for small responses. Of course, these leaps of faith must not begin and end with faith: They must be tempered by continual data generation regarding their effectiveness—which, of course, will occur if they are embedded in a systematical QI system. If they do not work, they should be modified or abandoned.
- *Look outside medicine.* Dentistry, for example, has been an amazingly successful profession in the last 10 years, and L. L. Bean has developed superlative phone systems. Honda has also implemented a range of QI strategies (Liker, 2004). Although each of these industries is not as clearly related to behavioral healthcare as is medicine, each may have important, albeit relatively specific, lessons to teach us.
- *Set aims and show constancy of purpose.* Constantly improving quality is foremost. An important part of leadership is setting quality goals.
- *Understand systems.* Improvements in quality cannot be achieved without what Deming (1986) has referred to as "deep knowledge." One must understand the processes—that is, the causal chains—that are producing low-quality goods and services. For example, we might find that problematic therapies can be traced back, at least in part, to problematic graduate training, which would suggest that improvements need to be made early in the chain.
- *Make action lists.* For example, reduce waste in all forms, reduce demand, plot measurements related to aims over time, and cooperate.
- *Never—ever—lose sight of the patient as the central figure.* The consumer (or patient), not our professional prerogatives, must be king. We need improved tools to increase patients' knowledge and input, as well as shared decision making.

Reform 3

The behavioral healthcare field needs to become more consumer-centric: We must remember that we would not exist without our consumers. Further, we are in business to help them. Therefore, we need to continually ask our patients the following questions: What are their concerns with quality?

What do they want, and how are we doing in delivering it? How can we improve? These questions need to be our ever present concerns. We need much more research on what our consumers want because these data may help to shed light on ways to overcome treatment noncompliance. For example, gathering information on the preferred duration, formats (e.g., group versus individual), and location (e.g., primary care clinics versus mental health clinics) of treatment may be particularly informative. Of course, we must sometimes deliver interventions that our clients find unpleasant in the short term (e.g., exposure and response prevention for obsessive-compulsive disorder), although even in these cases we must do so with full informed consent and with our clients' long-term needs in mind.

The British National Health Service attempts to improve quality by what it calls "understanding the whole patient journey" (http://www.institute.nhs.uk/images/stories/CreativityTools/Cause%20and%20Effect%203.jpg). It recommends that an organization create a map that identifies each step a patient experiences from the initial contact to the last contact. This map can then help the organization to see itself from the perspective of the consumer. Further, by asking a set of key questions related to the quality of services offered, organizations can determine how the consumer's experience might be improved. Key questions may include the following:

- How many steps are there?
- How many handoffs are there? Are any unnecessary?
- Could some tasks be carried out by one person instead of several?
- Is there any duplication of work?
- Are there any bottlenecks?
- How much error correction or rework is being carried out?
- What is the approximate time between each step?
- Which tasks help to achieve the purpose and which do not? Can we eliminate those that do not add value to patients?
- Are we doing the right things in the process?
- Are we doing things in the right order? Is the right/best person doing it?
- What information do we give to patients and at what stage? Is the information useful?

- Should some tasks that are performed in another process be performed here?

These questions can be asked about a patient seen in an outpatient private practice, a patient treated on an inpatient unit, or even a graduate student entering a graduate program in behavioral healthcare.

Reform 4

Our services need to be as safe as possible. We have insufficiently embraced the Hippocratic ethic of "first, do no harm" (Lilienfeld, 2007) and therefore need to make it a priority. The British National Health Service has adopted a quality improvement process called "Patient Safety Planning." It is based on the well-established finding in human factors research that we all make mistakes, and it emphasizes that an organization's goal should be to acquire a better understanding of why healthcare staff make errors and which "systems factors" threaten patient safety. The British National Health Service suggests building a "safety culture" that possesses the following characteristics:

- *Open culture:* staff members feel comfortable discussing patient safety incidents and raising safety issues with both colleagues and senior managers.
- *Just culture:* staff members and patients are treated fairly, with empathy and consideration, when they have been involved in a patient safety incident or have raised a safety issue.
- *Reporting culture:* staff members have confidence in the local incident reporting system and use it to notify healthcare managers of incidents that are occurring, including near misses.
- *Barriers to incident reporting have been identified and removed:* the reporting process is made easy, and staff members are not blamed or punished when they report incidents; instead, they receive constructive feedback after submitting an incident report.
- *Learning culture:* the organization is committed to learning more about safety, to communicating lessons to colleagues, and to remembering what is learned over time.
- *Informed culture:* the organization has learned from past experience and can identify and mitigate future

incidents because it learns from events that have already happened.

Reform 5
We need leaders who are well versed in taking a QI approach to behavioral healthcare. Currently, most of our leaders have little or no formal education in key skill sets needed for management. These skills include the ability to engage in strategic planning, human resources management, marketing, entrepreneurship, and finance. We need to use the QI cycle previously identified and to generate hypotheses about how to improve the leadership and management in our field. Improving the quality of our management will undoubtedly help to improve the quality of our work.

Reform 6
We need to increase transparency. Specifically, it will be important to create more open systems so that consumers can make more informed choices. We need transparent report cards that compare organizations on patient satisfaction, adherence to evidence-based protocols, price, and safety. O'Donohue (in preparation) devised a clinician report card that increases transparency to potential patients (see Table 9.1). The goal of this report card is to go beyond the informal means that are currently used to gain information about a prospective therapist. By providing information about training, price, ethical complaints, and past consumer ratings, potential patients can obtain important information upon which to base their decisions.

Reform 7
We need to strive constantly to produce a better value proposition for our consumers and to consider how to lower prices rather than to increase them. Although it may seem counterintuitive, this does not necessarily mean that practitioners will earn less. If we increase our productivity and the demand for our product, we will probably earn more. It is a basic law of economics that demand increases as price drops.

An important question to ask ourselves is how we can meet client demand in the most productive ways possible. For example, group therapies have been shown to be as effective as individual therapies for a number of mental health problems (e.g., McDermut, Miller, & Brown, 2001). Because many managed care organizations will pay about 40% or so of the price

Table 9.1 Clinician Transparency Report

Basic Information

Name:

Photo:

Contact information:

Emergency contact info:

Education/degrees:

A brief personal statement or info:

Statement of therapeutic approach (brief description, particularly in reference to evidence-based assessment and protocols):

Additional training/achievements (possible to attach vita):

Specialties, including total number of clients seen in each (e.g., adult depression, approximately 400 cases):

Current Licenses and Professional Standing

Public disciplinary actions against license:

Agreements and stipulations to cease medical practice temporarily:

Criminal convictions or plea arrangements for felonies and "crimes of moral turpitude" dating back to initial licensure in any state or country:

Judgments, settlements, and arbitration awards for malpractice claims dating back to 1990:

Refusal by an insurance carrier to issue professional liability insurance:

Financial Information

Rates:

General hourly rate:

Intake:

Any special rates (sliding scales or increased rates for special activities):

Types of third-party payments accepted:

Former Client Ratings and Comments

One to five stars and then anonymous comments:

For client ratings:

What type of problem did you see the therapist for (e.g., depression, marital problem)?

For how many sessions did you see the therapist?

What was your total cost?

How satisfied were you (1–5)?

How much did your problem remit (1–5)?

Would you recommend this therapist for a person with a similar problem?

What did you like least and most?

of individual therapy for an hour of group therapy (xxx), the clinician may actually start to make more money running an hour of group therapy versus an hour of individual therapy. A situation of this nature represents a win–win scenario for both practitioners and patients (as well as managed care organizations): Patients pay less for treatment, therapists may make more money, and managed care organizations pay less for treatment.

Reform 8

We need to integrate healthcare so that a patient can get physical and behavioral healthcare needs met in one setting by one team. Integrated care (Cummings, 2004) ought not to be seen as an isolated innovation, but rather as a key move to be made in a QI process for both behavioral and physical healthcare. Patients have already "voted with their feet" and shown that they want a large portion of their behavioral healthcare to take place in the primary care setting. Here, the patient can be seen holistically and the team can look simultaneously for behavioral drivers of medical problems and medical drivers of behavioral problems. The patient will no longer be seen as a divided individual composed of separate behavioral and physical components.

CONCLUSIONS

As we have demonstrated, there are significant quality problems in behavioral healthcare. Our clients are not consistently receiving high-quality assessments or interventions, and some are probably being harmed as a consequence. Therefore, we sorely need a transformational framework to improve our system across many dimensions. Fortunately, such a framework exists. QI, like science, is based on the principle that knowledge advances slowly but surely through the process of self-correction (see Schulz, 2010).

Unfortunately, with precious few exceptions (e.g., APA, 2009), quality improvement's potential for behavioral healthcare has been largely ignored. We have relied largely on the relatively unproductive "bad apples approach" to identifying errors and have been met with disappointing results as a consequence. Our field is falling behind physical medicine, which is rapidly embracing QI technology (see Berwick, 2004). With only a few notable exceptions, the field of behavioral healthcare has also been surprisingly defensive in the face of clear evidence that it could and should do better (Lilienfeld, 2010). A QI philosophy implies that we should welcome and even embrace criticisms of our field, rather than ignore or dismiss them.

We have pointed out that QI shares important commonalities with the process of scientific inquiry. Both call for humility in acknowledging that we are all prone to error, and both see mistakes as valuable opportunities for learning and improvement. As we have pointed out, there are a host of opportunities for the transformative power of QI in behavioral healthcare. We have also outlined several broad reforms that are long overdue, and we believe that we need to move to a system of behavioral healthcare based on continual growth and improvement. In the interest of being fully committed to the well-being of our patients and to reducing their suffering as efficiently and effectively as possible, we hope that our field soon embraces a systematic QI perspective.

REFERENCES

American Psychological Association. (2009). Criteria for evaluation of quality improvement programs and the use of quality improvement data. *American Psychologist, 64*(6), 551–557.

Andrulis, D. P. (1998). Access to care is the centerpiece in the elimination of socioeconomic disparities in health. *Annals of Internal Medicine, 129,* 412–416.

Ayanian, J. Z., Weissman, J. S., Schneider, E. C., Ginsburg, J. A., & Zaslavsky, A. M. (2000). Unmet health needs of uninsured adults in the United States. *Journal of the American Medical Association, 284,* 2061–2069.

Baker, T. B., McFall, R. M., & Shoham, V. (2009). Current status and future prospects of clinical psychology: Toward a scientifically principled approach to mental and behavioral health care. *Psychological Science in the Public Interest, 9,* 67–103.

Balluz, L. S., Okoro, C. A., & Strine, T. W. (2005). Access to health-care and preventive services among Hispanics and non-Hispanics, United States, 2001–2002. *Epidemiology, 16,* S18–S19.

Barlow, D. H. (2004). Psychological treatments. *American Psychologist, 59,* 869–878.

Becker, C. B., Zayfert, C., & Anderson, E. (2004). Survey of psychologists' use and attitudes towards exposure therapy for PTSD. *Behavior Research and Therapy, 42,* 277–292.

Berwick, D. M. (2004). *Escape fire: Designs for the future of healthcare.* New York, NY: John Wiley & Sons.

Bledsoe, S., Weissman, M., Mullen, E., Ponniah, K., Gameroff, M., Verdeli, H. et al. (2007). Empirically supported psychotherapy in social work training programs: Does the definition of evidence matter? *Research on Social Work Practice, 17*(4), 449–455.

Bloom, P., & Weisberg, D. (2007). Childhood origins of adult resistance to science. *Science, 316*(5827), 996–997.

CDC (Centers for Disease Control and Prevention). (December, 2009). *Chronic disease prevention and health promotion: Chronic disease cost calculator.* Retrieved from http://www.cdc.gov/chronicdisease/resources/calculator/index.htm

Chambless, D. L., Sanderson, W. C., Shoham, V., Bennett-Johnson, S., Pope, K. S., Crits-Christoph, P., Baker, M., Johnson, B., Woody, S. R., Sue, S., Beutler, L., Williams, D. A., & McCurry, S. (1996). An update on empirically validated therapies. *The Clinical Psychologist, 49*, 5–18.

Chambless, D., & Ollendick, T. (2001). Empirically supported psychological interventions: Controversies and evidence. *Annual Review of Psychology, 52*, 685–716.

Cooper, S. E., Benton, S. A., Benton, S. L., & Phillips, J. C. (2008). Evidence-based practice in psychology among college counseling center clinicians. *Journal of College Student Psychotherapy, 22*, 28–50.

Crits-Christoph, P., Chambless, D. L., Frank, E., & Brody, C. (1995). Training in empirically validated treatments: What are clinical psychology students learning? *Professional Psychology: Research and Practice, 26*, 514–522.

Cummings, N., O'Donohue, W., & Ferguson, K. (2003). Behavioral health as primary care: Beyond efficacy to effectivess: A report of the Third Reno Conference on the integration of behavioral health in primary care. Reno, NV: Context Press.

Deming, W. E. (1982). *Quality, productivity, and competitive position.* Cambridge, MA: MIT Press.

Deming, W. E. (1986). *Out of the crisis.* Cambridge, MA: MIT Press.

Fisher, J. E., & O'Donohue, W. (2006). *A practitioner's guide to evidence-based psychotherapy.* New York, NY: Springer.

Fitterling, H., & Wickramaratne, P. (2007). Empirically supported psychotherapy in social work training programs: Does the definition of evidence matter? *Research on Social Work Practice, 17,* 449–455.

Goin-Kochel, R. P., Myers, B. J., & Mackintosh, V. H. (2007). Parental reports on the use of treatments and therapies for children with autism spectrum disorders. *Research in Autism Spectrum Disorders, 1,* 195–209.

Goodheart, C. D., Kazdin, A. E., & Sternberg, R. J. (Eds.). (2006). *Evidence-based psychotherapy: Where practice and research meet.* Washington, DC: American Psychological Association.

Hays, K., Rardin, D., Jarvis, P., Taylor, N., Moorman, A., & Armstead, C. (2002). An exploratory survey on empirically supported treatments: Implications for internship training. *Professional Psychology: Research and Practice, 33,* 207–211.

Heppner, P., Carter, J., Claiborn, C., & Brooks, L. (1992). A proposal to integrate science and practice in counseling psychology. *Counseling Psychologist, 20,* 107–122.

Horan, W. P., & Blanchard, J. J. (2001). Training opportunities in empirically supported treatments and their relationship to intern recruitment and post-internship placement: A survey of directors of internship training. *Clinical Science (Winter),* 1–10.

Hunt, S. L., & Wisocki, P. A. (2008). Balancing science and practice in clinical psychology training programs: A survey of training directors. *Behavior Therapist, 31,* 91–96.

Institute of Medicine. (2001). *Crossing the quality chasm: A new health system for the 21st century.* Washington, DC: National Academy Press.

Karekla, M., Lundgren, J., & Forsyth, J. (2004). A survey of graduate training in empirically supported and manualized treatments: A preliminary report. *Cognitive and Behavioral Practice, 11,* 230–242.

Kessler, R. C., Soukup, J., Davis, R., Foster, D., Wilkey, S., Van Rompay, M., & Eisenberg, D. (2001). The use of complementary and alternative therapies to treat anxiety and depression in the United States. *American Journal of Psychiatry, 158,* 289–294.

Kuhn, T. (1977). *The essential tension.* Chicago, IL: University of Chicago Press.

Kuller, A. M., Ott, B. D., Goisman, R. M., Wainwright, L. D., & Rabin, R. J. (2010). Cognitive behavioral therapy and schizophrenia: A survey of clinical practices and views on efficacy in the United States and United Kingdom. *Community Mental Health Journal, 46,* 2–9.

Liker, J. K. (2004). *The Toyota way: 14 management principles from the world's greatest manufacturer.* New York, NY: McGraw-Hill.

Lilienfeld, S. O. (2007). Psychological treatments that cause harm. *Perspectives on Psychological Science, 2,* 53–70.

Lilienfeld, S. O. (2010, February 2). Is there a research-practice gap? Not if you listen to APA...Psychotherapy brownbag. Retrieved from http://www.psychotherapybrownbag.com/psychotherapy_brown_bag_a/2010/02/february-2010-psychotherapy-brown-bag-featured-article-is-there-a-researchpractice-gap-not-if-you-li.html

Lilienfeld, S. O., Lynn, S. J., & Lohr, J. M. (Eds.). (2003). *Science and pseudoscience in clinical psychology.* New York, NY: Guilford.

Luebbe, A. M., Radcliffe, A. M., Callands, T. A., Green, D., & Thorn, B. E. (2007). Evidence-based practice in psychology: Perceptions of graduate students in scientist-practitioner programs. *Journal of Clinical Psychology, 63,* 643–655.

McDermut, W., Miller, I. W., & Brown, R. A. (2001). The efficacy of group psychotherapy for depression: A meta-analysis and review of the literature. *Clinical Psychology: Science and Practice, 8,* 98–116.

McFall, R. M. (1991). A manifesto for a science of clinical psychology. *Clinical Psychologist, 44,* 75–88.

McFall, R. M. (2006). Doctoral training in clinical psychology. *Annual Review of Clinical Psychology, 2,* 21–49.

Mischel, W. (2009). Connecting clinical practice to scientific progress. *Psychological Science in the Public Interest, 9,* i–ii.

Nelson, T. D., & Steele, R. G. (2007). Predictors of practitioner self-reported use of evidence-based practices: Practitioner training, clinical setting, and attitudes toward research. *Administration and Policy in Mental Health and Mental Health Services Research, 34,* 319–330.

O'Donohue, W., & Cummings, N. A. (2008). *Evidence-based adjunctive treatments.* New York, NY: Academic Press.

O'Donohue, W., & Draper, C. (In press). *Evidence-based ehealth.* New York, NY: Academic Press.

O'Donohue, W., Moore, B., & Scott, B. (2007). *Handbook of pediatric and adolescent obesity treatment.* New York, NY: Routledge.

O'Donohue, W., & Rummel, C. (2010). The major dimensions of the healthcare crisis and key reforms. *American Psychologist,* under review.

Pidano, A. E., Kurowski, E. C., & McEvoy, K. M. (2010). The next generation: How are clinical child psychologists being trained? *Training and Education in Professional Psychology, 4,* 121–127.

Pignotti, M., & Thyer, B. A. (2009). Use of novel unsupported and empirically supported therapies by licensed clinical social workers: An exploratory study. *Social Work Research, 33,* 5–17.

Popper, K. R. (1957). *The logic of scientific discovery.* New York, NY: Routledge.

Russell, M., & Silver, S. M. (2007). Training needs for the treatment of combat-related posttraumatic stress disorder: A survey of Department of Defense clinicians. *Traumatology, 13,* 4–10.

Saha, S., Arbelaez, J. J., & Cooper, L. A. (2003). Patient–physician relationships and racial disparities in the quality of health care. *American Journal of Public Health, 98,* 1713–1719.

Saunders, R. R., & Saunders, J. L. (1994). W. Edwards Deming, quality analysis, and total behavior management. *Behavior Analyst, 17,* 115–125.

Schulz, K. (2010). *On being wrong: Adventures in the margin of error.* New York, NY: Ecco.

Shapiro, A., & Wiggins, J. (1994). A PsyD degree for every practitioner: Truth in labeling. *American Psychologist, 49,* 207–210.

Sheehan, A. K., Walrath, C. M., & Holden, E. W. (2007). Evidence-based practice use, training and implementation in the community-based service setting: A survey of children's mental health service providers. *Journal of Child and Family Studies, 16,* 169–182.

Weissman, M., Verdeli, H., Gameroff, M., Bledsoe, S., Betts, K., Mufson, L., Fitterling, H., & Wickramaratne, P. (2006). National survey of psychotherapy training in psychiatry, psychology, and social work. *Archives of General Psychiatry, 63,* 925–934.

Westen, D., Novotny, C., & Thompson-Brenner, H. (2004). The emperical status of empirically supported psychotherapies: Assumptions, findings, and reporting in controlled clinical trials. *Psychological Bulletin, 130*(4), 631–663.

Ten

The Behavioral Health Medical Home

DENNIS FREEMAN

BLENDING BEHAVIORISTS INTO THE PATIENT-CENTERED HEALTHCARE HOME

The debate over the most effective and prudent strategies to reform the U.S. healthcare system rages on. There is virtual consensus over the desired goals: expand insurance coverage to the millions currently without coverage, assure access to appropriate and timely care, achieve higher quality of care with improved outcomes, and reduce overall costs. The problems are easy to see; the solutions are not so readily apparent.

Various sectors of the healthcare marketplace have been implicated as contributors to the system's excessive costs and unacceptable outcomes. The insurance industry is criticized for high administrative costs and exclusionary policies. The profit margins of the pharmaceutical companies have been questioned. The proliferation of high-tech diagnostic options augments the bottom line for the tertiary care systems and lines the pockets of medical specialists, but do the outcomes justify the cost? Some argue that the prevailing fee-for-service payment methodology is the culprit, incenting unnecessary services and procedures. Proponents of pay-for-performance reimbursement schemes appear to be gaining converts. Despite the perspective or vantage point, there is universal agreement that the healthcare industry is exceedingly complex, with an array of interdependent and interactive sectors; that it suffers from fragmentation, duplication, and inefficiency; and that reform will prove to be challenging.

The behavioral health component of the industry is rarely mentioned in any analysis of what is right or what is amiss in healthcare. Direct expenditures for behavioral health services comprise only about 5% of the total healthcare bill in this country and that percentage continues to decline. Much as the services of mental health professionals are generally isolated from mainstream healthcare, their relevance seems peripheral to the healthcare reform conversation despite the energetic advocacy of the trade associations that represent them (American Psychological Association, 2009).

Parallel to the critique of the healthcare industry in the reform debate is an active, ongoing conversation about the American public's contribution to the problem. Poor health habits lead to poor health outcomes. Consumer demand and choice drive utilization and, thereby, cost. Delays in seeking necessary care are also a factor. And when afflicted with chronic medical conditions that require self-management and lifestyle change for effective care to occur, many patients do not embrace the recommendations of their providers. Sedentary lifestyles, unhealthy diets, and tobacco use have a deleterious impact on the health status of the nation. Healthcare may ameliorate, but cannot completely counteract, the consequences of these poor health habits. Most expensive chronic medical conditions could have been prevented, or at least postponed, if patients suffering these conditions had committed to better health habits earlier in life.

Obviously, the delivery of healthcare goods and services is in response to consumer presentation and demand. Every provider of healthcare can cite numerous examples of inappropriate demand. Every health service system can identify those who overutilize and are overly reliant on care. Half of the visits to hospital emergency departments could have been handled more appropriately in a primary care setting at a fraction of the cost.

On the other hand, avoidance of appropriate care also contributes to poor outcomes and increased cost. Advice to avail oneself of age-appropriate screenings and even simple blood pressure checks is often ignored. Low health literacy is a factor for some. More often, maintenance of health does not appear to be an acknowledged personal responsibility.

Along the life span, almost everyone will endure one or multiple chronic medical conditions. Established, evidence-based treatment protocols that will alter, suspend, or at least retard the disease process are available for almost all of these conditions. However, most of these protocols depend on the patient's adherence to medication regimen and lifestyle modifications. Regrettably, many of these recommendations require behavior change and the medical advice to make these changes is not followed. All too often, then, these conditions get out of hand and these patients reenter the medical system in crisis.

Our healthcare delivery system is geared to respond to acute care needs, although most of the conditions requiring extensive and costly care are chronic in nature. Therefore, ongoing, continuous management of these conditions, including patient self-management, would be a better match for most of the healthcare needs of the population. On balance, the clinical focus of the system is on sickness rather than wellness, giving prevention little beyond lip service. This is also true for the mental health sector. "Care" is an unfortunate choice of words to depict health services. It suggests a passive and one-directional process when, in fact, the patient's active participation is necessary in order to obtain the desired results.

A savvy, motivated, informed population of healthcare consumers who access the healthcare system only when appropriate and accept personal responsibility for their health maintenance would enhance the health status of the country, improve health outcomes, and bend the cost curve of healthcare expenses in a favorable direction. Pro-health behaviors in the population are significant factors in the prevention of, etiology of, and response to treatment of medical conditions. Thus, it would seem that behavioral professionals who are knowledgeable in behavior analysis and behavior change strategies would have a key role to play in a reformed healthcare system. To date, however, they have neither been assigned nor claimed much of a role in the projected healthcare system of the future.

THE PATIENT-CENTERED HEALTHCARE HOME

The patient-centered healthcare home is arguably the centerpiece of strategies to reform health service delivery in this country. Generally referred to as a medical home, depicting this innovation as a healthcare home is preferred here because it signifies a broader scope that includes maximizing health status, rather than just the provision of medical services. A healthcare home is an approach to providing patient-centered, continuous, and comprehensive primary care. The scope of

Table 10.1 Key Components of the Healthcare Home

Ongoing relationship with a personal physician who is trained to provide first contact, continuous and comprehensive care
An informed and activated patient
Whole-person orientation
Care is comanaged by a team who collectively take responsibility to provide or arrange for care
Levels of care include acute, chronic, and preventive
Span of life care
Care interfaces with family and community context as appropriate

care delivered is prevention oriented and includes treatment for both acute and chronic conditions.

Central to the healthcare home is an ongoing relationship with a personal physician who is the primary caregiver for the patient and also guides the patient to access other resources of the healthcare system as appropriate. An informed and activated patient is key, and the physician and other members of the healthcare team commit to improve the health literacy of the patient. The healthcare home is conceptualized as providing span-of-life care, interfacing with other family members and the community context as appropriate (Table 10.1).

Although the widespread discussion about the promise of healthcare homes has only come to the forefront over the last decade, it is far from a new concept. The American Academy of Pediatrics introduced the concept in 1967 as a care model that could coordinate the multiple resources necessary to provide better care for children with special needs (Sia, Tonniges, Osterhus, & Taba, 2004). The academy published a statement further defining the medical home in 1992 and operationalized the definition 10 years later (American Academy of Pediatrics, 1992, 2002).

In 2002, in an all too rare spirit of collaboration among the trade associations representing the health professions, seven organizations representing primary care providers came together and formed a work group that produced a consensus document, "The Future of Family Medicine: A Collaborative Project of the Family Medicine Community" (Martin et al., 2004). The intent of this project was to provide leadership that would transform and renew the specialties of family medicine, including family physicians, internists, and pediatricians. The clarion call from the project was that every American should have a "personal medical home" through which he or she would receive core management for chronic medical conditions as well as preventive services. These services should be "accessible, accountable, comprehensive, integrated, patient-centered, safe, scientifically valid, and satisfying to both patients and physicians." (p. 14)

Building on earlier work, the American College of Physicians produced a policy monograph, "The Advanced Medical Home: A Patient-Centered, Physician-Guided Model of Health Care" (Barr & Ginsberg, 2006). This model features clinical decision support tools and quantitative indicators of quality, incorporates principles of Wagner's (1998) chronic care model, and stresses the importance of health information technology to undergird the medical home. In the monograph, the American College campaigns for the advanced medical home as the solution for the problems facing the U.S. healthcare system. The college recommends several public policy positions, including reimbursement, workforce, and research on the advanced medical home model.

These policies support a fundamental change in the way primary care is delivered (Table 10.2). In 2007, the American Academy of Family Physicians, American Academy of Pediatrics, American College of Physicians, and American Osteopathic Association jointly released the "Joint Principles" (Table 10.3). This consensus statement by the most prominent primary care organizations serves as the current blueprint for the healthcare home movement. The document continues to place a personal physician as the principle provider of "whole-person care." A physician-directed team of professionals at the

Table 10.2 American College of Physicians (ACP) Advanced Medical Home Policy Position

Position 1. ACP calls for a comprehensive public policy initiative that would fundamentally change the way that primary care and principal care (whether provided by primary care or specialty care physicians) are delivered to patients by linking patients to a personal physician in a practice that qualifies as an advanced medical home.

Position 2. Fundamental changes should be made in third-party financing, reimbursement, coding, and coverage policies to support practices that qualify as advanced medical homes.

Position 3. Fundamental changes should be made in workforce and training policies to assure an adequate supply of physicians who are trained to deliver care consistent with the advanced medical home model, including internists and family physicians.

Position 4. Further research on the advanced medical home model and a revised reimbursement system to support practices structured according to this model should be conducted and should include national pilot testing.

Table 10.3 Joint Principles of the Patient-Centered Medical Home

Personal physicians
Physician-directed medical practice
Whole-person orientation
Care is coordinated and/or integrated
Quality on safety
Enhanced access
Payment reform

practice level collectively take responsibility for the ongoing and coordinated care of individual patients. Other than the physician, members of the team are not specified.

Widespread support of the healthcare home concept exists outside the medical profession. Health policy experts, legislators, politicians, corporate executives, and the health insurance industry generally tout the promise of the concept. The National Committee for Quality Assurance (NCQA) has developed a voluntary multitiered certification process, the "Medical Home Recognition Program," for primary care practices implementing the model. Medicare has designed an eight-state patient-centered medical home pilot and a number of state Medicaid programs have implemented innovative initiatives projected to improve health outcomes and reduce cost by organizing and coordinating care through enrollment of Medicaid recipients in healthcare homes.

Five hundred major U.S. corporations, insurers, consumer groups, and physician organizations came together in 2006 in an enterprise known as the "Patient-Centered Primary Care Collaborative" in order to promote the concept. Provisions favorable to the healthcare home dot the pages of the healthcare reform legislation passed by Congress, and President Obama has specifically endorsed the concept of the patient-centered medical home on a number of occasions.

The members of the physician-led healthcare team cited in the joint principles are not specified, nor are they prominently listed in other policy statements on healthcare homes. The assumption is that the authors are conceptualizing the customary staffing of a primary care practice: physician, nursing support, lab, and possibly an x-ray technician. Certainly, outside the journals and policy statements coming from the behavioral health professions, there is scant reference to behaviorists as participants on these teams. Despite the prevalence of mental health issues in every primary care practice and the significant role of behavioral factors in the etiology, the response to treatment, and the prognosis of most chronic medical conditions, behaviorists are not typically included as primary care team members. Rather, those writing about healthcare homes view behavioral health professionals as providing specialty services. Behaviorists, then, are considered external to the healthcare home by the chief architects of the concept.

THE BEHAVIORAL NATURE OF PRIMARY CARE

It has been established for years that more people seek and receive assistance for their mental health concerns in primary care than from the array of mental health specialty sector options. Most psychotropic prescriptions are written by primary care providers (PCPs). For these reasons, primary care has been referred to as the de facto mental health delivery system in this country (Regier et al., 1993).

A number of factors influence this pattern of service utilization. The widespread prevalence of mental disorders clearly exceeds the capacity of the mental health specialty sector. The National Comorbidity Survey Replication, the most recent comprehensive epidemiological study of mental disorders in the United States, reported an annual prevalence of around a quarter of the population and a lifetime prevalence of 48% (Kessler et al., 1994). As presently configured, the mental healthcare system is an inadequate match for the demand for services, let alone the unpresented need these percentages reflect. Currently, the mental health system is overloaded, access is an issue almost everywhere, and waiting lists abound.

The gap between demand for mental health services and the existing need in the U.S. population for services further exposes the existing significant access issue. The majority of those who need mental health services (59%) do not present those concerns for assistance anywhere. Of the 41% who do go for help, more seek help in primary care than from a mental health professional (Wang et al., 2005). In consideration of those who do not present their mental health dilemma anywhere for care, it should be noted that around 80% of the U.S. population with a behavioral health disorder cross the primary care threshold in a year's time (Narrow, Regier, Rae, Manderscheid, & Locke, 1993). So the majority of those in need who do not seek out a mental health service are available for mental health intervention in primary care. Primary care, then, is the gathering place for the population with mental health treatment needs. It is logical for mental health professionals to consider locating in the environment where the greatest number of those in need present.

Stigma about mental health treatment persists and is another factor determining the choice of primary care as the preferred site for the presentation of mental health problems. Stigma remains a barrier, frequently blocking primary care referrals to specialty mental health providers outside the primary care environment. A low percentage of referrals make a successful connection with a mental health professional (Fisher & Ransom, 1997; Hoge, Auchterlonie, & Milliken, 2006). It remains true that the majority of the U.S. population will not agree to enter a mental health specialty setting for treatment. Primary care providers struggle to overcome both the access and stigma barriers when they detect the need for mental health treatment in their patients and they attempt to refer for care. Even when patients are willing to accept the PCP's referral and go for mental health services, obtaining an appointment is often a challenge. Two thirds of primary care physicians in a recent study (Cunningham, 2009) reported they were unable to access outpatient behavioral healthcare for their patients. Health plan limitations and a shortage of mental health providers were listed as significant barriers. Typically, PCPs are left with trying to provide the best intervention they can in their offices. Usually, this means pulling out a prescription pad.

Clearly, patients prefer to receive their mental intervention in primary care. Often, there is a longitudinal, continuing relationship with the primary care provider and the primary care team, which engenders trust. It is easier to discuss mental health concerns in the context of this comfortable and trusting relationship than with an unknown professional.

An abundance of data suggests that the typical primary care intervention for patients with mental health problems falls short of the mark. This is not surprising, considering the limited preparation that primary care providers receive in their training and the stunning variety of medical problems they are called upon to address in a very short time on any given clinical day. Having a behaviorist handy to provide assessments and interventions with these patients enhances the competency of the primary care team.

Once mental health professionals enter the world of primary care, they are almost always surprised about the behavioral health nature of primary care practice. Every day patients with psychiatric conditions pack the schedules of primary care providers. Over and above these patients with clear-cut psychiatric diagnoses, psychological distress drives a good share of primary care utilization (Kroenke & Mangelsdorff, 1989). Often, an organic basis cannot be established for common somatic complaints. Psychosocial factors drive many visits (Strosahl, 1998). Cherokee Health Systems, a community-based provider of integrated care, has found similar levels of psychological distress when comparing primary care and community mental health center patients on standardized self-report measures such as the SF-36 health survey (Ware & Sherbourne, 1992). Thus, the primary care population often presents in distress and the majority of visits include a psychosocial component.

The organically based conditions that patients bring into primary care are often chronic in nature. Primary care providers frequently assist patients in the management of diabetes, cardiovascular problems, asthma, and hypertension. Successful management of these conditions is longitudinal and requires periodic visits in order to assess the condition and encourage self-management between visits by the patient. A major impetus to the patient-centered healthcare home movement is to provide this level of continuity and generate better outcomes for these high-cost and debilitating conditions.

Patient self-management requires the articulation, selection, and promotion of health-enhancing behaviors. Skill sets frequently mastered by behavioral health providers have direct applicability to the initial negotiation with patients over the selection of self-management goals, and to the ongoing lifestyle management these challenging conditions present. Assessing patients in accord with the readiness-to-change framework (Prochaska et al., 1994) and employing supportive and encouraging techniques like motivational interviewing (Rollnick, Miller, & Butler, 2007) add structure and strategies to the process of patients coping with chronic disease. Many behaviorists are equipped to facilitate the prepared and activated patient prescribed by the healthcare home model.

Comorbidities are the rule rather than the exception in primary care patients, especially as patients reach middle age. Patients with complex comorbid and interactive medical and psychiatric conditions are common in medical as well as psychiatric practice. Neither treatment setting is generally equipped to deal with the complexity. George Rust, professor of family medicine and director at the National Center for Primary Care at Morehouse School of Medicine, reported that over half the Medicaid enrollees in Georgia had three or more co-occurring disorders, including over 40% with a psychiatric or substance use disorder. Of enrollees with a substance use disorder, 73% had three or more co-occurring chronic medical problems (Rust, 2009).

These numbers are not surprising to clinicians working with similar populations. The profusion of medical comorbidities furthers the argument for multidisciplinary teams to address the complex needs in evidence during many patient presentations. The frequency of psychiatric diagnoses co-occurring with chronic medical conditions and the importance of behavioral self-management in all chronic conditions—psychiatric as well as medical—support the inclusion of behaviorists on the primary care team. A team of health professionals is often necessary to provide appropriate care. No single treating professional is an expert with all these conditions and their behavioral ramifications.

The mental health problems of patients in medical settings inflate costs and impede outcomes. One health plan reported that the cost for treating a chronic medical condition in Medicare patients who have a comorbid psychiatric condition is 22% higher than the cost for those without a psychiatric disorder, even excluding any direct costs of treating the psychiatric disorder (Harrington, 2008). Those entities responsible for paying for care, especially state Medicaid plans, have noticed this and a niche managed care industry has arisen targeting these expensive dually diagnosed health plan enrollees.

PARADIGM SHIFT: LOCUS AND MODE OF BEHAVIORAL HEALTH INTERVENTION

A significant paradigm shift is emerging with respect to the manner of delivery of behavioral health interventions and the locus of those interventions throughout the healthcare system. Not only is there widespread acknowledgment that primary care is the most frequent site of intervention for individuals who need treatment for mental health problems, but there is also general acceptance that this is an appropriate, and even preferred, environment for the treatment of many psychiatric problems. Relatedly, there is a focus on enhancing the capabilities of the primary care team to treat these conditions effectively. A second component of the paradigm shift is occurring within the primary care service model as behaviorists are becoming members of the primary care team. Both of these trends are fully compatible with the concept of the healthcare home, and healthcare reform can be expected to accelerate both.

A rapidly increasing number of behavioral health professionals are providing services in primary care settings. This is especially true in safety-net organizations. The delivery of mental health services is a program expectation placed upon federally qualified health centers (FQHCs) by the Bureau of Primary Health Care, U.S. Department of Health and Human Services. Over the past few years, the number of FQHC patients treated for mental health problems, the number of mental health services delivered by these organizations, and the number of mental health providers they employ have each increased fourfold or more (Druss et al., 2006; Lardiere, 2009).

Mental health providers have become more aware of the general health status of their patients. This interest has been fueled, in part, by the evidence that persons with serious psychiatric problems have a much shorter life expectancy than average and that this reduced longevity is primarily due to undetected or undertreated chronic medical conditions (Parks, Svendsen, Singer, Foti, & Mauer, 2006). Most of these medical conditions could have been moderated or even prevented if common risk factors such as poor nutrition, lack of exercise, and smoking had been addressed. The isolation of mental health services from the rest of the healthcare system has had disastrous consequences for this high-need population. This population, especially, needs the prevention, health screenings, treatment, and ongoing support and monitoring of a healthcare home.

The shocking health disparity suffered by this population has generated a groundswell of concern among the nation's community mental health centers (CMHCs)—the delivery system providing mental health services to many of these individuals. Many of these organizations are seeking linkages with primary care systems in order to secure medical care for their patients. A few CMHCs are trying to import or develop primary care services within their organization, although this is a formidable task and the effort generally falls short of the criteria customarily used to define the patient-centered healthcare home model. The National

Council for Community Behavioral Healthcare, the trade association for the CMHCs, has provided strong leadership for this paradigm shift among behavioral health safety-net providers (NCCBH, 2009).

There is also an expanding appreciation among mental health professionals of the volume of mental health problems seen in primary care. Taking note of the findings from epidemiological studies detailing the gap between prevalence and access and the discouraging barrier stigma continues to present, some mental health professionals are leaving traditional specialty environments and setting up shop in primary care.

Although these trends are emerging from the experience of clinicians at the practice level, the echo is beginning to be heard by the academic community. A few psychology graduate programs are providing some preparation for professional practice in primary care settings through health-related course work and training placements in the primary care milieu. A handful of psychology internship programs have taken on the cause of preparing psychologists for work in primary care. The U.S. Air Force has mounted a notable effort to blend its psychologists into its medical clinics and Alexander Blount (2007) has developed a certification program in primary care behavioral health at the Department of Family Medicine and Community Health, University of Massachusetts Medical School (www.integratedprimarycare.com/Certificate%20Program%20fall%2007.htm).

The American Psychological Association convened a Primary Care Psychology Curriculum Interdivisional Task Force, which recommended curricula for training at the graduate, intern, and postdoctoral levels (2002). The curriculum is posted on the APA Web site (www.apa.org/ed/primarycare2.pdf), but in a recent article on primary care psychology and the patient-centered medical home (McDaniel & Fogarty, 2009), the authors report that many psychology faculty and training programs have not, as yet, adopted these curricula.

Despite a few exceptions here and there, the academic world has yet to embrace the paradigm shift that is occurring. The Annapolis Coalition, a not-for-profit organization dedicated to the study of the mental health workforce, reported that providers are typically trained for a world that no longer exists (www.annapoliscoalition.org). At this point in time, the majority of behaviorists who are making clinical contributions within primary care settings are self-taught.

INTEGRATION OF PRIMARY CARE AND BEHAVIORAL HEALTH

When healthcare professionals discuss integrated care or collaborative care, it is clear they do not all have the same definitions or models in mind. Some describe integration as merely tightening up referral relationships so that patients get back and forth effectively between primary care and mental health providers. Others implement screening instruments for conditions like depression, substance abuse, or a chronic medical condition and call this identification process integration. Screening may be a first step toward integration but it achieves little without appropriate intervention after conditions are identified.

Often, the initial approach to integration is the colocation of providers—generally bringing a mental health professional into primary care but occasionally bringing primary care into a behavioral healthcare facility. This strategy improves access and allows some opportunity for providers to consult with one another about their respective care plans for patients they are both seeing. However, the increased access that colocation provides often generates a stream of referrals that will exceed the capacity of the mental health professional pursuing a traditional psychotherapy practice model in primary care.

Furthermore, this is not really integration at the clinical level. It does not change what happens in either the primary care exam room or the colocated therapist's office. It is simply an internal referral system with some opportunity for face-to-face conversation between providers about mutual patients. Traditional specialty mental health services are not a very good fit for the primary care environment.

Disease management strategies are commonplace in primary care practice. Typically, there is a registry or some tracking procedure for a population of patients with the same chronic condition. The goal is to improve outcomes by ongoing, periodic monitoring of specific markers of the condition. Enlisting the collaboration of the patient is key. Improving outcomes for chronic conditions like diabetes, asthma, and cardiovascular problems is generally dependent on lifestyle modifications by the patient.

Disease management approaches in primary care have been extended to include psychiatric disorders, especially depression. Depression is common in primary care, often as a presenting concern and even more frequently identified by providers as underlying somatic complaints such as fatigue, generalized tension, and disrupted sleep. Depression is a frequent companion of diabetes, cardiovascular disorders, and other chronic medical conditions.

The effectiveness of the treatment of depression in primary care has been well researched and documented in the professional literature (Gilbody, Bower, Fletcher, Richards, & Sutton, 2006) with the generous support of the Robert Wood Johnson Foundation, the MacArthur Foundation, and the pharmaceutical industry. Generally, these studies have reported on a "stepped" approach to the treatment of depression, beginning with a prescription for an antidepressant and then monitoring of effectiveness by a care manager, often a nurse, who is added to the primary care team to fulfill this role. If treatment is not effective, care is "stepped up" to include specialty mental health services and providers.

Disease management programs have exposed the inadequacy of simply monitoring and recording measures that track the status of a chronic medical condition. Reporting on the status of the measures to patients and providers does not necessarily translate into improved treatment adherence or lifestyle modification. Also, focusing on a single disease state has its limitations, given the high probability of comorbid, interacting conditions. It is not feasible to have a care manager for each condition nor is it practical to maintain a registry for every chronic disease presented in primary care.

The contributions that behaviorists bring to the healthcare home are best realized when they become integrated into the primary care team. With experience trying to collaborate, both primary care providers and behavioral health professionals generally gravitate toward this embedded behaviorist model. The strategies listed in Table 10.4 can be considered the developmental progression of the integration of behavioral health and primary care.

Table 10.4 Primary and Behavioral Healthcare Integration Strategies in Search of a Model

Preferential referral relationship
Formalized screening procedures
Colocation of services
Disease management
Behaviorist on primary care team

Table 10.5 Comparison of Clinical Integration and Colocation Models

Integrated Care	Colocated Mental Health
Embedded member of primary care team	Ancillary service provider
Comanagement of care	Autonomous provider
Verbal communication within team predominate	Written communication to primary care team predominates
Patient contact via handoff	Patient contact via referral
Brief, aperiodic interventions	Regular schedule of sessions
Flexible schedule	Fixed schedule
Generalist orientation	Specialty orientation
Behavior medicine scope	Psychiatric disorders scope

The practice of a behaviorist who is integrated into the primary care team differs in many ways from that of a mental health clinician colocated in a medical setting. The differences between these two models are summarized in Table 10.5. In the colocation model, the mental health professional provides services that are ancillary, albeit more convenient, to the primary care practice. In distinct contrast, when it is clinically integrated, the work of the behaviorist is a vital and routine component of the primary care visit, just as lab, x-ray, and nursing support are part of the visit. In clinical integration the behaviorist and the primary care provider share a clinical record and develop a common treatment plan for the patients they both see. In the integrated model, care is comanaged by the members of the treatment team.

In contrast, colocated providers are independent providers who may communicate about their clinical impressions and treatment plan with the primary care provider only upon gaining the patient's consent. These communications are more likely to be written than verbal. Primary care providers and integrated behaviorists "hand off" patients to one another during the visit when the services of their colleague are indicated. Colocation is an internal referral model in which the mental health provider typically maintains a regular, fixed schedule of appointments in the customary manner of specialty mental health providers. The schedule of the integrated behaviorist is much more flexible and similar to that of primary care colleagues in terms of pace, flow, and collaborative interactions.

Colocated providers generally maintain a scope of practice focused on psychiatric disorders. Integrated behaviorists adopt the generalist orientation of the primary care practice and their work draws upon a broader health-oriented, behavioral medicine framework. Their scope of practice must include a wide range of presenting issues, rather than just the conditions that accord with the diagnostic criteria outlined in the *Diagnostic and Statistical Manual of Mental Disorders* (DSM-IV TR).

Most behaviorists have trained in mental health settings, mentored by those of their own profession. Until recently, few behaviorists had been trained or had work experience in a primary care environment. Adapting to the medical treatment culture requires some appreciation of the differences and accommodation of those differences.

The pace of primary care is usually hectic. Provider schedules are typically amended many times over the course of the day with walk-ins and work-ins. The work flow is frequently disrupted by phone calls, e-mails, and emergencies. In contrast, mental health professionals typically work from a relatively rigid schedule with neat, uninterrupted blocks of time. PCPs see themselves as generalists and deal with a wide range of presenting problems every day. Most mental health professionals see themselves as specialists. Primary care promises life-long, birth-to-grave treatment relationships, whereas most mental healthcare is episodic in nature. Primary care documentation is succinct and problem focused. Mental health documentation is generally quite extensive, often theoretical, and even speculative. Primary care is delivered by a team; communication about the care of individual patients may be free flowing and is common within that team-based care model. Mental health providers are often not accustomed to this level of communication and shared responsibility.

Not every behaviorist will be comfortable or effective working in primary care. Few have had any academic preparation to do so. In order for behaviorists to become accepted and productive team members in the healthcare home of the future, some personality characteristics and professional skill sets are important (Table 10.6). Embedded behaviorists need to be comfortable with the pace of primary care, be good communicators, and enjoy working within a team. It is a demanding role requiring solid clinical skills, the ability to formulate patient presentations quickly, and arrive at some practical recommendations that are helpful to the primary care provider and will be embraced by the patient.

Table 10.6 The Behavioral Health Consultant in Primary Care: Characteristics, Skills, and Orientation to Practice

Personal Characteristics
Flexible, high energy level
Team player
Interest in health and fitness

Professional Skills
Finely honed clinical assessment skills
Behavioral medicine knowledge base
Cognitive behavioral intervention skills

Orientation to Practice
Action oriented, directive, focus on patient functioning
Emphasis on prevention and building resiliency
Utilizes clinical protocols and pathways
Invested in educating patients, improving health literacy

THE BEHAVIOR-FOCUSED HEALTHCARE HOME: THE CHEROKEE HEALTH SYSTEMS MODEL

For three decades, Cherokee Health Systems has focused on the clinical blending of behavioral health perspectives and interventions into primary care practice. The quest has always been to maximize the interplay between and among primary care providers, behavioral health consultants (BHCs) and their patients in order to achieve excellent clinical outcomes while maximizing access to underserved populations. The Cherokee care model embraces the tenets and goals of the patient-centered healthcare home and enhances that model through the presence of BHCs who are embedded in the primary care team.

Cherokee Health Systems is a community-based, not-for-profit Tennessee corporation providing a service mix that merges the missions of FQHCs and community mental health centers (CMHCs). Rooted in the population-based, outreach-oriented community mental health ideology of the 1960s, Cherokee has evolved a clinical care system that combines the skills and knowledge bases of primary care providers and behavioral health practitioners, thereby reducing the customary isolation of mental health services and blending in behavioral interventions to address the multitude of behavioral issues that patients present in primary care.

Table 10.7 Blending Behavioral Health Into Primary Care: Cherokee Health Systems' Clinical Model

Behaviorists on the Primary Team

The behavioral health consultant (BHC) is an embedded, full-time member of the primary care team. The BHC is a licensed health service provider in psychology. Psychiatric consultation is available to primary care providers (PCPs) and BHCs.

Service Description

The BHC provides brief, targeted, real-time assessments and interventions to address the psychosocial aspects of primary care.

Typical Service Scenario

The primary care provider determines that psychosocial factors underlie the patient's presenting complaints or are adversely impacting the response to treatment. During the visit, the PCP "hands off" the patient to the BHC for assessment or intervention.

At Cherokee Health Systems, behavioral health consultants work as core members of the primary care team, following a flexible schedule very similar to that of their primary care colleagues (Table 10.7). The behavioral health consultant, generally a psychologist with a behavioral medicine orientation, is available at the time of the primary care visit for assessment, triage, and intervention for the mental health, stress-related, and family problems that flood primary care practices. Over 80% of the mental health problems are managed in the healthcare home without referral on to specialty mental health services. Often, behavioral alternatives to psychopharmaceutical interventions are utilized. When these medications are necessary, behavioral strategies are also employed, enhancing the effectiveness of care.

The behavioral health consultant (Figure 10.1) is involved in a wide range of patient presentations, rather than just when mental health or substance use disorders are detected. These behaviorists assist in chronic disease management by providing support and teaching patients to modify their behavior in accord with their readiness to change their lifestyle. They help patients select and monitor self-management goals. The overarching aim of this integrated practice model is to enhance the skills and resiliency of patients in Cherokee practices. This clinical model has a high degree of both patient and provider satisfaction. Patients declare their strong preference for the convenience of receiving assistance for their mental health concerns in the comfort of their primary care provider's office. Primary care providers relish

The Behavioral Health Medical Home

Cherokee Health Systems
Job Description

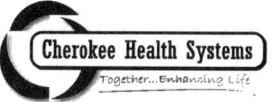

Job Title: Behavioral Health Consultant
Education/License: Licensed Clinical Social Worker (Masters) or a Licensed Clinical Psychologist (Doctoral)
Position Requirements:
Excellent working knowledge of behavioral medicine and evidence-based treatments for medical and mental health conditions.
Ability to work through brief patient contacts as well as to make quick and accurate clinical assessments of mental and behavioral conditions.
Should be comfortable with the pace of primary care, working with an interdisciplinary team, and have strong communication skills.
Good knowledge of psycho-pharmacology
Ability to design and implement clinical pathways and protocols for treatment of selected chronic conditions.

Figure 10.1   The behavioral health consultant.

the complementary skills a behaviorist adds to the practice. Access to behavioral health interventions is increased, stigma is averted, and the effectiveness of the primary care visit is enhanced (Table 10.8).

Consultation by a psychiatrist is also available on a real-time basis to Cherokee's primary care providers and BHCs. This consultation plays a key role in the care model. Psychiatrists are in short supply throughout the country and access to a psychiatrist is a problem almost everywhere for every population. In the Cherokee model, the overriding goal of the integrated care psychiatrist is to enhance the practice skills of his or her primary care colleagues. Thus, the psychiatrist practices within the primary care team and the healthcare home framework instead of assuming all the referrals into his or her own

Table 10.8   The Behavioral Health Consultant (BHC) in Primary Care

Management of psychosocial aspects of chronic and acute diseases
Application of behavioral principles to address lifestyle and health risk issues
Emphasis on prevention and self-help approaches
Build resiliency and encourage personal responsibility for health
Consultation and comanagement in the treatment of mental disorders and psychosocial issues

clinical caseload. Even when it is clinically necessary for the psychiatrist to provide direct clinical care for an acutely ill or destabilized patient, the goal is always to stabilize the patient and return them to the care of the primary care provider.

Primary care physicians have an increased comfort level in accepting these patients back knowing that psychiatric consultation is only a quick call away. In this comanagement care model, the PCP, the BHC, and the psychiatrist step forward when their special expertise is required. The model significantly reduces the rate of referral outside the healthcare home to the overtaxed mental health system and provides care that addresses both the physical and behavioral needs of patients.

Training health service providers in the integrated care model is at the core of Cherokee's mission. Training affiliations with nearby universities provides a steady stream of health professionals in training, including physicians, nurse practitioners, social workers, nurses, healthcare administrators, and psychologists. Preinternship doctoral candidates in clinical, counseling, and school psychology are assigned 16 hours per week in year-long rotations. All trainees experience the multidisciplinary clinical services model of Cherokee. In the past 6 years, Cherokee has offered an APA-approved internship in clinical psychology that features training in primary care psychology. In addition, Cherokee has participated in a consortium for many years that provides an APA-approved school psychology internship.

As Cherokee's behaviorists find their footing in the primary care suite, new service opportunities continue to emerge: coordinating group medical visits for patients with chronic medical conditions like diabetes, participating in well-child checks and kindergarten readiness groups with pediatricians, tackling childhood obesity, and designing and implementing smoking cessation efforts. The opportunities to address the behavioral aspects of primary care and thereby improve treatment outcomes are endless. Cherokee's behavioral health consultants and integrated care psychiatrists have become indispensable members of the primary care team. In effect, through collaboration with their primary care colleagues, these behaviorists are reengineering the primary care visit to respond to the complex needs that patients frequently bring to the clinical encounter.

The Cherokee Health Systems care model is a behaviorally enhanced healthcare home with an embedded BHC and readily available psychiatric consultation. Most behavioral interventions take place in the healthcare home. Patients are

Table 10.9 Cherokee's Blended Behavioral Health and Primary Care Clinical Model: A Behaviorally Enhanced Healthcare Home

Embedded behaviorist on primary care team
Real-time behavioral and psychiatric consultation to PCP
Focused behavioral intervention *in* primary care
Behavioral medicine scope of practice
Encourage patient responsibility for healthful living
A behaviorally enhanced healthcare home

encouraged and supported in healthful living. The model provides focus on the behavioral aspects of every primary care visit (Table 10.9).

The effectiveness of the healthcare home model has been clearly demonstrated. In a recent review of over 200 publications, the accumulated evidence indicated that healthcare homes produced improved health outcomes, reduced overall healthcare costs, and generated higher patient and provider satisfaction (Rosenthal, 2008). The addition of a BHC to the primary care team should lead to even better outcomes. The effectiveness of Cherokee's care model has been recognized by payers who have been willing to consider some unique and creative reimbursement methodologies and have solicited consultation in order to spread the model to other primary care systems.

Blue Cross Blue Shield compared the service utilization of Cherokee patients with patients of other primary care systems in the same region and found that Cherokee patients were more likely to rely on their healthcare home for care (Figure 10.2). Utilization of emergency rooms, medical specialists, and hospital care by patients in Cherokee's healthcare homes was substantially below the rate of use by other Blue Cross enrollees. Overall healthcare costs were only 78% of the average cost per enrollee. The fundamental difference between Cherokee and the other primary care practices was the BHC on the treatment team. The data suggest that the presence of a behaviorist in the healthcare home makes a significant difference in the utilization of healthcare and the overall cost of care.

REFORMING PAYMENT SYSTEMS TO SUPPORT BEHAVIORISTS IN HEALTHCARE HOMES

Although the benefits of blending behaviorists into healthcare homes seem obvious, existing payment methodologies do not

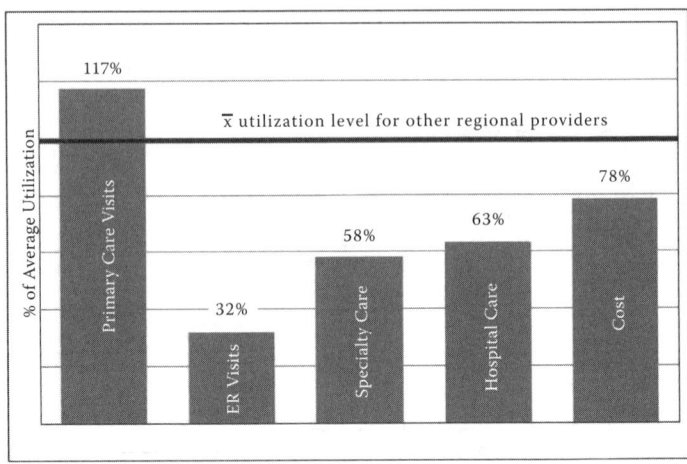

Figure 10.2 Healthcare utilization of Cherokee Health Systems patients compared to those of other regional providers.

always encourage this service innovation. Variations in the service models that behaviorists are attempting to implement have been a complicating factor. No single reimbursement scheme fits all the diverse integration programs providers are putting into place. An even greater source of complexity is imposed by payers who vary in terms of their appreciation and understanding of clinical integration and, subsequently, their willingness and flexibility to provide payment for new or relocated services. As is true of innovations, the idealistic trailblazers and the risk takers have demonstrated that concept. Widespread implementation, however, will be dependent upon continuing to demonstrate the financial viability of the concept and general use of some commonly applied payment methodologies.

Financing Integrated Care: Disincentives and Barriers

Some current payment systems for behavioral health services offer disincentives for the provision of behavioral services that are adapted to the healthcare home model (Table 10.10). Mental health carve-outs in health plans are a formidable barrier to the entry of behaviorists into healthcare homes. In the past, many mental health sector advocates have argued vehemently for carving out a separate payment stream in order to preserve an established level of financial support for mental health service delivery. Carve-outs attempt to divide the indivisible, ignoring the interplay of psyche and soma and the frequency of psychiatric and medical comorbidities. Regrettably,

Table 10.10 Payment Disincentives for Behaviorists Practicing in Healthcare Homes

Mental health carve-outs
Excessive documentation requirements
Encounter-based reimbursement
Same-day billing prohibition
Antiquated coding requirements

mental health carve-outs have served to further isolate the behavioral health world from the rest of healthcare. Separate funding streams are disincentives for both providers and payers to collaborate.

The usual documentation of clinical work expected of mental health professionals is another potential barrier to integration. The mental health sector is notorious for oppressive documentation requirements. A behaviorist working in tandem with a primary care provider will not have time for extensive charting, nor will long narrative reports be of any interest to the behaviorist's primary care colleagues. Total reliance on encounter-based reimbursement is another disincentive to integrate behaviorists into primary care. When integrated care is effective, patient encounters are prevented. The efficiencies are found in the consultation activities, which are often brief hallway conversations between providers that are neither easily documented nor considered reimbursable activities by most payers. Some payers will not reimburse two services on the same day, effectively preventing PCPs from handing off patients to behaviorists for quick, relatively inexpensive and cost-reducing interventions.

Finally, it can be anticipated that clinical innovation will always precede the necessary financing mechanisms and bureaucratic support to encourage and sustain them. Thus, the billing codes listed in the annual current procedural terminology (CPT) edition—the reimbursement bible—always lag behind the delivery system to some extent, retarding implementation of effective new services and procedures while punishing innovators. New service models usually do not fit into the existing coding and payment structures.

Financing Integrated Care: Building Blocks for the Foundation to Support Integration

The behavioral health consultant model (the preferred model of primary care and behavioral health integration) is a unique

Table 10.11 Financing Structure for Integration of BHCs Into Healthcare Homes

Health and behavior assessment/intervention
CPT codes 96150–96155
Same-day billing by PCP and BHC
Valuing consultation and case coordination
Pmpm care management rates
Global funding streams
Value-based contracting

care model with unique provider activities and services. It stands to reason that the usual reimbursement structures might not be a good fit for the interventions of a BHC.

Table 10.11 lays out some building blocks to support the foundation of BHC work in healthcare homes. The health behavior assessment/intervention CPT codes 96150–96155 first appeared in the 2002 edition of the CPT code book. These codes are a good match for the services provided by BHCs working in primary care. It is critical that same-day billings by the PCP and the BHC be permitted in order to gain the full benefit of the collaboration while the patient is still in the primary suite. Also, payers must appreciate and value all the professional staff time that is not face-to-face time with the patients. Not every helpful clinical activity translates to an available CPT code. This is especially true within a well functioning patient-center healthcare home. Provider-to-provider hallway consultations, case coordination, clinical team meetings, and outreach activities all contribute mightily to good patient care and positive clinical outcomes. These nonclinical efforts are the core of the workings of the healthcare home and the services of behaviorists on the primary care team.

Global funding streams allow providers the most flexibility to manage care clinically without being fettered by a restrictive fee-for-service mentality. Clinicians have enough to worry about taking care of their patients without always considering the reimbursement potential of the variety of activities they perform. A monthly case rate for the care of an individual and a per-member-per month (pmpm) payment for the care of an identified population are examples of global funding streams. Partnering in risk sharing arrangements like percent of premium agreements aligns incentives between payers and provider organizations. The efficiencies and cost savings realized by integrating behaviorists into the healthcare home spring from a care model that features consultative, collaborative, and coordinating activities in addition to direct clinical contact with patients. Global funding mechanisms pay providers to take care of patients, permitting clinicians more autonomy in how this is accomplished. They incent efficient management of care rather than reward overutilization or the provision of unnecessary services.

Payment of a pmpm rate to support the care management and the care coordination expected of a healthcare home is a financing strategy that is gaining momentum around the country. A number of commercial insurance plans and state Medicaid programs are using this payment mechanism to incent primary care providers to adopt the healthcare home model. These programs pay a monthly care management fee to physician practices that agree to provide a defined level of care management and coordination for patients in the program. The common underlying assumptions in these pilot programs are that the healthcare home will yield better health outcomes and save money.

Behaviorists and behavioral services are not specifically included in these healthcare home demonstration efforts. If behaviorists are to become part and parcel of the healthcare home movement, they will need to demonstrate that they contribute to the dual goals of improved health outcomes and reduced overall costs. Return on investment will be the most prominent criterion by which services will be judged in the reformed healthcare system. The seminal medical cost offset work by Nicholas Cummings and later reviews by others (Childs, Lambert, & Hatch, 1999; Cummings, O'Donohue, & Ferguson, 2002) offer some hope for behaviorists in this regard and point the way toward models for cost-effective behavioral programming in medical settings.

A VISION OF THE FUTURE

Healthcare reform will change the relationship between payers and providers in significant ways. At long last, value-driven contracting and financing will come to the fore. Payers and provider groups will partner in the care of identified populations based on mutual financial interest, as evidenced in improved clinical outcomes, practice efficiencies, and overall cost of care. Organized systems of care will predominate and independent practitioners, including mental health professionals, will struggle to compete in the healthcare marketplace.

Reimbursement will be for the accomplishments of a team rather than payment for individual services rendered. Pay for performance will be the norm and reliance on encounter-based, fee-for-service financing of healthcare will decline as a result.

In the reformed healthcare system, more behaviorists will realize that primary care provides the best platform for mental health interventions and the number of behaviorists working in medical settings will increase exponentially. Blended behavioral health and primary care teams will significantly increase penetration into members of the population who need mental health services and will meet this population with timely, appropriate, and more effective interventions. As a consequence of these earlier interventions and the broader vantage primary care provides, more mental health professionals will focus their work on prevention and the promotion of health. Gradually, university-based training programs will begin preparing behavioral professionals for this rapidly expanding job market; however, most practitioners will continue to learn these skills at the community level.

The patient-centered healthcare home (PCHH) will be the centerpiece of the reformed healthcare system. In concept, the PCHH addresses many of the problems of the current system. Advocates of the PCHH promise reduced fragmentation, duplications, and overall cost of care. They foresee a population of engaged, health-literate patients in the health services system who are active participants in their own care. Empowered by the guidance that their healthcare home provides, patients will become informed and responsible consumers of healthcare goods and services and more likely to adopt a healthier lifestyle.

As envisioned, the PCHH will provide acute and preventive care as well as assist the patient in the management of chronic medical conditions throughout the patient's life span. The patient's personal physician will coordinate the appropriate utilization of other healthcare resources beyond the healthcare home and assure that care is delivered that is culturally relevant for the patient and takes into consideration both the patient's family and community context. All of this is a tall order, given the current staffing, practice pattern, and resources of most primary care offices; the primary care sector can be expected to struggle to meet the expanded expectations.

Appropriately trained, primary-care-oriented behaviorists will bring unique, complementary perspectives and skills to many PCHHs. The diagnostic acumen and array of interventions that behaviorists bring to the primary care team will enhance the ability of the PCHH to meet the ambitious goals envisioned for the care model. Behaviorists will not only provide an in-house answer for the frequent presentations of psychiatric disorders, but will also contribute behavioral expertise in the promotion of health-enhancing behaviors. Health-oriented behaviorists will coach and encourage patients to accept personal responsibility for their health.

Much is expected of the patient-centered healthcare home. The promise is much more likely to be achieved with a behavioral health consultant as a full-fledged member of the primary care team.

REFERENCES

American Academy of Family Physicians, American Academy of Pediatrics, American College of Physicians, and American Osteopathic Association. (2007). Joint principles of the patient-centered medical home.

American Academy of Pediatrics, Ad Hoc Task Force on Definitions of the Medical Home. (1992). The medical home. *Pediatrics, 90,* 774.

American Academy of Pediatrics, Medical Home Initiatives for Children with Special Needs Project Advisory Committee. (2002). The medical home. *Pediatrics, 110,* 184–186.

American Psychological Association Practice Association. (2009). Health care reform: Congress should ensure that psychologists' services are key in primary care initiatives. http//www.apapractice.org/apo/legislative_advocacy/health_care_reform.html#

American Psychology Association Interdivisional Task Force for a Primary Care Curriculum. Members S. H. McDaniel, C. D. Belar, E. L. Freeman, D. S. Hargrove, & C. Schroeder. (2002). hhtp://www.apa.org/ed/primarycare2.pdf

Barr, M., & Ginsberg, J. (2006). The advanced medical home: A patient-centered, physician-guided model of health care. A policy monograph of the American College of Physicians.

Blount, A. (2007). Certificate program in primary care behavioral health. www.integratedprimarycare.com/Certificate%20Program%20i

Childs, J. A., Lambert, M. J., & Hatch, A. L. (1999). The impact of psychological interventions on medical cost offset: A meta-analytic review. *Clinical Psychology Science and Practice, 6,* 204–220.

Cummings, N. A., O'Donohue, W. T., & Ferguson, K. E. (2002). *The impact of medical cost offset on practice and research: Making it work for you.* Part of the foundation for behavioral health: Healthcare utilization and cost series, Reno, NV: Context Press, 5.

Cunningham, P. J. (2009). Beyond parity: Primary care physicians' perspectives on access to mental health care. *Health Affairs, 28*(3), 490–501.

Druss, B. G., Bornemann, T., Fry-Johnson, Y. W., McCombs, H. G., Politzer, R. M. & Rust, G. (2006). Trends in mental health and substance abuse services at the nation's community health centers. *American Journal of Public Health, 96*(10), 1778–1784.

Fisher, L., & Ransom, D. C. (1997). Developing a strategy for managing behavioral health care within the context of primary care. *Archives of Internal Medicine, 6,* 324–333.

Gilbody, S., Bower, P., Fletcher, J., Richards, D., & Sutton, A. J. (2006). Collaborative care for depression: A cumulative meta-analysis and review of longer-term outcomes. *Archives of Internal Medicine, 166,* 2314–2321.

Harrington, J. (2008). Presented at behavioral health symposium: Integrating mental health services and physical health services. Windsor MedicareExtra Symposium, Spartanburg, SC, October 29, 2008.

Hoge, C. W., Auchterlonie, J. L., & Milliken, C. S. (2006). Mental health problems, use of mental health services, and attrition from military service after returning from deployment to Iraq and Afghanistan. *JAMA, 295,* 1023–1032.

Kessler, R. C., McGonagle, K. A., Zhao, S., Nelson, C. B., Hughs, M., Eshelman, S.,...Kendler, K. S. (1994). Lifetime and 12-month prevalence of DSM-III-R psychiatric disorders in the United States. *Archives of General Psychiatry, 51,* 8–19.

Kroenke, K., & Mangelsdorff, D. (1989). Common symptoms in ambulatory care: Incidence, evaluation, therapy and outcome. *American Journal of Medicine, 86,* 262–266.

Lardiere, M. R. (2009). Enhancing the continuum of care: Integrating behavioral health into your health center program. Presented to the National Association of Community Health Centers Community Health Institute.

Martin, J. C., Avant, R. F., Bowman, M. A., Bucholtz, J. R., Dickinson, J. R., Evans, K. L.,...Weber, C. W. (2004). Future of Family Medicine Project Leadership Committee. The future of family medicine: A collaborative project of the family medicine community. *Annals of Family Medicine, 2*(1, Suppl), 3–32.

McDaniel, S. H., & Fogarty, C. T. (2009). What primary care psychology has to offer the patient-centered medical home. *Professional Psychology: Research and Practice, 40*(5), 483–492.

Narrow, W. E., Regier, D. A., Rae, D. S., Manderscheid, R. W., & Locke, B. Z. (1993). Use of services by persons with mental and addictive disorders: Findings from the National Institute of Mental Health Epidemiologic Catchment Area Program. *Archives of General Psychiatry, 50,* 95–107.

National Committee for Quality Assurance. (2010). PPC—Patient-centered medical home. www.ncqu.org/tabid/948/Default.aspx

NCCBH (National Council for Community Behavioral Healthcare). (2009). Behavioral health/primary care integration and the person-centered healthcare home. http://www.integratedprimarycare.com/Integration%20and%20HealthcareHome-Final.pdf

Parks, J., Svendsen, D., Singer, P., Foti, M., & Mauer, B. (2006). Morbidity and mortality in people with serious mental illness. National Association of State Mental Health Program Directors (www.nasmhpd.org).

Prochaska, J. O., Velicer, W. F., Rossi, J. S., Goldstein, M. G., Marcus, B. H., Rakowski, W.,...Rossi, S. R. (1994). Stages of change and decisional balance for 12 problem behaviors. *Health Psychology, 13,* 39–46.

Regier, D. A., Narrow, W. E., Rae, D. S., Manderscheid, R. W., Locke, B. Z. & Goodwin, F. K. (1993). The de facto U.S. mental and addictive disorder service systems. *Archives of General Psychiatry, 50,* 85–94.

Rollnick, S., Miller, W. R., & Butler, C. C. (2007). *Motivational interviewing in health care: Helping patients change behavior.* New York, NY: Guilford Press.

Rosenthal, T. C. (2008). The medical home: Growing evidence to support a new approach to primary care. *Journal of the American Board of Family Medicine, 21,* 427–440.

Rust, G. (2009). The concept of the healthcare home. Presented at the Smoky Mountain Integrated Care Conference II: The Behaviorally Enhanced Healthcare Home. Cherokee Health Systems, Knoxville, TN, April 23, 2009.

Sia, C., Tonniges, T. F., Osterhus, E., & Taba, S. (2004). History of the medical home concept. *Pediatrics, 113*(5), 1473–1478.

Strosahl, K. (1998). Integrating behavioral health and primary care services: The primary mental health care model. In A. Blount (Ed.), *Integrated primary care: The future of medical and mental health collaboration* (pp. 139–166). New York, NY: W. W. Norton.

Wagner, E. H. (1998). Chronic disease management: What will it take to improve care for chronic illness? *Effective Clinical Practice, 1*(1), 2–4.

Wang, P. S., Lane, M., Kessler, R. C., Olfson, M., Pincus, H. A., & Wells, K. B. (2005). Twelve-month use of mental health services in the United States. *Archives of General Psychiatry, 62,* 629–640.

Ware, J. E., & Sherbourne, C. D. (1992). The MOS 36-item short-form health survey (SF-36). I. Conceptual framework and item selection. *Medical Care, 30*(6), 473–483.

Eleven

Reforms in Professional Education

RONALD R. O'DONNELL

INTRODUCTION

The historic healthcare reform bill makes clear that the focus of the twenty-first century healthcare system is cost control. A major mechanism to achieve cost control is integrated care: improved cost effectiveness by better prevention and management of chronic disease, improved delivery of these services in primary care, increased use of evidence-based practices, and new payment mechanisms such as pay-for-performance incentives to encourage best practices (see Chapter 12, this volume). Providers are urged to be more accountable for healthcare costs and results and to demonstrate cost effectiveness (Antos et al., 2009). In addition, cost control will be achieved by reduced reimbursement rates for Medicare and Medicaid programs. The writing is on the wall: Integrated care, accountability, and cost savings are the focus of healthcare reform.

If you were an educator, what grade would you give to the current model of educating and training behavioral clinicians to prepare them to meet these demands of twenty-first century healthcare? How well prepared are recent graduates to provide evidence-based care in primary care settings? How well prepared are they to enter into negotiations for pay-for-performance contracts with payers based on evidence of cost savings? How well prepared are they to absorb yet another cut in fee-for-service reimbursement? A recent article by O'Donohue, Cummings, and Cummings (2008) concluded that the field has failed to adequately prepare behavioral care providers with the clinical competencies necessary to provide integrated care or with the business skills necessary to navigate healthcare economics, finance, and reimbursement or to demonstrate cost effectiveness. The authors concluded that the unmet education and training needs in these areas result in an educational deficit for behavioral care providers from all disciplines.

This unmet need to prepare for twenty-first century behavioral healthcare is exacerbated by another factor: the glut of therapists providing traditional mental health and substance abuse services. Graduate training programs continue to churn out new master's and doctoral level therapists. Meanwhile, the number of patients seeking traditional psychotherapy is declining as more patients turn to medication for relief of behavioral problems (Olfson & Marcus, 2009). U.S. spending on mental health other than medications has remained nearly flat from 1996 to 2006 (Frank et al., 2009). For psychologists, the trend for health plans and carve-outs to reimburse all providers at master's level rates will continue. Neither consumers nor payers of behavioral healthcare recognize the value added for doctoral level providers that will justify higher reimbursement.

Meanwhile, there is a growing demand from physicians for integrated behavioral health and a shortage of providers with these skills (Blount & Miller, 2009). Physicians recognize the adverse impact of behavioral issues on medical problems and the need for integrated care. Demand is also influenced by patient preference for integrated care. When referred from their physician to an outside, traditional behavioral health clinician office, only 15% of patients follow through. When offered behavioral intervention onsite in the physician office, about 90% accept the referral (Chaffee, O'Donohue, & Cummings, in preparation; Strosahl, 1998). The combination of high demand by physicians and patients and low supply of behavioral clinicians is in striking contrast to traditional settings.

The premise of this chapter is that radical reform in educating and training is needed to prepare a new workforce of *applied, doctoral level* behavioral care providers specializing in integrated care. The new doctor of behavioral health degree program at Arizona State University will serve as a case study to highlight failures of the current doctoral education programs for psychologists, solutions to these failings, and opportunities and challenges for the twenty-first century doctoral level, behavioral care provider. The recommendations for reform include:

Reforms in Professional Education 259

- A new applied, professional doctorate degree in integrated behavioral health
- A new professional accreditation body for the degree
- A flexible course curriculum that eliminates courses irrelevant to practicing clinicians and adds courses essential to meet the demands of healthcare reform (which will be continual)
- Elimination of the dissertation, replacing it with a research project that focuses on the skills needed to demonstrate cost effectiveness in healthcare
- Upgrading master's level licensed clinicians for enrollment in order to deliver more doctoral level integrated care clinicians in medical settings
- Approving distance learning and distance supervision for practicum training
- Incorporating e-health and telehealth into practice training
- Adopting the competency model recommended by the APA Task Force (APA, 2006)
- Creating a new national examination specific to competencies of applied practitioners

Cummings and O'Donohue (2008) have outlined major blunders that cripple psychology in America. Many of these arguments are relevant to education reform and are summarized next.

BLUNDERS IN EDUCATION AND TRAINING

Irrelevant Course Curriculum

The course curriculum of PhD and PsyD programs is inflexible, limited, and irrelevant to the needs of applied behavioral clinicians in healthcare reform. Multiple courses in research design and statistics necessary for academics are irrelevant for applied behavioral care providers who will not be conducting academic research. Similarly, while the doctoral dissertation is clearly appropriate in preparing academic psychologists for careers in research, it is not relevant for applied clinicians.

Courses in non-evidence-based psychological tests, such as the Rorschach, are still mandated in many programs. Every time an APA task force adds a new required course in a topic such as cultural diversity, no course is subtracted. Conversely, essential courses on evidence-based integrated behavioral care interventions and medical literacy courses such as clinical medicine, pathophysiology, and neurology are not included in the curriculum. This results in inefficient training, which takes too long (nearly 10 years to become licensed as a doctoral level clinical psychologist; see O'Donohue & Boland, in preparation).

Antibusiness, Antihealthcare Agenda

Cummings and O'Donohue (2008) conclude that most behavioral clinicians are economic illiterates. Traditional education for clinicians does not include courses on healthcare economics, the healthcare system, and basic business entrepreneurship skills that are essential for success in integrated care settings. A course in healthcare systems should include policy, economics and finance, contracting, billing, and reimbursement in order to understand and navigate the system. A course in business entrepreneurship is necessary to provide the applied clinician with the skills necessary to develop and present proposals for healthcare payers that seek reimbursement beyond traditional fee-for-service models.

In addition, many leaders in education demonize and take adversarial stances toward health plans, carve-outs, and vendors. Behavioral clinicians are not prepared for the utilization review, quality oversight, and, in general, the increased accountability expected by the very organizations that are *paying* for healthcare. While overall healthcare costs have increased as a percentage of GDP from about 7 to 15% since 1970, mental health spending as a percentage of GDP has remained flat at less than 1% (Frank, Goldman, & McGuire, 2009). The twenty-first century behavioral care provider needs to join and embrace the medical healthcare system, rather than ignore or fight it.

Credentialing

Accreditation requirement for doctoral behavioral clinicians is the responsibility of the American Psychological Association (APA), which comprises two competing constituencies: academics based in university psychology departments and practicing professional psychologists. This is contrary to nearly every other healthcare profession, such as nursing, medicine, pharmacy, social work, and many others, in which professional schools use a relevant professional society to determine training and practice standards.

Cummings and O'Donohue (2008) traced the history of the APA "house divided" between research and clinical psychologists and provided a short list of many concerted efforts by academic psychologists to block advances favored by practicing psychologists. Due to this continued in-fighting, the APA struggles to advance the agenda of practicing psychologists, and initiatives are frozen as endless committees struggle over years and even decades to complete reforms. Healthcare reform is happening *now,* and a professional credentialing organization that is solely devoted and responsive to the needs of practicing doctoral clinicians is overdue.

Clinical Training and Competence

Traditional models for clinical training for psychologists have relied upon completion of coursework, exams, graduate degrees, hours of supervised experience, and performance on the multiple-choice examination for professional practice in psychology (EPPP) to determine proficiency to practice. The criteria for competence have not included objective measures of performance other than supervisor ratings and recommendations. A number of authors have raised concerns about the failure of this model to address professional competency and a trend to move students with competency issues to graduation and practice due to lack of a clear process and mechanism to address these problems (DeMers, Van Horen, & Rodolfa, 2008).

The supervision model is often based on academic psychologists with little or no direct clinical experience training applied clinicians for practice. In addition, many departments still indoctrinate clinicians into a specific school of treatment often led by charismatic "gurus" (Cummings & O'Donhoue, 2008) rather than a balanced overview of evidence-based practice. The predominant treatment modality is individual therapy delivered in a traditional 50-minute hour, with lack of accountability in terms of measuring outcome, treatment alliance, or patient satisfaction. Indeed, efforts to evaluate individual psychotherapy are deemed intrusive or are met with resistance such as arguments that, as a field, we are not yet ready to measure behavioral health outcomes. This model is at odds with the needs of the healthcare system for providers who can deliver *efficient* interventions in busy medical settings such as group therapy, disease management, e-health, and case management. It is at odds with the calls for *accountability* in healthcare.

Licensure

The state licensure requirements for clinical psychologists are largely based on the APA accreditation standards (APA, 2007) as well as the Association of State and Provincial Psychology Boards (ASPPB, 2009). These organizations, in turn, institutionalize the blunders noted earlier. The national exam for psychologists, the EPPP, is based on many items that, while relevant for academic researchers, are not for applied doctoral clinicians (O'Donohue & Buchannan, 2003). In addition, the APA, ASPPB, and individual states are grappling with challenges such as portability of licensure, distance learning, telehealth, e-health, and supervision requirements (DeMers et al., 2008). Competencies for entry-level proficiency to practice are based on outdated benchmarks rather than objective assessment of actual competency.

Controversies and Emerging Reforms

The traditional models of training doctoral level behavioral care providers—primarily clinical psychologists—are under assault. After decades of inflexibility and active opposition to reform, significant challenges from within and outside the APA and ASPPB, which provide oversight and accreditation for training of psychologists, are raising controversy and gaining ground. Examples in recent years include the following:

- The National Alliance of Professional Psychology Providers (NAPPP) was formed in 2006 as a professional organization for practicing psychologists solely dedicated to the advocacy of practicing doctoral clinicians.
- The Association for Psychological Science (APS) announced a new accreditation system for clinical science, the psychological clinical science accreditation system (PCSAS), with a series of media releases highly critical of the APA and psychologists for not incorporating empirically supported research into clinical practice.
- The APA has announced several significant changes relevant to education and training, such as
  - Defining psychology as part of rather than separate from the healthcare system
  - Promoting integrated care as a career path for psychologists
  - Published new standards for professional competency assessment

- The APA and ASPPB have recommended dropping the requirement of postdoctoral training and replacing it with 2 years of combined practicum and internship experience.

"UNBLUNDERING": THE DOCTOR OF BEHAVIORAL HEALTH

In 2008 Nicholas Cummings, in collaboration with leadership in Arizona State University, developed the doctor of behavioral health (DBH) program. The DBH is a new doctoral degree in behavioral health designed to train behavioral clinicians to provide integrated care in medical settings. The program is based on models of professional training and credentialing typical of most other healthcare professions. The first cohort of students enrolled in the program in the fall semester of 2009. The DBH program is cosponsored by the Nicholas and Dorothy Cummings Foundation. The DBH program reform is *radical* in that it

- is founded on a knowledge base that incorporates clinical skills in integrated care, medical literacy, healthcare economics, and entrepreneurship
- relies on a small core of nontenured faculty complemented with adjunct faculty and clinical supervisors who are practicing clinicians
- provides hands-on practicum experience in primary care and related settings
- systematically collects individual and program outcome data in order to evaluate competency
- embraces the mission of producing behavioral care providers who have the ability to produce and document medical cost offset in their clinical practice
- has received provisional accreditation by a new entity, the National Institute of Behavioral Health Quality, formed under the auspices of the National Alliance of Professional Psychology Providers

The DBH is *traditional* in that it is designed to meet

- the requirements for accreditation as a program of psychology by the APA
- the guidelines on practicum experience endorsed by the ASPPB

anticipated requirements for doctoral licensure as APA and ASPPB recommendations are adopted by state licensing boards

The DBH program is *progressive* in that it

- has already incorporated a comprehensive competency assessment program
- replaces the dissertation with a rigorous yet relevant research project
- uses distance learning in order to make courses and supervision available to students around the world
- incorporates innovative e-health approaches as an adjunct to treatment

The DBH program is currently designed as an upgrade for licensed, master's level behavioral clinicians. The program requires 84 credit hours for completion, 30 of which are credited from the clinician's master's degree program. The remaining 54 credit hours include 10 core courses, four elective courses, a culminating research project, and practicum. The practicum program begins the first semester of the program and is based on a sequential, stage-based training with students completing an average of one 8-hour day per week in each semester for a total of 500 hours of practicum experience. The program requires 2 years of study after the master's degree, or it may be completed in 18 months in an accelerated program that includes summer sessions.

The DBH core faculty is small and comprises clinical psychologists with experience as practitioners in integrated care. Adjunct faculty members are typically contracted psychologists with excellent teaching skills and full-time professional experience in the area in which they are teaching. The adjunct faculty all make a living doing what they are teaching. In addition, the faculty includes representatives of other healthcare graduate programs in the university, such as nursing, a doctoral health and wellness program, a behavioral health research department, the school of business healthcare administration, and public health.

The Macrocurriculum

The integrated behavioral care provider will need a thorough understanding of the healthcare system in order to grasp the implications of healthcare reform, as well as business entrepreneur skills to be able to respond proactively to pursue career and economic opportunities in the changing healthcare environment (O'Donohue et al., 2008). The DBH course on healthcare systems and economics includes healthcare policy and reform, financing and reimbursement, and quality and accreditation. The behavioral entrepreneurship course includes:

- Personality factors and attitudes that contribute to success
- How market forces enhance or limit success
- Steps and resources needed for a "start-up" company
- Venture capital and investment
- Compensation
- Business law and regulation
- How to write, present, implement, and evaluate a business plan
- Exit strategy

The objective is to increase the ability of the behavioral care provider to demonstrate added value to healthcare payers as a means of expanding his or her economic base.

The Clinical Curriculum

The clinical skills necessary for effective delivery of integrated behavioral care are not the same as those necessary for traditional mental health and substance abuse treatment settings. McDaniel, Schroeder, Belar, Hargrove, and Freeman (2002) noted that the provider must be a generalist who is responsive to a wide range of medical and behavioral problems for diverse populations across the life span. Principles of population-based management and stepped care are essential, yet foreign, to most behavioral clinicians (Strosahl, 2005). In addition, the behavioral provider must be able to function as a member of a multidisciplinary medical team, usually headed by a primary care physician, and in consultation with other specialists.

The shift from traditional behavioral health into the medical culture—the values, beliefs, norms, and behaviors that comprise the medical mind-set—is a dramatic challenge because they run directly counter to how traditional psychotherapy is delivered: Visits are brief, the therapist is on the floor interacting with the team and ready for a "hallway handoff" at any time, sessions may be interrupted for crises, and verbal and written communication must be concrete, action oriented, symptom focused, and evidence based. There is substantial pressure to summarize and distill a large amount of essential information, which can be a source of stress that overwhelms the unprepared trainee (Satterfield, 2003).

Strosahl (2005) provides an excellent summary of core domains and practice competencies required for integrated behavioral care:

- The first domain, clinical practice skills, includes rapid problem identification and patient engagement, a strengths model, ability to help the client focus on specific problems and functional outcomes, medical literacy, health psychology, preventive health, and lifestyle change interventions.
- The domain of practice management skills includes effective use of brief sessions, screening and outcomes measurement, time management, knowledge of community-based resources, flexible and creative scheduling, contact strategies (e.g., phone, e-mail), and case management.
- The consultation skills domain includes the ability to focus on the referral question and provide effective feedback to the medical team, expertise in psychopharmacology in order to consult effectively with prescribers, leading efforts to develop behavioral health clinical pathways, and recommendations that help reduce the physician's workload and improve productivity.
- Documentation skills include recording the referral question and timely, clear, and concise notes on the treatment plan and progress.
- Team performance skills include awareness of team roles and functions effectively within the medical culture, frequent rounds on the floor in order to enhance awareness of behavioral services, readily responding to consultation by cell phone, and willingness to provide in-service training.
- Administrative skills include understanding and following policies, procedures, and protocols.

France et al. (2008) also provide an excellent summary of core knowledge-based and applied competencies based on APA task force recommendations. The DBH program has incorporated these core competencies into the curriculum and practicum.

The Critical Ingredients: Efficiency and Medical Cost Offset

A distinguishing feature of the DBH clinical curriculum is clinical training on the *Biodyne* model of integrated care and psychotherapy, which is described in detail by Cummings and Sayama (1995) and Cummings and Cummings (2000). The model was developed by Nicholas Cummings beginning in the late 1950s in Kaiser Permanente and subsequently refined over the course of five decades in the Hawaii Medicaid Project (Cummings, 2002) and in the training and supervision of hundreds of psychologists in the American Biodyne managed care company.

The Biodyne model is seen as critical for two key reasons. First, the model is based on *efficient* delivery of clinical services. Efficiency is achieved largely through the use of therapeutic strategies and techniques designed to manage patient resistance effectively and achieve rapid therapeutic alliance. In addition, the service delivery model focuses on clinician productivity and efficiency using group treatment protocols. Second, the Biodyne model has consistently demonstrated what Cummings and associates termed "medical cost offset." Medical cost offset is used to describe how focused, targeted behavioral interventions delivered in primary care lead to reductions in medical cost that are greater than or offset the cost of delivering the behavioral intervention (Cummings, 2002).

The reductions in medical cost are due to decreased overuse of medical services such as primary care physician visits, specialist referrals, labs, and imaging. These savings are achieved by the combination of efficient provision of effective psychotherapy plus population-based management of high-utilizing patients via telephonic outreach, behavioral interventions, and case management. For example, a recent integrated care study by O'Donohue, Laygo, and Cummings (2010) found a 21% reduction in total medical costs in integrated care settings compared to utilization the prior year.

The service delivery model based on clinician time in the primary care setting consists of 25% individual appointments, 50% in group disease and population programs, and 25% group psychotherapy. The group disease programs include conditions such as asthma, diabetes, hypertension, obesity, and fibromyalgia. The psychotherapy groups include phobias, bereavement, borderline personality disorder, depression, schizophrenia, anxiety, and panic (Cummings & Cummings, 2005). The group culture greatly facilitates treatment progress. Each group program is based on

- Treatment of the behavioral and medical aspects of each condition
- Facilitating patient self-management of chronic aspects of their illness
- Prevention of relapse or worsening of outcomes due to poor condition self-management

The group protocols share common characteristics that are interchangeable between specific groups, such as patient education, pain management, relaxation and stress management, homework assignments, and a self-management component in which patients learn to self-monitor and manage biomedical and behavioral indicators.

The Biodyne model of psychotherapy and service delivery is an *anagram* in that current and emerging evidence-based practice is continuously added to the individual and group protocols in a Biodyne treatment manual. For example, many of the protocols in James and O'Donohue (2008) and O'Donohue, Byrd, Cummings, and Henderson (2005) are in use. The manual is designed to be modified easily based on the unique characteristics of the treatment setting. A treatment protocol for depression will be different for American Indians in a reservation in Arizona, for rural patients in a small PCP office in Iowa, or for urban Latino patients in downtown Phoenix. The modular formatting of these treatment manual components enables each group protocol to serve different populations with similar treatment needs by inserting or substituting modules, further contributing to efficiency.

Medical Literacy Courses

Three courses are designed to prepare the behavioral clinicians with a broad survey of clinical medicine and pathophysiology, psychopharmacology, and clinical neuropathophysiolgy. These courses are designed to present a survey of disease etiology, course, and progression; medical treatment; and outcome. The objective is for the behavioral clinician to understand and consult with medical providers within a multidisciplinary team setting and converse in the language of these providers.

Research Courses and the Culminating Research Project

The DBH program includes a sequence of three courses and a culminating research project that are designed to train the behavioral clinician as an educated consumer of science. This means that the clinician will understand how to identify, evaluate, and incorporate current and emerging evidence-based practice research into his ongoing professional development. First, the population-based health management course includes a survey of epidemiology and approaches such as disease management, screening, outcomes management, medical cost offset, and return on investment. A course on research design in healthcare is focused on quality improvement, performance measurement, and value-based and pay-for-performance incentive programs. The health statistics course includes a survey of statistics commonly used in population-based care, quality improvement programs, and return on investment analyses.

The culminating research project is designed to demonstrate the student's ability to design an integrated behavioral care intervention, including a literature review, appropriate research design and analysis, and reporting of results and discussion. While the project is completed in the final semester, the student actively begins to develop the project with his advisor in each of the sequential courses described before. In this manner, the research project is developed as part of a comprehensive, sequential learning experience.

THE DBH PRACTICUM PROGRAM

Overview

The DBH practicum program affords students the opportunity to function as behavioral care providers in a functioning medical setting. The practicum program is based on a sequential model that includes competency levels tied to the course curriculum progression. In the novice stage, the students learn about the culture of primary care, the role of the behavioral care provider, and the model of targeted, focused behavioral interventions. In the intermediate phase, in the first semester, the student focuses on screening, assessment, and treatment of the most common behavioral conditions in primary care, such as depression, anxiety, substance abuse, and somatizers. Students begin to focus on comorbid medical and behavioral chronic conditions and lifestyle interventions designed to enhance health and wellness.

In the advanced phase, which continues into the third semester, the student integrates course material on more challenging conditions, such as schizophrenia and psychotic disorders, borderline personality disorders, and suicide prevention. In the third and fourth semesters, the student moves to the proficient level, with a focus on couples and family interventions and specialization in areas such as pediatrics.

DBH Program Practicum Supervision

The DBH program practicum supervision is provided by licensed psychologists who are DBH faculty or contracted with the program. Supervisors are experienced in the Biodyne model and integrated care, and they are trained in the DBH competency model described later. Students meet in small group supervision for 75 minutes per week. Group size is kept small to facilitate discussion (typically five to eight students). Online students meet in groups with Webcams that enable a streaming image of each participant on the computer.

Audio recordings of clinician–patient sessions are reviewed routinely during the program, and students are encouraged to record sessions by mini-videocameras or cell phone when possible. The audio and video recordings are reviewed by the group for discussion and feedback. Practicum supervisors routinely integrate relevant course content into supervision in order to help students practice new skills. The practicum supervisor is the key liaison between the DBH program and the practicum site preceptor for student performance feedback on an as-needed basis and during regular student performance evaluations.

DBH Practicum Sites

The DBH program contracts with primary care offices using an affiliation agreement that defines responsibilities of the clinic, the DBH program, and the practicum student. Sites vary in size and complexity—from integrated delivery systems to solo practices and from sites serving largely commercial insurance products to federally qualified health centers. Unlike traditional doctoral training clinics, these sites generally do not have dedicated behavioral clinicians affiliated with the office to provide supervision and oversight. These arrangements simply do not exist today, and this is the gap the DBH program aims to fill.

Instead, each practicum site identifies a preceptor to oversee each student and serve as liaison with the DBH program. Ideally, the preceptor is a medical health provider. Responsibilities of the preceptor include orientation of the student to office policy and procedures and the work environment, facilitating introduction of the student to the medical team and support staff, and facilitation of collection of measures of student performance.

Competency Assessment

The DBH program is based on a comprehensive model of competency assessment based on a developmentally informed, multimethod, and multi-informant process using established evaluation tools. Assessment results are reviewed sequentially in the program in order to obtain formative and summative results matched to training goals. Assessment results are incorporated into supervision in the program and in the practicum site, and they are reviewed with the student advisor over the course of the program.

First, a rating scale of integrated care knowledge and applied competencies (Robinson & Reiter, 2007) is used to evaluate student performance. The assessment dimensions are (1) clinical practice skills, (2) practice management, (3) consultation, (4) documentation, (5) team performance, and (6) administrative. The ratings are completed by the student as a self-assessment, by the DBH practicum supervisor, and by clinicians at the practicum site. Near the end of each semester, these forms are administered, collected, analyzed, and reviewed with each student, DBH supervisor, practicum supervisor, and advisor.

Second, an outcomes management program is used to collect and evaluate patient progress based on measures of clinical outcome and treatment alliance. The measures are the outcome rating scale (ORS) and the session rating scale (SRS) developed by Barry Duncan and Scott Miller (Miller, Duncan, Brown, Sorrell, & Chalk, 2006). Research has demonstrated that the systematic collection and review of patient outcomes feedback by clinicians during the course of behavioral treatment has positive effects on treatment outcome (Harmon et al., 2007). Reviewing outcomes and alliance in real time allows the clinician to adjust the treatment plan for patients who are deteriorating or not making expected progress in treatment.

Research on the ORS and SRS demonstrated that outcomes and treatment alliance feedback resulted in a significant improvement in clinical effectiveness and improved treatment retention (Miller et al., 2006). The DBH program contracted with the company MyOutcomes (www.myoutcomes.com) to provide Internet access to and real-time scoring and feedback of the ORS and SRS. The system automatically tracks and reports patient progress and the students review these results in supervision. In addition, MyOutcomes will generate reports that summarize effect size and other measures for each student, for each practicum site, and for the DBH program in aggregate.

Third, the DBH program has contracted with ProChange Behavior Systems (www.prochange.com), a company founded by James Prochaska, in order to make a suite of Internet-based, patient behavior change computer programs based on the transtheoretical model of behavior change available to DBH students and their patients. The ProChange system uses patient self-assessment based on the patient's stage of change to develop individually tailored behavior change interventions (Prochaska, Redding, & Evers, 2008). Patients complete these assessments at monthly intervals and receive individually tailored feedback.

These approaches have demonstrated significant improvement for many behavioral conditions, including diet, exercise, stress, and depression (Prochaska et al., 2008). The DBH student will assign patients to work on specific ProChange programs outside sessions as a means of using homework to extend the benefits of treatment. The contract with ProChange will make program-level, aggregate reports available for all users. The individual student will need to review and collect individual patient reports manually in order to incorporate these data into treatment planning.

Fourth, the program incorporates measures of clinician productivity and efficiency necessary for calculating medical cost offset. The Biodyne criterion for effectiveness is reduction in patient medical and surgical service utilization from the start of treatment compared to a full year's utilization in a 1-year period prior to the start of treatment. Efficiency is measured based on the number of weighted sessions per treatment episode (Cummings, 2002). For example, individual sessions are counted based on the number of minutes of contact, whereas a 2-hour group session with one therapist and eight patients is weighted a quarter of an hour per patient. The cost-effectiveness ratio is the average number of medical services for 1 year prior to the start of treatment divided by the average medical utilization in the year after treatment initiation plus the number of weighted behavioral treatment sessions for that group of patients (Cummings, 2002).

Fifth, students will routinely administer a measure of work productivity: the health performance questionnaire (HPQ) (http://www.hcp.med.harvard.edu/hpq/) (Kessler et al., 2003). Employers are increasingly aware of the adverse impact of chronic medical and behavioral conditions on workforce productivity and they are searching for health promotion and disease management programs in an effort to rein in the increasing costs of lost productivity and disability. Practicum students administer the HPQ at the beginning of treatment and at 6-month intervals after treatment initiation. The HPQ data can be used to calculate the dollars saved by employers based on improvements in productivity.

Credentials

The DBH program limits enrollment to master's level, licensed behavioral clinicians, such as social workers, counselors, and marital and family therapists. The rationale for this criterion is that, as a new doctoral degree in behavioral health, the DBH has not yet been recognized for licensure in any state. Requiring that each student already has a license to practice the program ensures that, upon graduation, students will have a doctoral degree from an accredited university and a master's license to practice integrated behavioral care. In addition, the supply of existing therapists far exceeds the demand for patients in traditional settings. Upgrading master's level providers to integrated care doctoral care providers shifts clinicians from the oversupply in traditional settings to meet the demand to treat patients who are currently *not* being treated in primary care. This is good for patients, the healthcare system, and DBH graduates.

The DBH program is provisionally accredited by the National Institute of Behavioral Health Quality (NIBHQ), an accreditation developed by the National Alliance of Professional Psychology Providers. The vision is that other universities or professional schools adopt the DBH as a new applied doctoral degree for behavioral providers in integrated care settings, and that the NIBHQ becomes the professional accreditation organization for these emerging programs. In addition to giving clinicians credit for their master's degree credits toward the DBH degree, the program also gives clinicians credit for between 1,500 and 3,000 hours of supervised practicum experience that were part of their master's degree and master's license. The DBH is designed to build on existing competencies in psychotherapy, with specific new competencies for a doctoral level behavioral care provider in an integrated care setting. The DBH practicum hours (500) on top of the prior supervised practicum hours are seen as sufficient for achieving proficiency, provided the student achieves the benchmarks based on assessment of competency in the program.

In addition, the DBH program curriculum and practicum program is designed largely to meet current and emerging APA and ASPPB standards for both a doctoral psychology program and practicum experience. This includes the APA Guidelines and Principles for Accreditation of Programs in Professional Psychology, the recommendations of the APA Task Force on the Assessment of Competence in Professional Psychology, and the ASPPB Guidelines on Practicum Experience for Licensure. Admittedly, it may a long and winding trajectory from establishment and credentialing of a new program to state licensure. Designing a program that largely meets existing state license board requirements for a doctoral degree license in behavioral care is prudent and logical.

Career Opportunities for the DBH Behavioral Care Provider

The key career path for the DBH behavioral care provider is the primary care or related medical setting. However, a number of other career paths seem appropriate for the provision of integrated behavioral care:

- The Substance Abuse and Mental Health Services Administration is awarding grants for pilot projects to locate primary care and nursing providers in traditional mental health and substance abuse treatment settings.
- Health plans, carve-outs, and other vendors continue to offer disease management and case management programs using telephonic outreach to engage high-cost, high-risk patients with comorbid medical and behavioral conditions.
- Large employer groups are searching for solutions to address the high cost of lost productivity and disability due to behavioral conditions. The use of employee assistance program services is on the rise and a potential career path.
- There is a proliferation of companies developing e-health interventions for behavioral and medical

conditions. Clinicians familiar with e-health and integrated care are likely to contribute significantly to design and evaluation of such programs.

Finally, traditional education in behavioral health leaves clinicians with the perception that their only options are to accept relatively low, fee-for-service reimbursement from payers or to opt out of insurance panels. The DBH program emphasis on behavioral entrepreneurship is designed to help clinicians think outside the box for new business start-up opportunities.

SUMMARY

The doctor of behavioral health degree represents a model for radical reform in the education of doctoral level, behavioral care providers. The program is designed to meet the emerging needs of healthcare reform to produce clinicians who are able to provide clinical services in integrated care settings with the explicit goal of improved clinical outcome and demonstrating medical cost offset. The DBH curriculum and training progression are based on a cohesive, sequential program of study that will prepare graduates with the clinical and medical literacy and entrepreneurial skills necessary to thrive in the twenty-first century healthcare system.

Significant challenges and barriers lie ahead for the program and DBH graduates. The path to DBH licensure will be controversial. Even though DBH graduates may be reimbursed based on their master's license, some payers require a doctoral license to practice in certain settings. Reimbursement for behavioral health in primary care is often difficult. The use of available codes for reimbursement in primary care is often not recognized by payers, with significant variation both within and between states across the country.

A key advantage is that the success of the DBH program and its graduates will be largely determined by the healthcare marketplace. The entities responsible for paying for healthcare are searching for providers that can improve the health of current patients and prevent future chronic conditions in order to reduce the cost of healthcare and support reform. Employers are interested in working with providers that can improve workplace productivity and reduce disability related to behavioral and medical illnesses. These types of providers are currently a rarity in the workforce. They are also the future graduates of the DBH program.

REFERENCES

APA (American Psychological Association). (2006). APA Task Force on the Assessment of Competence in Professional Psychology: Final report. Retrieved April 2, 2010, from http://www.apa.org/ed/resources/competency-revised.pdf

APA (American Psychological Association) Commission on Accreditation. (2007). *Guidelines and principles for accreditation of programs in professional psychology.* Washington, DC: American Psychological Association.

Antos, J., Bertko, J., et al. (2009). Bending the curve: Effective steps to address long-term healthcare spending growth. *American Journal of Managed Care, 15,* 676–680.

ASPPB (Association of State and Provincial Psychology Boards). (2009). *Guidelines on practicum experience for licensure.* Retrieved April 2, 2010, from http://www.asppb.net/files/public/Final_Prac_Guidelines_1_31_09.pdf

Blount, F. A., & Miller, B. F. (2009). Addressing the workforce crisis in integrated primary care. *Journal of Clinical Psychology in Medical Settings, 16,* 113–119.

Chaffee, B., O'Donohue, W. T., & Cummings, N. A. (In preparation). A military integrated-care project demonstration.

Cummings, N. A. (2002). Medical cost offset as a roadmap to behavioral entrepreneurship: Lessons from the Hawaii project. In N. A. Cummings, W. T. O'Donohue, & K. E. Ferguson (Eds.), *The impact of medical cost offset on practice and research: Making it work for you* (pp. 27–45). Reno, NV: Context Press.

Cummings, N. A., & Cummings, J. L. (2000). *The essence of psychotherapy: Reinventing the art for the new era of data.* San Diego, CA: Harcourt Press.

Cummings, N. A., & Cummings, J. L. (2005). Behavioral interventions for somatizers within the primary care setting. In N. A. Cummings, W. T. O'Donohue, & E. V. Naylor (Eds.), *Psychological approaches to chronic disease management* (pp. 49–70). Reno, NV: Context Press.

Cummings, N. A., & O'Donohue, W. T. (2008). *Eleven blunders that cripple psychotherapy in America: A remedial unblundering.* New York, NY: Routledge.

Cummings, N. A., & Sayama, M. (1995). *Focused psychotherapy: A casebook of brief intermittent psychotherapy throughout the life cycle.* Madison, CT: Psychological Press.

DeMers, S. T., Van Horen, B. A., & Rodolfa, E. R. (2008). Changes in training and practice of psychologists: Current challenges for licensing boards. *Professional Psychology: Practice and Research, 39,* 473–479.

France, C. R., Belar, C. D., et al. (2008). Application of the competency model to clinical health psychology. *Professional Psychology: Research and Practice, 39,* 573–580.

Frank, R. G., Goldman, H. H., & McGuire, T. G. (2009). Trends in mental health cost growth: An expanded role for management? *Health Affairs, 28,* 649–659.

Harmon, S. C., Lambert, M. J., Smart, D. M., et al. (2007). Enhancing outcome for potential treatment failures: Therapist–client feedback and clinical support tools. *Psychotherapy Research, 17,* 379–392.

James, L., & O'Donohue, W. T. (2008). *The primary care toolkit: Practical resources for the integrated behavioral care provider.* New York, NY: Springer.

Kessler, R. C., Barber, C., Beck, A., Berglund, P., Cleary, P. D., McKenas, D.,...Wang, P. (2003). The World Health Organization health and work performance questionnaire (HPQ). *Journal of Occupational and Environmental Medicine, 45,* 156.

McDaniel, S. H., Schroeder, C., Belar, C. D., Hargrove, D. S., & Freeman, E. L. (2002). A training curriculum for professional psychologists in primary care. *Professional Psychology: Research and Practice, 33,* 65–72.

Miller, S. D., Duncan, B. L., Brown, J., Sorrell, R., & Chalk, M. B. (2006). Using formal client feedback to improve retention and outcome: Making ongoing, real-time assessment feasible. *Journal of Brief Therapy, 5,* 5–22.

O'Donohue, W. T., & Boland, J. P. (In preparation). The Rube Goldberg model of clinical training: Toward the explication of core competencies.

O'Donohue, W. T., & Buchanan, J. A. (2003). The mismeasure of psychologists: A review of the psychometrics of licensing requirements. In W. T. O'Donohue & K. Ferguson (Eds.), *The handbook of professional ethics for psychologists.* Thousand Oaks, CA: Sage Publications.

O'Donohue, W. T., Byrd, M. R., Cummings, N. A., & Henderson, D. A. (2005). *Behavioral integrative care: Treatments that work in the primary care setting.* New York, NY: Brunner-Routledge.

O'Donohue, W. T., Cummings, N. A., & Cummings, J. L. (2008). The unmet educational agenda in integrated care. *Journal of Clinical Psychology in Medical Settings, 16,* 94–100.

O'Donohue, W. T., Laygo, R., & Cummings, N. (2010). *Hawaii integrated health care demonstration project.* Reno, NV: The Cummings Foundation for Behavioral Health.

Olfson, M., & Marcus, S. C. (2009). National patterns of antidepressant medication treatment. *Archives of General Psychiatry, 66,* 848–856.

Prochaska, J. O., Redding, C. A., & Evers, K. E. (2008). The transtheoretical model of behavior change. In K. Glanz, F. M. Lewis, & B. K. Rimer (Eds.), *Health behavior and health education: Theory, research and practice* (3rd ed.) (pp. 97–121). San Francisco, CA: Jossey–Bass.

Robinson, P., & Reiter, J. (2007). *Behavioral consultation and primary care: A guide to integration.* New York, NY: Springer.

Satterfield, J. M. (2003). Core competencies of the primary care provider in an integrated team. In N. A. Cummings, W. T. O'Donohue, & K. E. Ferguson (Eds.), *Behavioral health as primary care: Beyond efficacy to effectiveness.* Reno, NV: Context Press.

Strosahl, K. (1998). The dissemination of manual-based psychotherapies in managed care: Promises, problems, and prospects. *Clinical Psychology: Science and Practice, 5,* 382–386.

Strosahl, K. (2005). Training behavioral health and primary care providers for integrated care: A core competencies approach. In W. T. O'Donohue, M. R. Byrd, N. A. Cummings, & D. A. Henderson (Eds.), *Behavioral integrative care: Treatments that work in the primary care setting.* New York, NY: Brunner-Routledge.

Twelve

Pay for Performance and Other Innovations in Reimbursement for Behavioral Care Services

NICHOLAS A. CUMMINGS AND JANET L. CUMMINGS

INTRODUCTION

It is painfully apparent that for the past two decades reimbursement for psychotherapy has suffered in the following ways:

- The reimbursement scales reflect master's level providers who comprise the majority of provider networks and are willing to work for a lower fee.
- When there is a differential payment for doctoral level psychologists, it is often paltry.
- In most networks, any increases in payment over the years have been small, and when inflation is taken into account, fees have actually declined in real dollars.
- Established psychotherapists who can attract a clientele able and willing to pay out of pocket are opting out of the networks.

More recently, a number of payers have sought to reward the efficient and effective provider with a higher rate of reimbursement on the expectation that these providers in the long run save the company money by doing the job well and in a timely fashion. A number of systems have emerged, and although they differ, they all fall under the general name or designation "pay for performance," with the rubric of "P4P."

In a number of P4P arrangements, the paperwork to qualify is so daunting and the higher differential paid so small that most practitioners do not bother to qualify.

This chapter will examine the P4P arrangement currently extant, as well as those that are in process of implementation and likely to emerge in healthcare reform, and then propose P4P mechanisms not yet developed that would likely benefit both the payer and the provider. We are proposing that the practice profession seize the opportunities accorded by the changing times and design and present payment approaches that would be of mutual benefit to payers, providers, and patients alike.

HOW DID P4P COME ABOUT?

Pay for performance, mostly in the form of bonuses, has been successfully employed in industry for a number of decades. The American International Group (AIG), Fannie Mae/Freddie Mac, Merrill Lynch, and other monumental financial scandals of 2008 and 2009 would belie the fact that, in the overwhelming number of companies over the years, P4P has worked very well, increasing assets and retaining top-performing employees. Because of widespread abuses, the U.S. Treasury Department moved in 2009 to restrict the amount of and qualification for such compensation in distressed corporations receiving government "bailout" money, and we may be witnessing a highly restricted, if not totally disappearing, P4P in industry.

The rising costs in healthcare that brought about its industrialization also modestly introduced some forms of P4P in the 1980s, but in that era the new managed care companies that were rapidly proliferating were relying on diagnosis related groups (DRGs) and a number of private sector restrictions (e.g., prior authorization, fee restrictions on providers, caps on benefits) to lower costs. Enhanced compensation lagged behind in spite of the fact that Kaiser Permanente, the nation's first and consistently most efficient health maintenance organization (HMO), had been paying bonuses to its physicians since its inception in 1946.

The manner in which this early P4P system operated was ingenious and has seldom been replicated by other healthcare companies. The Permanente Medical Group received from the Kaiser Health Plan a fixed amount of money per year, based on a capitated system of per member, per month (pmpm). The medical staff received a monthly salary, which varied in accordance with specialty and longevity. If, at the end of the fiscal year, the cost of providing services exceeded the amount received, the doctors would have to bear the loss. However, if the doctors were able to provide efficient, effective services for less than the fixed capitation, there would be a "devisable surplus" that would be divided among the medical staff and distributed in the form of a bonus at the end of the year. For the exception of a few years when the surplus was plowed back into the medical group for expansion, the bonus consistently and appreciably exceeded the physician's base salary (Cummings & VandenBos, 1981).

Beginning with the inception of Blue Cross and Blue Shield, along with other forms of health insurance introduced in the 1930s, healthcare has been subjected to varying forms of accountability. Mental healthcare, on the other hand, was regarded as being beyond any kind of accountability—a widespread perception that prevented its becoming a covered benefit until decades after insurance reimbursement for physical healthcare was common. During World War II employer-sponsored healthcare increased rapidly until it became the mode in America, but mental health coverage was conspicuously absent. It was not until the discovery of the medical cost offset phenomenon (Cummings & Follette, 1967; Follette & Cummings, 1966) that showed that brief behavioral interventions reduced *medical* costs impressively, as well as a series of government-sponsored replications, confirmed the phenomenon (Jones & Vischi, 1979) that third-party payers seriously began extending coverage to include psychotherapy.

When healthcare industrialized in the 1980s and the managed behavioral health organizations (MBHOs) were launched, it was quickly demonstrated that managed care could apply to behavioral care as it did to physical care. Having just recently achieved widespread third-party reimbursement and having stubbornly ignored all the warnings that managed care would also morph into managed behavioral care, the psychological practitioners were blindsided and have never quite recovered. Now, as of this writing and in spite of the rapid growth of P4P in general healthcare, behavioral care seems to be all but oblivious to the emergence of P4P as the future standard for reimbursement. This is especially probable because healthcare reform is certain to change drastically how healthcare is financed and dispensed (Fisher & Chamberlin, 2005; Godbole, 2005; Kennedy, 2004).

WHERE IS P4P NOW?

In 2006, the most recent year for which survey data exist, there were 42 states with a total of 85 state Medicaid pay-for-performance programs functioning (Kuhmerker, 2006). In 2007, there were more than 150 private sector P4P programs in the United States (*Business Wire*, 2007) and 70% of all such programs were working to expand the scope and number of performance measures they use. Furthermore, within 2 years, 30% of these programs were able to document increased provider performance along with significant cost savings. During the 3-year period of 2003–2006, seven California health plans made $145 million in bonus payments to 40,000 California physicians (HIA, 2007) and plan to continue to provide such incentives to the practitioners.

Unquestionably, behavioral healthcare has lagged behind the P4P trend growing within general healthcare, given the following considerations:

- The care management industry has decided that most of the cost savings in mental healthcare have been realized, and further cost containment efforts may not be worth the trouble.
- The percentage of the national healthcare budget of $2 trillion has shrunk from an all-time high of 9% in 1985 to 4.5% in 2008. In other words, behavioral care has ceased to be a significant player in the healthcare scene.
- Referrals for psychotherapy have declined precipitously as psychotropic medication has become the standard treatment for mental health disorders. When medication costs are removed from the 4.5% of the healthcare budget for mental health, the portion attributed to behavioral care services shrunk to 1.5% in 2008 and is expected to decline to 1.2% in 2009 (Carnahan, 2002; Cummings, O'Donohue, & Cummings, 2008; Nemko, 2006).
- Between 80 and 85% of the mental health services (medication as well as counseling) are provided by nonpsychiatric physicians, making primary care the de facto mental health system of the nation.
- There are a few P4P programs in the private sector and in Medicare, but the differential in pay is so small and the paperwork so extensive that most practitioners are ignoring the slightly higher pay scale.

Historically, when managed behavioral healthcare networks were formed, any differential compensation was unnecessary inasmuch as the MBHOs chose the potentially best applicants for their networks. Practitioners fought back by the successful enactment of "every willing provider" laws, which mandated that the MBHOs had to accept every qualified applicant as defined by state licensure and certification laws. The MBHOs adjusted by sending most of their referrals to a select group within the network whom the company's record keeping demonstrated had shown effective and efficient resolution of patients' problems. This worked well for a time, but eventually these silently "preferred" practitioners became overloaded and declined any further referrals. Furthermore, these high-performing psychotherapists discovered that their well-deserved reputations in the community enabled them to attract patients who could afford and were willing to pay out of pocket (Cummings, 2006).

It soon became apparent that some system had to be developed that would result in retaining the best performers, who, in turn, were saving the MBHO money by effective and efficient treatment. They looked to industry, which had long ago instituted various forms of P4P for the answers. But before doing so, let us look at the emergence of research evidence as the basis for reimbursement and participation in the healthcare system.

EVIDENCE-BASED TREATMENT

Every successful industry is dependent upon sound, proven modes of operation, whether it is bridge building, with its necessity for the best in engineering, or banking, which requires established economic stability. Violation of the latter, prompted by well-intentioned government relaxing of subprime mortgage rules so as to put persons who could not afford a home into one—multiplied by the greed of derivative-based lenders who climbed on the precarious but highly remunerative bandwagon—resulted in the economic meltdown of 2008.

To the MBHOs, the less devastating but costly practice of long-term psychotherapy based on various and often conflicting schools had to be reined in. Early use of "bean counter" methods such as preauthorization, session limits, therapist profiling, and denial of reimbursement created a cat-and-mouse game between the MBHO and practitioner. This was unsatisfactory because a savvy, wily practitioner often pulled it off, while in other cases the MBHO came off looking as if it were harming a needy patient. A national populist revolt soon restricted the heavy hand of the MBHO, raising the need for a sound basis for reimbursement.

During this period (the late 1990s and early 2000), the movement promoting evidence-based treatments (EBTs) was gaining momentum (Chambless et al., 1996). This ostensibly provided a sound basis for reimbursement and case managers began to look for EBTs in the treatment plans that were required. Practitioners cried foul, regarded EBTs as a kind of psychotherapy practice homogenization, and disdained treatment manuals as "cookbooks" that stifled therapist acumen and flexibility. They complained that much of psychotherapy is an art and cannot be reduced to protocols. Nonetheless, medicine and healthcare, spurred by the prestigious and well-documented report of the Institute of Medicine (IOM, 2001), are moving steadily into evidence bases for all practice. The President's Freedom Commission on Mental Health (Hogan, 2003) and subsequent reports by the IOM (Godbole, 2005), which directly address EBTs in mental health, make the continued trend toward EBTs in behavioral interventions inevitable.

As the controversy continues within psychology, Barlow (2004) has proposed that only interventions based on research evidence be eligible for healthcare reimbursement. These would be called "psychological treatment," and everything else would continue as is and retain the title psychotherapy. Most psychotherapists reject the Barlow designations; nonetheless, there is a rush by each "school" of psychotherapy to produce evidence for the ostensible legitimacy of its particular methods. Often this research is questionable, prompting Barlow to state that a psychological treatment must not only show research validity (efficacy), but should also demonstrate that it works outside the laboratory (effectiveness). Cummings, Cummings, and O'Donohue (2008) would propose that it must also show efficiency—that is, that it works not only better, but also more rapidly in its effectiveness. Thus there is emerging the "three Es" of behavioral interventions (our preferred term to "psychological treatments"): efficacy (Chambless), effectiveness (Barlow), and efficiency (Cummings).

WHAT WE ARE LEARNING FROM P4P IN THE HEALTHCARE INDUSTRY

As previously stated, industry has led the way in instituting various forms of P4P. Some would argue, erroneously, that programs successful in industry do not translate to healthcare. This is the same kind of short-sightedness that, in the 1980s, declared healthcare was incapable of industrializing because health practice is based on the doctor–patient relationship and defies the economics that would apply to already industrialized sectors of our economy (in sequence): manufacturing, mining, transportation, and retail industries. In this erroneous belief, all the warnings and harbingers were ignored as healthcare, including mental healthcare, industrialized big time (Dranove, 2000). Belatedly, those professional leaders who assured their rank-and-file colleagues that it was impossible have now seen healthcare fully industrialized.

By 2008, there were more than 150 P4P programs in the private sector and over 80 in state Medicaid programs (*Business Wire,* August 29, 2008). The *Business Wire* survey of these programs revealed the following:

- Over 70% of all P4P programs are working to expand the scope or number of performance measures they use.
- More than 60% of these respondents have now evaluated their programs and at least half find their clinical performance has improved significantly.
- Over 30% of all P4P respondents posted information on provider performance publicly in their provider directories.
- Over 30% of all P4P survey respondents have been able to demonstrate cost savings.

In perhaps the only study of its kind, the Integrated Healthcare Association (IHA) reported that between 2003 and 2008, seven California health plans encompassing 40,000 doctors made bonus payments of $145 million (*Medical News Today,* May 7, 2008). If this were equally distributed, it would average $3,375 per physician. However, it was differentially distributed according to performance, and the report conveys no further information in this regard. The survey also does not describe the performance rating systems that were employed to make the distribution.

BEHAVIORAL HEALTH P4P LAGS BEHIND

Not surprisingly, P4P is rare in behavioral health. Of the 150 P4P healthcare programs in existence in 2008, only 24 (16%)

included any measurement of quality of care for mental or substance abuse disorders (Morgan, 2009). Of these programs, only nine included measures providing incentives tied to outcomes. The National Committee for Quality Assurance (NCQA) identified four factors contributing to the minor role played by behavioral health in P4P programs (Morgan, 2009):

- There is a lag in the development of reporting infrastructure and electronic record keeping among behavioral healthcare providers relative to general healthcare.
- There is difficulty in achieving consensus on standardized measures. This is further complicated by the large number of disciplines licensed to diagnose and treat behavioral health patients.
- The dominant role is played by state public sector programs, which are less likely to respond to market pressures for increasing quality and efficiency.
- The complex clinical profile of behavioral health consumers also defies consensus.

In summary, it will take advances in electronic record keeping and increased cross-disciplinary collaboration within behavioral health before there will be an improvement and an increase in the number of P4P programs within behavioral care.

Additionally, two other problems plague behavioral care systems when they are able to accomplish a provider rating based on outcomes and then use it preferentially to refer and reward these high performers: (1) The preferred providers soon find their practices overloaded and refuse to accept additional referrals; (2) the increased prestige in the community places these providers in such demand that it is more lucrative for them to move into strictly out-of-pocket practice. Consequently, to prevent this, the P4P rate has to be raised regularly. P4P does not increase the number of top performers as do approaches yet to be discussed.

Stating it bluntly, a health policy expert says, "For many psychologists the idea of pay-for-performance programs is like fingernails on a chalkboard" (Doucette, 2008, p. 2). But mental health providers have always been touchy about accountability, usually hiding behind concern for privacy even when patient protection can be built into the system. Furthermore, according to Doucette, some practitioners may focus on earning an incentive rather than providing good care. Emphasis on meeting program criteria may obscure other areas that contribute to good care. Finally, in some instances, in order to make themselves look good, some providers select only patients who are likely to do well. Excellent psychotherapists who are willing to treat the very difficult patients may be unjustly penalized by P4P measures.

In looking for a way around such considerations, an interesting switch to the usual P4P programs is to reward the consumer with reduced premiums and lower copayments for selecting providers who meet quality standards. Directing P4P toward consumers is more recent than rewarding practitioners, but indications are that this practice will increase.

In spite of the P4P lag in behavioral care, however, it is moving forward in physical care. A study by the American Association for Retired Persons (AARP) revealed that 30% of primary care physicians already have some kind of pay-for-performance incentives written into their plan contracts, and 28% of group practices include performance benchmarks (Kluger, 2009).

ARE WE PAYING DOCTORS TOO MUCH?

Two perennial questions reverberate throughout the healthcare system: (1) Do we pay doctors too much? (2) Do we pay doctors the wrong way? Most authorities are reluctant to state the first, but in actuality this seems to be the prevailing sentiment, as shown by a consistent reduction of scales, first by Medicare and Medicaid, and then by the private sector, which feels empowered by the reductions and then emulates the government's example. It is difficult to feel sorry for a profession that is earning an average of $179,000 annually, but when one factors the 12–15 years of education and training and adds the burden of debt shouldered by medical graduates (generally, in excess of $200,000 on average), the envy is hardly justifiable. But more importantly, now that cost-cost-cost is the overriding concern, the easy way out is to slash provider fees. Medicare and Medicaid continue to lead the way with a repeated ratcheting down of fee scales; the private sector then takes the cue and follows suit.

But there is a limit. Three years ago, Cummings asked an undersecretary of health how long the government intends to do this, and the surprising reply was, "Until most providers begin opting out of these programs. Then we will know we have reached the appropriate fee scale." This may already have occurred: Seniors are having difficulty finding a primary care physician who accepts Medicare and, in several states (principally Texas among them), it is nigh impossible. The Mayo Clinic in Scottsdale, Arizona, announced in January 2010 that it would no longer accept Medicare. This is surprising inasmuch as Mayo is not famous for primary care, but rather for secondary and tertiary care that is overwhelmingly for older adults.

Psychotherapy is particularly vulnerable to the ratcheting of fees inasmuch as it performs no procedures and is paid an hourly rate. Physicians can load additional revenue producers (e.g., various tests, vaccines, bone density scans, ancillary services) onto a visit, but the behavioral care provider is pretty well limited to the hourly rate that, when lowered, immediately results in markedly reduced total income. Additionally, nondoctoral providers seem willing to work for less, so doctoral psychologists are forced to accept a fee ratcheted down from the already low master's level practitioner fee schedule. This is not likely to improve inasmuch as licensed nondoctoral behavioral care providers are being accorded full diagnostic and treatment privileges.

More recently, there is a growing sentiment that we pay doctors the wrong way. In a stinging indictment before the U.S. Senate, one member stated, "Today, Medicare pays the same regardless of quality of care. Some people would argue that in fact, the current Medicare payment system rewards poor quality. This situation just doesn't make sense to me, nor should it to beneficiaries" (Senator Charles Grassley, introducing the Medicare Value Purchasing Act of 2005). The growing recognition that this is generally true in healthcare continues to propel P4P programs as well as emerging systems that go even beyond.

ARE SALARIES A SOLUTION TO THE PAYMENT DILEMMA?

Recently, APA leaders predicted that salaried psychologists will likely replace our current fee-for-service system (Hartman-Stein, 2009). According to U.S. Representative Brian Baird, himself a doctoral level psychologist, who gave the opening address at the APA's 2009 convention in Toronto:

> The fee-for-service model is likely to change quite dramatically. What will be more likely is a fixed salary model for healthcare practitioners in the foreseeable future because fee for service is coming under great scrutiny in terms of cost containment. Fee for service has every incentive to order more procedures,

one more MRI or one more therapy session. (Hartman-Stein, 2009, p. 1)

A similar message was echoed by a number of other psychologist leaders, among them the then current APA president James Bray and past president Patrick DeLeon. Certainly, this would be the aim of government-sponsored healthcare (termed the "public option" during the 2009 healthcare reform debate in Congress) and is the method of provider reimbursement in nations having single-payer (government) healthcare. But the salaried system heralded by the APA is naïve, inasmuch as the examples frequently touted by both the APA and the present administration in Washington are anything but mere salaried positions. Furthermore, such a system in nations having it has resulted in a shortage of doctors, with undue reliance on foreign physicians; doctor dissatisfaction; long waiting lists for specialty services; and healthcare rationing. (France, where there are sufficient numbers of physicians, is the notable exception.)

Geisinger Health System (Danville, Pennsylvania), frequently touted by both the APA and the Washington administration (Novotney, 2010), has a self-determined set of incentives that render it both cost effective and therapeutically effective—in our estimation, conditions that are necessary for salaries to succeed. The Geisinger Health System owns three hospitals and serves 2.6 million people in its core 31-county market, where it has captured 30% of the population. Within this, 30% belong to the Geisinger Health Plan, its own insurance company; however, it also treats patients belonging to other health plans (Nash, 2009).

Three cost-cutting approaches are applied in some measure at Geisinger: pay-for-performance compensation, episode care (a fixed price for an entire procedure, such as heart bypass surgery, from beginning to end), and, most broadly, global care. The latter provides access to a diverse team of caregivers who cover all of a patient's needs for a single premium over the length of a policy. "A doctor's pay is not fixed in advance. Salaries are pegged so that they stay within 80% of the national average, but up to 20% of income is based on teams' achieving performance goals" (Nash, 2009, p. 38).

Similarly, Kaiser Permanente, founded in 1946 and providing care principally on the West Coast as well as in regions in Texas and on the East Coast, is several times larger than Geisinger. Because it is regarded as the largest, most successful physician-owned health plan in the world, it is often touted as a model (Cummings & VandenBos, 1981). Its approximately 15 million enrollees belong to the nonprofit Kaiser Foundation Health Plan, and the for-profit Permanente medical corporations (semiautonomous from region to region) service only these members. The physicians are on a fixed salary, but, at the end of the year, share in the "divisible surplus" accrued by achieving high performance standards that save money above the capitation rate paid by the Kaiser Health Plan. Within the divisible surplus, a differential amount from physician to physician is determined by peers in accordance with perceived individual performance. Thus, Kaiser Permanente not only goes beyond mere salary, but also has incentives within incentives.

The Kaiser Permanente System inadvertently provides other important information. Optometrists, who do not share in the divisible surplus, are out of their offices within seconds after 5:00 p.m.; ophthalmologists, who do share in that incentive, are often still seeing patients long after. So pervasive seems to be the 9:00–5:00 mentality of the salaried individual that European countries with universal healthcare have had to mandate unpaid overtime as necessary, resulting in what has been thought to be anger and a reduction in productivity as the response from physicians.

The inevitable conclusion from these large, long-standing, and successful "salaried" provider groups that the expectation salaries without further incentives will not only replace fee for service, but also cure all of its ills, is unrealistic.

PROCESS VERSUS OUTCOMES: THE NEXT DEBATE

Credentialing of practitioners and/or their training programs by a plethora of organizations (e.g., state licensing boards, specialty boards, professional societies) has dominated as the right to practice ever since the Flexner Report, which spurred rigid standards for medical practice and its training in only qualified medical schools. Recently, in an attempt to address the rapidly escalating cost of healthcare, there has been a proliferation of new certification bodies, most often self-generated, purporting to reduce costs where their predecessors have failed, by imposing stricter standards or by identifying the best providers. Some are challenging existing credentialing, as the Association for Psychological Science (APS) is doing with what it regards as a failed accrediting system by the APA. Others, such as the NCQA, which has appointed itself to rate the performance of physicians, or the newer American Board of Behavioral Healthcare Practice (ABBHP), which would be the first to do the same for the new practice of behavioral care within primary care, seek to fill gaps in defining practitioner performance.

The proliferation of these bodies would seem to be clear evidence that such a process has not and probably will not impact costs positively. The very nature of certification is that, once they have been certified, all certified practitioners are thereby "created equal."

Recently, Miller and his colleagues (Miller, Duncan, Brown, Sorrell, & Chalk, 2006; Miller, Duncan, Sorrell, & Brown, 2005) have demonstrated the efficacy of outcomes over process—specifically, ongoing and systematic feedback of consumer evaluation and outcome. Consider the following (Miller et al., 2006, p. 21):

- Instead of assuming that identifying and utilizing the "right" process leads to favorable results, there is the use of outcome—specifically, client feedback—to inform and construct treatment as well as inspire innovation.
- Other than *evidence-based practice,* therapists tailor services to the individual client via *practice-based evidence.*
- Instead of empirically supported *therapies,* consumers would have access to empirically validated *therapists.*
- With perpetual client/peer feedback, poorest therapists often become high performers.

These psychologists have developed an outcome and rating scale manual (Miller & Duncan, 2004) and their method is just beginning to be heard in P4P circles. They have developed electronic aids and are actively marketing a proprietary company. In spite of its rapid, new departure from traditional process modes, positive corroboration by other researchers has recently been published (Reese, Norsworthy, & Rowlands, 2009).

Given its current and historical emphasis on identifying and codifying methods of treatment, it remains to be seen whether the field can put outcome ahead of process. But one national, large-scale system (American Biodyne with 25 million enrollees in all 50 states) successfully employed outcomes over process for over a decade (Cummings, Cummings, & Johnson, 1997). That system's innovations (to name only a few) included:

- Psychotherapists were chosen for their skills, rather than their credentials or discipline.
- Consumer and peer feedback was ongoing, with 15% of practitioners' time devoted to such quality assurance.
- A culture of openness and acceptance was established in which practitioners eagerly sought feedback, especially for their failures.
- Consumer feedback was perpetually sought and obtained.
- Pedantic processes were eliminated to the extent that psychotherapists were rewarded and promoted by high performance, regardless of discipline (i.e., psychiatrists were not in charge by virtue of their usual "rank" in the overwhelming number of our nation's mental health systems).

WHAT DOES THE FUTURE PORTEND?

At this juncture, it is difficult to foretell where healthcare is heading. Because the future of P4P essentially depends on the form of healthcare delivery itself, it is not possible to predict which P4P system will prevail. One thing is certain: Within most scenarios, P4P is bound to increase in response in the face of escalating healthcare costs.

Scenario A: Continuation of Present System

The percentage of practitioners that will be accorded some kind of monetary incentive for high performance will undoubtedly increase from its present 30% of providers to the majority. Unable to address adequately its IT problems of a lack of interface with healthcare in general, behavioral health will continue to lag behind. Consequently, other systems will be more applicable for behavioral care. More payers will realize the need to train the disparate psychotherapists, but they will continue to believe that ongoing supervision is unnecessary. In time, it will be recognized that training plus pay alone is of minimal benefit, and in many systems the slightly positive results will be negated by the cost of implementing and maintaining the so-called incentives. Within these P4P systems, there will be a continuing increase of rewarding the patient, through reduced copayments or other incentives, for choosing a highly rated performer.

Scenario B: Universal Healthcare or Lesser Public Ownership of Healthcare Delivery

The health reform debates of 2009 and 2010 have demonstrated that American voters are sharply and contentiously divided on what role, if any, the so-called "public option" will play. In European style universal healthcare, the providers are on salary and any incentives are those characteristic of the bureaucracy: regulation, possible promotion, shorter hours, increased pay, retirement benefits, or the fear of punitive action. Pay for performance as defined in this chapter is unknown, resulting in a shortage of doctors, defections to nations with free-market systems, a reluctance of the brightest students to go into medicine, reliance on foreign-trained doctors, and long waits for services, especially for specialty care.

Interestingly, however, where most of the physicians chafe at the thought of being on salary alone, the current generation of mental health providers is on a master's degree level and not only prefer to be, but also are on salary in various public and private agencies. This may number as much as 80% of the nation's practicing (as opposed to teaching or administering) psychotherapists and is likely to grow. Of course, P4P is not likely to grow within this sector and, as seen throughout this chapter, it is the obtuse nature of behavioral healthcare that defies involvement in P4P. There are indications that psychology is attempting to move closer to the general healthcare system, and if that is accomplished, participation in P4P is more of a possibility because communication would be adequate once physical and behavioral healthcare are one system.

Scenario C: Continuation of Present Free-Market Healthcare

The Geisinger and Kaiser Permanente healthcare models have been so successful in controlling costs through their unique incentives that physicians are emulating them on a smaller scale, usually with group practices of 8–15 doctor-owners. Typical is LifeScape, a group practice in Scottsdale, Arizona, whose physicians came out of Scottsdale's Mayo Clinic. It consists of five primary care physicians, two pediatricians, one psychologist, two nurse practitioners, laboratory and radiology technicians, and the support staff. Because of its excellent reputation, it has garnered an appreciative patient population, which it keeps limited so that it can offer same-day service, holistic medicine, 24-hour on-call contact, and other niceties that seem to have disappeared in most settings. The doctors are owners, are paid a salary, and share in the profits in accordance with performance feedback from patients as well as peer evaluation.

The continued proliferation of these group practices with their internal P4P incentives depends on the continuation of our current free-market health system. But to date no other form of pay for performance has been as successful as doctors working for themselves in group practices as small as LifeScape or as large as Geisinger and Kaiser Permanente.

Scenario D: Further Emergence of the "Cleveland Clinic" Model

The question arises as to who would be willing to see the intractable patients, inasmuch as the very difficult nature of the cases reduces the probability of high performance. The answer, of course, lies in having high-performing specialty centers that are paid accordingly for caring for these difficult cases. In cardiac surgery, the Cleveland Clinic's reputation is unmatched—no wonder, inasmuch as its motto is that one is not a skilled heart surgeon until he or she has performed 1,000 such surgeries. We would add that one is not a skilled psychotherapist until he or she has seen 1,000 patients in psychotherapy. Along with treatment efficacy, there is no substitute for experience. Unfortunately, too many psychotherapists do a little therapy, along with a little teaching, and a little supervision, along with a little research, with prestige in the field being measured by how far away the practitioner is from direct, hands-on treatment.

Years ago, Nicholas Cummings and his colleagues created such a psychotherapy center in San Francisco; it came to be regarded as the treatment of last resort in Northern California. Fees were high and third-party payers were more than willing to pay, inasmuch as it was far cheaper than the interminable treatment and successive hospitalizations for which they had been paying.

Scenario E: Empirically Validated Psychotherapists

It may seem far off before a credentialing-oriented psychology culture makes a shift to the "empirically validated psychotherapists" that Miller and his colleagues (2006) describe. Surprisingly, however, such a marketable system has already been developed, a company has been formed, and managed care companies are seriously looking at it (Scott Miller, Brendan Madden, and Enda Madden, personal communication, January

2010). Using continuous client feedback and peer supervision, managed care companies have been able to identify high performers; the procedure can also lift low performers to become high performers.

SUMMARY AND CONCLUSIONS

Attempts to rein in healthcare costs by improving practitioner performance have led to a variety of "doctor incentives" called pay for performance, or P4P. Although forms of P4P vary widely in form and application, it is estimated that one third of physicians are now involved in some form of P4P incentives, and these promise to continue to increase in form and number. On the other hand, behavioral health practice is lagging woefully behind physical healthcare because of difficulties peculiar to mental health delivery, as well as because of resistance from behavioral practitioners.

While P4P programs are increasing in number, there is also a proliferation of new or reformulated accreditation and certification systems hoping to impact costs by improving practitioner performance. Although gaining attention among academic circles, these strategies have not been significant within delivery systems.

Among adherents of government-sponsored healthcare, the substitution of salaries for fee-for-service payment is being heralded, but the successful plans they tout in promoting such a method (e.g., Geisinger and Kaiser Permanente) are very much salary plus financial incentives—a combination that is not extant in government single-payer systems in countries that have these.

There are promising beginnings of an emphasis on outcomes, particularly continued consumer–practitioner feedback, as differentiated from the preceding process approaches. This is the only approach that has demonstrated the rapid improvement of low performers to the status of high performers. Although it has been extensively demonstrated as successful in one large national health plan, it remains to be seen whether our traditionally process-oriented system will be able to make that shift.

REFERENCES

Barlow, D. H. (2004). Psychological treatments. *American Psychologist, 59,* 869–876.

Business Wire (2007, August 29). There are more than 150 pay-for-performance plans.

Carnahan, I. (2002, January 21). Asylum for the insane. *Forbes,* 33–34.

Chambless, D. L., Sanderson, W. C., Shoham, V., Johnson, S. B., Pope, K. S., Crits-Christoph, P., et al. (1996). An update on empirically validated therapies. *Clinical Psychologist, 49,* 5–18.

Cummings, N. A. (2006). Psychology, the stalwart profession, faces new challenges and opportunities. *Professional Psychology: Research and Practice, 27*(6), 598–605.

Cummings, N. A., Cummings, J. L., & Johnson, J. N. (Eds.). (1997). *Behavioral health in primary care: A guide for clinical integration.* Madison, CT: Psychosocial Press.

Cummings, N. A., Cummings, J. L., & O'Donohue, W. T. (2008). We are not a healthcare business: Our inadvertent vow of poverty. *Journal of Contemporary Psychotherapy, 5*(2), 7–15.

Cummings, N. A., O'Donohue, W. T., & Cummings, J. L. (2008). The financial dimensions of integrated behavioral/primary care. *Journal of Clinical Psychology in Medical Settings, 16*(1), 74–82.

Cummings, N. A., & Follette, W. T. (1967). Psychiatric services and medical utilization in a prepaid health plan setting: Part 2. *Medical Care, 6,* 31–41.

Cummings, N. A., & VandenBos, G. R. (1981). The twenty year Kaiser Permanente experience with psychotherapy and medical utilization: Implications for national health policy and national health insurance. *Health Policy Quarterly, 1,* 159–175.

Doucette, A. (2008). As quoted by the APA Practice Organization. *Practice Update,* March 27.

Dranove, D. (2000). *The economic revolution of American healthcare: From Marcus Welby to managed care.* Princeton, NJ: Princeton University Press.

Fisher, D. B., & Chamberlin, J. (2005). The role of mental health consumers in leading the recovery transformation in mental health. In N. A. Cummings, W. T. O'Donohue, & M. A Cucciare, (Eds.), *Universal healthcare: Readings for mental health professionals* (pp. 219–242). Cummings Foundation for Behavioral Health: Healthcare Utilization and Cost Series, vol. 9. Reno, NV: Context Press.

Follete, W. T., & Cummings, N. A. (1967). Psychiatric services and medical utilization in a prepaid health plan setting. *Medical Care, 5,* 25–35.

Godbole, A. (2005). Evidence-based practices and behavioral healthcare policy. In N. A. Cummings, W. T. O'Donohue, & M. A. Cucciarre (Eds.), *Universal healthcare: Readings for mental health professionals* (pp. 163–193). Cummings Foundation for Behavioral health: Healthcare Utilization and Cost Series, vol. 9. Reno, NV: Context Press.

Hartman-Stein, P. E. (2009). APA leaders say fixed salaries may replace fee-for-service billing. *National Psychologist, 18*(5), 1, 3.

HIA (Health Insurance Association (2007). *Pay-for-performance in California health plans.* New York, NY: HIA.

Hogan, M. F. (2003). New Freedom Commission Report: The President's New Freedom Commission—Recommendations to Transform Mental Health Care in America. *Psychiatric Services, 54,* 1467–1474.

Institute of Medicine (IOM). (2001). Crossing the quality chasm: A new health system for the 21st century. Washington, DC: National Academy of Sciences.

Jones, K. R., & Vischi, T. R. (1979). The impact of alcohol, drug abuse, and mental health treatment on medical care utilization: A review of the research literature. *Medical Care, 17* (suppl), 43–133.

Kennedy, E. (2004, October 9). Comments made on the U.S. Senate floor regarding healthcare. Washington, DC: C-Span Cable Network.

Kluger, J. (2009). A healthier way to pay doctors. *Time,* October 26, 36–40.

Kuhmerker Consulting Group LLC. (2006). The number of states and programs in state Medicaid pay-for-performance programs. As reported in *Business Wire,* August 29, 2007.

Medical News Today. (2008). Bonus payments to 7 California health plans. May 7.

Miller, S. D., & Duncan, B. L. (2004). *The outcome and session rating scales: Administration and scoring manual.* Chicago, IL: Authors.

Miller, S. D., Duncan, B. L., Brown, J., Sorrell, R., & Chalk, M. (2006). Using formal client feedback to improve outcome and retention: Making ongoing, realistic assessment feasible. *Journal of Brief Therapy, 5,* 5–22.

Miller, S. D., Duncan, B. L., Sorrell, R. F., & Brown, G. S. (2005). The partners for change outcome management system. *Journal of Clinical Psychology, 61*, 199–208.

Morgan, L. (2009). P4P rare in behavioral health due to lack of IT infrastructure and consensus on outcomes. *Open Minds Circle,* October 7.

Nash, D. (2009). Private health system touted in PA. *Philadelphia Inquirer,* October 18, A8–9.

Nemko, M. (2006, November 15). Overrated career: Psychologist. *U.S. News and World Report,* 51–52.

Novotney, A. (2010). Integrated care is nothing new for these psychologists. *Monitor on Psychology, 41*(1), 41–45.

Reese, R. J., Norsworthy, L. A., & Rowlands, S. R. (2009). Does a continuous feedback system improve psychotherapy outcomes? *Psychotherapy: Theory, Practice, Training, 46*(4), 418–431.

Thirteen

Trends in Behavioral Healthcare for an Aging America

CHRISTINA GARRISON-DIEHN, CLAIR RUMMEL,
CASEY CATLIN, AND JANE E. FISHER

INTRODUCTION

The population of the United States is on the edge of a major demographic transformation. The current system is on track to be overwhelmed by financial burden and a workforce of providers unprepared to meet the behavioral health needs of the largest group of older adults in U.S. history.

The behavioral health of older adults often compromises chronic disease, polypharmacy, and powerful life transitions including the deaths of family members and friends, retirement, and relocation. Rarely do graduate programs provide instruction or clinical training in evidence-based assessment and treatment of problems in late life. With the demographic transformation, training programs and behavioral health providers must become more responsive in preparing providers to address the behavioral health needs of older adults. This chapter will review the demographics of the U.S. aging population, explore prevalent age-associated physical and behavioral health problems, and discuss the implications of recent trends for identifying and prescribing needed treatment reforms.

THE DEMOGRAPHIC SHIFT

Currently, close to 39 million individuals are age 65 or over, comprising 12.8% of the total population (U.S. Administration on Aging [AoA], 2009); by 2030, there will be over 72 million older adults, accounting for 19.3% of the population. Individuals aged 85 or older will continue to comprise the most rapidly growing segment of the population (U.S. Administration on Aging, 2009).

The older adult population will also become more ethnically and racially diverse in the coming years. In 2003, 83% of older adults living in the United States were non-Hispanic White, 8% were non-Hispanic Black, 6% were Hispanic, and 3% were Asian. The projections for 2030 indicate a significant change, with 72% of older adults non-Hispanic White, 11% Hispanic, 10% non-Hispanic Black, and 5% Asian (Centers for Disease Control [CDC], 2007). This shift toward a more diverse older adult population highlights the importance of multicultural training for service providers, as well as the need for providers who are able to provide behavioral health services in languages other than English.

Rural areas have a higher proportion of older adults than the rest of the country. This has been attributed to a migration of younger populations to urban areas, along with an immigration of older, retired individuals (Crowther, Scogin, & Norton, 2010). Overall, 25% of the older adult population lives in rural areas (National Advisory Committee on Rural Health and Human Services, 2004), where it is common for behavioral health services to be limited or unavailable. In order to meet the needs of the older adult population living in rural areas, treatment reform in increasing accessibility to behavioral health services will be important. The increased penetration of the Internet within rural households and baby boomers' familiarity with computer technology and Web-based services point to an historically unprecedented means of delivering information and services to isolated older adults in rural communities.

HEALTHCARE SPENDING AND MEDICARE

As the population ages, the United States will be confronted with the greatest incidence of age-related health problems in history. With this increase in incidence will come a dramatic increase in healthcare spending. The cost of providing healthcare for an older American is 3.3 to 5.6 times greater than the cost for someone under the age of 65 (Centers for Medicare & Medicaid Services, 2010). Projections for the next 10 years reveal that, by the year 2019, spending growth for Medicare is expected to increase on average 6.9% annually (Centers for Medicare & Medicaid Services, 2010). Healthcare spending in the United States is projected to increase by 25% by 2030 due to these demographic shifts (CDC, 2003). Clearly, there is a strong economic incentive for action.

Access to healthcare providers in the Medicare system is currently an area of concern for Medicare beneficiaries. The Medicare Payment Advisory Commission (MEDPAC, 2010) reports that, in 2009, 22% of Medicare beneficiaries seeking a new primary care provider (PCP) reported problems finding physicians accepting new Medicare patients. The American Medical Association (AMA, 2009) labeled 21 states and the District of Columbia as "hot spots" for Medicare beneficiaries experiencing problems accessing Medicare physicians.

The AMA's objective measures of access problems included issues like low percentage of practicing physicians per 1,000 Medicare beneficiaries, a significant percentage of the Medicare population living under 150% of the poverty line, a significant percentage of the Medicare population living in an area with limited access to PCPs, low number of hospitals per 1,000 Medicare beneficiaries, and a lack of healthcare-seeking behavior of Medicare beneficiaries in the past 12 months due to cost (AMA, 2009). A survey of over 9,000 physicians found that 31% of PCPs reported restricting the number of Medicare patients they accept (AMA, 2010). Inadequate Medicare reimbursement was the primary reason physicians gave for limiting patients; the second most common reason was concern about the future instability of the Medicare system.

MEDPAC (2008), an advisory committee to Congress on Medicare issues, has suggested promoting the use of PCPs as a way to improve the Medicare healthcare system, citing studies that report positive performance outcomes in geographic areas with more PCPs per capita. MEDPAC (2008) also cites studies that conversely show that when an area is highly reliant on specialized healthcare providers, there is an increase of healthcare spending, without benefits such as improved access, health outcomes, or patient satisfaction.

The behavioral health field is also experiencing provider access problems within the Medicare system. The American Psychological Association (APA, 2010) reports that 50% of psychologists do not accept Medicare reimbursement, with low reimbursement rates specified by 23% of nonproviders as the reason why they did not accept Medicare (nonappropriate case load was cited by 30%). Chiles, Lambert, and Hatch (1999) conducted a meta-analysis of 91 studies of various behavioral health treatments in patients undergoing medical procedures, medically high-utilizing patients, and patients being treated only for behavioral health issues. The meta-analysis found that average savings to medical cost from the behavioral health intervention was 20%; one third of the studies reported significant savings even after the cost of the behavioral health treatment was taken into account. These findings indicate that behavioral health treatment can contribute to lower healthcare costs and should be taken into account in the Medicare system and healthcare system in general.

PHYSICAL HEALTH

Individuals are living longer with chronic diseases. The coupling of increased longevity and newer healthcare technologies that allow older adults to live for decades with chronic disease is a significant driver of healthcare costs. The average life expectancy at birth increased by 8.2 years between 1960 and 2010 (Organization for Economic Cooperation and Development, 2009). This boon in life expectancy is due in large part to advances in medical care and prevention efforts, which have also resulted in an epidemiologic shift of the leading causes of death, from infectious disease and acute illness to chronic disease and degenerative illness (CDC, 2003). In 2007 the top five causes of death for U.S. adults aged 65 or older were heart disease (28%), malignant neoplasms (22%), cerebrovascular diseases (6%), chronic lower respiratory diseases (6%), and Alzheimer's disease (4%) (Xu, Kochanek, & Tejada-Vera, 2009).

Close to half of all Americans suffer from one or more chronic diseases, which disproportionately affect older adults (CDC, 2009b). Approximately 80% of older adults in the United States are living with at least one chronic condition and 50% have at least two (CDC, 2003). The treatment of chronic disease within the older adult population accounts for almost 95% of their healthcare expenditures (CDC, 2003; Hoffman, Rice, & Sung, 1996). Approximately 1 in 5 U.S. healthcare dollars is spent caring for an individual with diabetes and approximately 1 in 10 healthcare dollars is attributed to diabetes (American Diabetes Association, 2008). Currently, close to a quarter (23.1%) of persons over the age of 60 have diabetes (CDC, 2008). Projections show that the incidence of diabetes will continue to grow with aging of the population; the largest increases are expected among persons 75 or older—from 1.2 million women and 0.8 million men in 2000 to 4.4 million women and 4.2 million men in 2050 (Boyle et al., 2001). On average, individuals with diabetes have medical expenditures approximately 2.3 times higher than individuals without diabetes (American Diabetes Association, 2008).

In addition to the increased healthcare costs, chronic diseases place a heavy burden on older adults with the condition and those caring for them. The risk of behavioral health issues such as depression increases when functioning is impaired by disease (National Institute of Mental Health, 2007). The CDC (2007) stated in a report on aging and health in America that "these conditions can cause years of pain, disability and loss of function and independence before resulting in death" (p. 4). Arthritis, the most common cause of disability in the United States, is a key example of a chronic disease that leads to a high rate of chronic pain, activity limitation, reduced quality of life, and high healthcare costs for older adults (CDC, 2006, 2009a). Currently, an estimated 21.6% (46.4 million) of the adult U.S. population have been diagnosed with arthritis (CDC, 2009b). Due to the aging of the U.S. population and an increase in the number of obese individuals, an estimated 67 million adults will be affected by arthritis by 2030 (CDC, 2007; Hootman & Helmick, 2006).

Behavioral medicine is a component of behavioral healthcare that focuses on improving health and preventing chronic disease (Oldenburg, 2002). Lifestyle changes are promoted to prevent or reduce chronic disease such as diabetes and heart disease. These often include behavior changes such as smoking cessation, diet modification, and promotion of exercise (Smith, Nealey, & Hamann, 2000). Given the preceding statistics on chronic disease prevalence, the reduction and/or prevention of excess disability in older adults with chronic disease will become even more important in improving older adults' overall health and reducing overall healthcare costs.

DEMENTIA

Over the past several decades, dementia has emerged as a major form of disability for older adults. In the United States, close to 5.3 million Americans have Alzheimer's disease (AD), the most common form of dementia (Alzheimer's Association, 2009). To put this number in perspective, one person in eight aged 65 or older in the United States is affected and the disease is the fifth leading cause of death for older adults (Xu et al., 2009). The direct costs of dementia amount to more than $112 billion dollars annually (Lewin Group, 2004); indirect costs exceed $35 million (Koppel, 2002; Alzheimer's Association, 2009).

Future projections reveal that the financial and emotional burdens of caring for individuals with dementia will continue to rise because the number of individuals aged 65 and older with AD is estimated to reach between 11 and 16 million by 2050, barring a breakthrough in prevention and treatment (Hebert, Beckett, Scherr, & Evans, 2001). The influx of individuals with dementia will put a vast strain on the healthcare system because older adults with AD use significantly more healthcare services, especially hospital stays, than older adults without AD (Alzheimer's Association, 2008).

LIFE-HISTORY FACTORS AND BEHAVIORAL HEALTH

Historically, older adults have utilized behavioral health services at lower rates than younger cohorts. The 1985 report of the National Institute of Mental Health Epidemiological Catchment Area Program found that just 4.2% of individuals aged 65–74 and 1.4% of individuals aged 75 and older received mental health treatment, in contrast to 8.7% of individuals aged 18–64 (German, Shapiro, & Skinner, 1985). This disparity in utilization rates has been diminishing and will continue over the next decades.

The National Comorbidity Survey Replication (NCS-R) is a population-based probability sample composed of 9,282 adult participants, collected between February 2001 and April 2003 (Byers, Yaffe, Covinsky, Friedman, & Bruce, 2010; Kessler et al., 2005; Wang et al., 2005). The findings of this sample indicate that individuals aged 45–59 were 2.5 times as likely to receive specialty behavioral health treatment as individuals aged 60 and older (Wang et al., 2005). Mackenzie, Popejoy, Petroski, Mehr, and Rantz (2008) found that within a subsample of the NCS-R ($N = 5,692$), only 0.6% of adults aged 75 and older had sought mental health services in their lifetime; the lifetime utilization rate increased with younger cohorts. The study found that 1.8% of adults aged 65–74, 3.6% of adults aged 55–64, and 5.7% of adults aged 45–54 had received mental health services over their lifetimes.

It is often hypothesized that lower utilization of services by older adults is due to stigmatization of behavioral health services (Quinn, Laidlaw, & Murray, 2009; Segal, Coolidge, Mincic, & O'Riley, 2005). The higher utilization rates in younger cohorts could indicate less stigmatization of behavioral health services, which would be expected to stay constant as the cohort ages. If this is the case, as younger cohorts age, they can be expected to utilize behavioral health services at similar rates across their life spans.

Importantly, older adults are more likely to discuss behavioral health problems with their PCP than with a behavioral health provider. Older adults are more likely to make an appointment with their PCP when experiencing behavioral health issues as they manifest in more physical symptoms (Blazer, 1996; Kravitz et al., 2006; Speer & Schneider, 2003). Unfortunately, PCPs often fail to identify 50% of behavioral health problems and only refer 40% of patients with such problems to behavioral health providers (Speer & Schneider, 2003). Pickard and Tang (2009) surveyed 317 older adults in a Midwestern community and found participants were more likely to make an appointment with a clergy person than with a clinician when seeking behavioral health counseling. In light of these findings, collaboration between PCPs and clergy is an apparent point of intervention in increasing appropriate behavioral health services among older adults.

The discrepancy between older and younger adult utilization of behavioral healthcare does not stem from a lack of need among older adults. Studies have indicated that 12% of community-dwelling older adults meet the criteria for at least one clinical diagnosis (Gatz, Kasl-Godley, & Karel, 1996; Regier, Boyd, Burke, & Rae, 1988). In examining the NCS-R findings, Byers and colleagues (2010) found that while the likelihood of having a mood or anxiety disorder decreased with age, still, 5% of older adults met diagnostic criteria for a mood disorder, and 12% met criteria for an anxiety disorder. Seitz, Purandare, and Conn (2010) conducted a meta-analysis of studies reporting on rates of behavioral health problems in long-term-care facilities and found that the average prevalence of major depressive disorder was 10% and the average prevalence of depressive symptoms was 29%.

Major depression declines with age, but depressive symptoms have been found to increase over the life span (American Association for Geriatric Psychiatry, 2008). Clinically significant depressive symptoms have an estimated prevalence rate of 15–25% in adults over 65 (Jeste et al., 1999). The risk of depression increases with the addition of illnesses that lead to functional impairments, such as the common occurrence of chronic disease in older adults. Depression in this population remains largely under-recognized and undertreated (National Institute of Mental Health, 2007), resulting in decreased quality of life and increases in healthcare spending. In a recent analysis of healthcare costs for close to 15,000 Medicare recipients with diabetes and/or congestive heart failure, individuals with depression had significantly higher total healthcare costs over a 12-month period than those without depression: $20,046 versus $11,956, respectively (Unützer et al., 2009). Interestingly, depressed individuals had higher healthcare costs across all categories except specialty mental health services, which accounted for less than 1% of total costs.

Substance abuse by older adults is expected to increase significantly in the coming decades. The Substance Abuse and Mental Health Services Administration (SAMHSA, 2010) reports this trend has already begun, citing that, in 1992, persons aged 50 and older represented 6.6% of all substance abuse admissions compared to 12.2% of all substance abuse admissions in 2008. Historically, alcohol abuse and prescription drug abuse have been the most common substances abused by older adults, with estimates of up to 17% (U.S. Department of Health and Human Services Treatment Improvement Protocol, 1998). The SAMHSA (2010) report shows a shift in what substances are being abused by older adults, indicating that the percentage of substance abuse admissions for alcohol abuse decreased from 84.6 to 59.9%, while all other substance types, including heroin, cocaine, and prescription pain relievers, increased in this time period. Illegal substance use by older adults has traditionally occurred at much lower rates, from less than 1% to 2.2%, but the rate is expected to increase to 3.3% by 2020 (Caracci & Miller, 1991; Colliver, Compton, Gfroerer, & Condon, 2006). Substance abuse of all types is projected to double in adults over the age of 50, from 2.5 million in 1999 to 5 million in 2020 (Gfroerer, Penne, Pemberton, & Folsom, 2002).

Suicide is also a critical issue in treating older adults due to the disproportionate percentage of completed suicides per year in this age group. In 2004, individuals aged 65 and older comprised 12% of the population, but accounted for 16% of completed suicides. Non-Hispanic White men were the most likely to die of suicide, with 49.8 out of 100,000 in that age group; this is significantly higher than the general population rate of 11 out of 100,000 (CDC, 2005). Risk factors for suicide in older adults include stressful life events, substance abuse, and physical illness; however, physical illness's effect appears to be mediated by depressive disorders—the greatest risk factor for suicide in older adults (Conwell, Duberstein, & Caine, 2002).

Other Issues Impacting Behavioral Health

The concepts of *primary* and *secondary* aging have been used to describe changes in physical and psychological functioning across the life span (Busse, 1969). Primary aging is defined as normal, disease-free, age-related changes in physical and psychological functioning. Secondary aging effects are those due to disease, environmental factors, disuse, or abuse (Busse, 1969). A large body of research has documented the risk factors for secondary aging effects and the benefits of programs that target these factors. Behavioral health problems often lead to (through diet, exercise, or lifestyle factors) or co-occur with secondary aging effects.

Preparing behavioral health specialists to discriminate accurately between primary aging and secondary aging effects is critical for the prevention or reversal of excess disability in older adults. For example, depression in older adults is commonly associated with cognitive declines, reduced activity, and poor health outcomes (Kertzman et al., 2010). If the symptoms of depression in an older adult are misinterpreted as normal aging and hence left untreated, the resultant poorer quality of life perpetuates the risk of depression.

Activity and secondary aging effects. The saying "use it or lose it" captures the relationship between physical and cognitive activity and the prevention of secondary aging effects. Research has shown that avoiding "disuse" of one's physical and cognitive capacity through physical and cognitive activity has protective effects against disease as well as physical and cognitive decline (e.g., Bean, Vora, & Frontera, 2004; Ben-Sira & Oliveira, 2007; Larson et al., 2006; Liu-Ambrose et al., 2010.).

Medication and secondary aging effects. Polypharmacy is standard practice within the medical care of older adults. The potential for misuse or abuse of medication in older adults is strikingly high. Qato and colleagues (2008) found that 29% of older adults were taking at least five prescription drugs concurrently in a nationally representative probability sample of persons aged 57–85. The complexity of polypharmacy increased with age in the sample, with 36% of women and 37.1% of men aged 75–85 taking five or more prescription drugs.

Qato and colleagues (2008) also examined the use of over-the-counter drugs and dietary supplements in conjunction with prescription drugs and found that 46% of the sample used at least one over-the-counter drug and 52% used at least one dietary supplement along with their prescription drugs. Their results indicate that 4% of the sample or nearly 1 in 25 individuals was at risk for a major drug–drug interaction, with half of those at risk due to the use of nonprescription medications.

Adverse drug reactions and events are common in older adults. Moore, Cohen, and Furberg (2007) found that of adverse drug events reported to the FDA from 1998 to 2005, more than one third occurred in older adults. Kongkaew, Noyce, and Ashcroft (2008) conducted a meta-analysis of hospital admissions associated with or due to adverse drug reactions and found that risk increased with age; an average of 10.7% of older adult hospital admissions were associated with or caused by adverse drug reactions, compared to 4.1% for children and 6.3% for adults. Increased risk factors for adverse drug reactions include depression, mobility issues, number of drugs prescribed, number of comorbidities, and specific drug types, including psychotropic, anti-infective, and anticoagulant (Cecile et al., 2009; Field et al., 2001; Field, Mazor, Briesacher, Debellis, & Gurwitz, 2007; Gurwitz et al., 2000).

According to Gurwitz and colleagues (2000), adverse drug events involve the physical domain, including rashes, falls, and hemorrhage, as well as the neuropsychiatric domain, including oversedation and delirium. They found that 51% of adverse drug events that occurred in their sample ($N = 28,839$) were preventable, with neuropsychiatric events being the most common types of preventable adverse drug event. Preventable adverse drug interactions include inappropriate prescription, suboptimal prescription of a drug, and misuse or abuse by the individual (Field et al., 2007; Gurwitz et al., 2000; Kaur, Mitchell, Vitetta, & Roberts, 2009). Field and colleagues (2007) found that there is an increased risk of adverse drug events due to misuse or abuse among older adults with the increased number of prescribed drugs and with a higher score on a comorbidity scale. Due to the prevalence and associated risks of polypharmacy, behavioral health clinicians should assume that medications will be an issue when working with the older adult population and assess for possible misuse or abuse of prescription drugs.

Excess Disability in Dementia
Excess disability occurs when an individual experiences functional impairment that is inconsistent with what can be directly attributed to disease (Dawson, Wells, & Kline, 1993).

This excessive deficit is more impairment than would be expected, given the person's history and current diagnosis (Fisher, Drossel, Yury, & Cherup, 2007), and can be caused by several conditions, including depression, medication side effects, delirium, and social isolation (Eastham & Jeste, 1996; Fick & Foreman, 2000; Ritchie, Touchon, & Ledésert, 1998; Yury & Fisher, 2007). Excess disability can also result from environmental factors like insufficient reinforcement for adaptive behaviors, punishment, or aversive consequences of adaptive behaviors (Buchanan & Fisher, 2002). An example of environmental factors causing excess disability is a nursing home resident who is socially avoided by staff due to a history of inappropriate statements and consequently loses verbal functioning due to misuse.

Excess disability may be avoided or treated if properly detected by caregivers or health professionals. It can be difficult for caregivers to distinguish between expected declines and excess disability, but progress has been made in monitoring stable, high-frequency adaptive behaviors, which, when suddenly absent, may indicate excess disability (Garrison-Diehn, Rummel, Catlin, & Fisher, 2009). Detecting and treating the cause of excess disability is an important area of increasing or maintaining the quality of life for a person with dementia.

SERVICE DELIVERY: IMPROVING ON TRADITIONAL MODELS

Evidence indicates that several empirically supported treatments, such as cognitive behavioral therapy for depression and anxiety, are just as effective in the older adult population as they are in the general adult population (Knight, Kaskie, Shurgot, & Dave, 2006). In addition to delivering empirically supported treatments, providers must consider health issues, such as pain status and medication use, that can affect the individual's behavioral health and quality of life. To adapt to the behavioral health needs of this population, providers should be flexible in moving away from the traditional 50-minute office session mode of service delivery. Mobility issues are common with medical comorbidities and age-associated visual changes.

Further, a large percentage of older adults reside in rural areas. Providing services in settings that are accessible, such as in an integrated-care model where the behavioral health professional is colocated in the primary care setting or within consumers' homes, will increase acceptability. Providing services in a consumer's residence—whether that is a home, a group home, assisted living facility, or long-term care facility—not only increases the likelihood that services will be received but also gives the professional a unique glimpse into the individual's home environment and the opportunity to observe environmental influences and behavioral responses.

Case Examples: Home-Based Services

The *Program to Encourage Active, Rewarding Lives for Seniors (PEARLS)* intervention is an empirically supported, home-based program aimed at the treatment of minor depression and dysthymia in older adults. The program is funded by the Centers for Disease Control and is tailored specifically for chronically ill, low-income, and homebound individuals. The program includes structured home visits to individuals by service providers, increasing activation in social and physical domains, problem-solving treatment, and recommendations to PCPs about psychotropic medication (Ciechanowski et al., 2004). A randomized controlled trial found that, compared to a treatment-as-usual group, individuals receiving the PEARLS intervention were more likely to experience a reduction or remission of depression symptoms and an increase in both emotional and functional well-being (Ciechanowski et al., 2004).

Case Examples: Integrated Care

A simple definition of integrated care is when behavioral health services are colocated and provided collaboratively with primary care services (Bartels et al., 2004). Integrated care of older adults has shown positive results in reducing overall healthcare costs (Chiles et al., 1999) and also shown positive evidence for reducing behavioral health issues. Unützer and colleagues (2002) compared an integrated-care model, *IMPACT* (*improving mood—promoting access to collaborative treatment*), with a treatment-as-usual condition in a randomized control study of 1,801 participants. Participants were tracked for 12 months after intervention began and the results showed that, in the IMPACT intervention group, 45% of participants had a 50% or greater reduction in their depressive symptoms, compared to 19% of participants in the treatment-as-usual condition. The IMPACT intervention group also showed higher rates of depression treatment, higher rates of satisfaction with depression care, less functional impairment, and higher quality-of-life ratings.

The PRISM-E study, a multisite, randomized trial, compared the effects of an integrated-care model versus an enhanced referral care model on depression, anxiety, and substance abuse in an older adult population (Bartels et al., 2004; Krahn et al., 2006; Levkoff et al., 2004; Oslin et al., 2006). The study randomized 2,022 participants who met the criteria for depression, anxiety, and/or at-risk drinking behavior into either an integrated-care group, where mental health specialists were colocated with the primary care office, or an enhanced-referral group, where transportation, case management, and other services to increase older adult service utilization were added to the traditional primary care referral system. Bartels and colleagues (2004) found that 71% of participants in the integrated-care condition engaged in mental health and substance abuse treatment, compared to 49% in the enhanced-referral condition. The integrated-care condition was also associated with higher rates of mental health and substance abuse visits per participant than was the enhanced referral condition (Bartels et al., 2004).

Gallo and colleagues (2004) surveyed 127 primary care clinicians, including PCPs, nurse practitioners, and physician's assistants, who took part of the PRISM-E study. The surveyed clinicians indicated that they strongly preferred the integrated-care model over the enhanced-referral model. They cited a greater convenience for patients and less stigma attached to mental health services when provided in the primary care location (Gallo et al., 2004).

The PRISM-E study found similar clinical outcomes for depression and substance abuse (Krahn et al., 2006; Oslin et al., 2006). Krahn and colleagues (2006) found that *participants across diagnostic groups* (dysthymia, minor depression, and depression not otherwise specified at baseline) experienced similar reductions in the severity of depression. Among participants who met criteria for major depression at baseline, the enhanced-referral condition was associated with slightly better symptomatic outcomes, but had similar remission rates and functional outcomes. Oslin and colleagues (2006) found that, across both conditions, participants who met criteria for at-risk alcohol use reported lower levels of weekly and binge drinking, with no significant difference between the conditions.

Bruce and colleagues (2004) conducted a randomized control trial of an integrated-care model, *prevention of suicide in primary care elderly: collaborative trial* (*PROSPECT*), versus a treatment-as-usual condition. The study found that participants in the integrated-care condition experienced faster declines in suicidal ideation than the treatment-as-usual group did. The study also found a positive impact on depression symptoms, response to depression treatment, and remission of depression in the integrated-care condition (Bruce et al., 2004).

Case Examples: Stepped Care

According to Bower and Gilbody (2005), stepped care is a model of service delivery that has been implemented and studied in healthcare as an answer to the problem of increased demand for services and limited supply of providers. They suggest that there are two fundamental features to stepped-care service delivery. First, recommended treatment within the model should be the least restrictive of the available choices, with "least restrictive" referring to cost and personal inconvenience to the patient. Second, the model corrects itself, in that treatment targets are systematically monitored and changes in service delivery ("stepping up") are made if the current level of service is not producing treatment targets. An example of a treatment "staircase" is self-help through computerized treatments and bibliotherapy, followed by guided self-help from a mental-health worker, followed by individual therapy from a mental-health professional (Bower & Gilbody, 2005).

Hegel and colleagues (2002) report on the stepped-care model for depression in the IMPACT study (see the preceding section on integrated care). In the IMPACT study, depression clinical specialists (DCSs) were assigned to each participant in the integrated-care condition. The DCSs coordinated and monitored the treatment delivery of the participants within the stepped-care model. The steps in the IMPACT study consisted of either antidepressant medication or problem-solving therapy for primary care (PST-PC), a modified problem-solving therapy that involves four to eight 30-minute sessions, after an initial 60-minute session. Participants were educated about the treatment options and chose which treatment they would like as their "step one." DCSs monitored treatment adherence and targets and, at the end of 8–12 weeks, participants not meeting treatment targets were given either the other treatment they did not choose or a combination of medication and PST-PC as "step two." After 10 weeks of step two, participants who were still not meeting targets were given a psychiatric consult and additional treatment changes (Hegel et al., 2002).

Van't Veer-Tazelaar and colleagues (2010) report on a randomized trial of the effectiveness of a stepped-care intervention for subthreshold anxiety and depression in older adults in the Netherlands. The "steps" in the trial included "watchful waiting," bibliotherapy, problem-solving treatment, and antidepressant medication. Outcomes of each step were monitored every 3 months to determine if the participant would "step up." Results indicated that the stepped-care intervention reduced the incidence rate of anxiety and depression by 50% compared to treatment as usual over a 12-month period.

E-health

Seeking health information online is popular among Internet users (Baker, Wagner, Singer, & Bundorf, 2003; Powell & Clarke, 2002). Computer and Internet usage in older adult households are becoming more common. The Pew Research Center conducted a survey in 2009 of Internet usage by demographics, finding that currently 38% of individuals aged 65 and older use the Internet, compared to 70% of individuals aged 50–64, a good portion of the baby boomer cohort (Pew Internet and American Life Project, 2009). Thousands of Web sites and forums offer treatment and diagnoses information, actual treatment, and social support. This surplus of accessibility has both benefits and drawbacks. Some benefits include fast access to information, increased access to service delivery, and opportunity for more informed treatment choices by the consumer. Some drawbacks are a lack of regulation of information quality and the services being offered and privacy concerns (Cleary, Walter, & Matheson, 2008; Eysenbach, Powell, Kuss, & Sa, 2002).

Since the late 1990s when Internet usage became more common, there has been much discussion about quality indicators for healthcare information Web sites (Boyer, Selby, Scherrer, & Appel, 1998; Monahan & Colthurst, 2001; Silberg, Lundberg, & Mussacchio, 1997). Currently, the Health on the Net Foundation offers Internet searches through its Web site that bring users to Web sites that have passed its inspection for ethical standards of information presentation and where the source and purpose of information are clear to the user (Boyer, Gaudinat, Baujard, & Geissbühler, 2007). Charnock, Shepperd, Needham, and Gann (1999) developed a tool for behavioral health providers to determine if an Internet publication contains low- or high-quality information. This type of regulation will be necessary for consumers searching for empirically based treatments and for behavioral health providers recommending Internet material for education or as a supplement to treatment.

Cleary and colleagues (2008) summarize findings in e-behavioral health services indicating that Internet-based treatments have been shown to improve some behavioral health issues, such as depression. With the increase of Internet usage in the older adult population, e-health services for behavioral health issues could be an answer to service delivery barriers such as rural populations and individuals with limited mobility.

Behavioral Health and Aging in Place

The majority of older adults prefer to stay in their homes for as long as possible, to "age in place" (Callahan, 1992) in the gerontology literature—a term used to refer to individuals staying in their home by modifying the environment with prosthetics and enhancing support to compensate for sensory, cognitive, and/or physical declines. There are both psychological and economic benefits to the individual in an "aging in place" model.

Economically, living in a skilled nursing facility is associated with the highest healthcare costs for older adults. At age 65, a married couple without chronic disease will spend, on average, $197,000 on uninsured healthcare cost for the remainder of their lives, including insurance premiums, out-of-pocket costs, and home-health costs, excluding nursing home care, with a 5% probability that cost will exceed $311,000. If nursing home care is included, the average cost jumps to $260,000, with a 5% probability that cost will exceed $570,000 (Webb & Zhivan, 2010).

Approximately 15% of skilled nursing facility residents have been estimated to have been placed inappropriately due to (1) public financing favoring nursing home placement, (2) state regulations that reduce options, and (3) a lack of agreement among decision makers about the best setting for the individual (Marek, Popejoy, Petroski, Mehr, & Rantz, 2005; Spector, Reschovsky, & Cohen, 1996). The national average of nursing facility costs is $198/day, while alternatives such as assisted living facilities cost $3,131/month and adult day care health centers cost $67/day. These figures have provided incentives for federal and state governments to provide services for older adults that prevent the need for more costly residential care (U.S. Department of Health and Human Services, 2009).

Marek and colleagues (2005) matched patients receiving community-based nursing services with patients living in a nursing home setting and found that the community patients showed stable or improved outcomes in areas such as cognitions, depression, activities of daily living, and incontinence;

the nursing-home patient group showed deteriorated outcomes. These functional outcomes provide the individual with quality-of-life incentives for staying in the home setting.

Behavioral health providers can play an important role in helping individuals age in place. Some of the important tools providers can offer include detection of excess disability, helping caregivers manage challenging behaviors of individuals with dementia, services that prevent or decrease common behavioral health problems, and behavioral management plans for lifestyle changes to reduce and prevent symptoms of chronic disease.

FUTURE DIRECTIONS

As the population shifts toward an aging society, it is necessary that the behavioral health field move away from traditional models of service delivery toward models that meet the needs of older adults. Evidence suggests this may be accomplished through integrated-care models, stepped-care models, and changing perspectives of where service is delivered, whether in the individual's home or through technology. Three important areas will make a difference in changing the way behavioral healthcare services are delivered: public policy, research resources, and education.

Public policy should prioritize the support of behavioral healthcare for older adults due to the benefits of reducing and/or preventing both behavioral health problems and healthcare costs. Research resources should be spent on identifying and improving service delivery systems for disseminating evidence-based behavioral healthcare to older adults. Finally, there must be an emphasis on educating behavioral health and healthcare workers and providers in behavioral healthcare for older adults in order to meet the needs of this soon to be substantial portion of the population.

REFERENCES

Alzheimer's Association. (2008). Alzheimer's disease facts and figures. *Alzheimer's & Dementia, 4*(2), 1–41.

Alzheimer's Association. (2009). 2009 Alzheimer's disease facts and figures. *Alzheimer's & Dementia, 5,* 234–270.

American Association for Geriatric Psychiatry. (2008). *Geriatrics and mental health—The facts.* Retrieved from http://www.aagponline.org/prof/facts_mh.asp

American Diabetes Association. (2008). Economic costs of diabetes in the U.S. in 2007. *Diabetes Care, 31*(3), 596–615.

AMA (American Medical Association). (2009). *AMA releases 22 new "patient access hot spots" nationwide—Medicare cuts to physicians will make problems works.* Retrieved from http://www.ama-assn.org/ama/pub/news/news/patient-access-hot-spots.shtml

AMA (American Medical Association). (2010). *AMA online survey of physicians: The impact of Medicare physician payment to seniors' access to care.* Retrieved from http://www.ama-assn.org/ama1/pub/upload/mm/399/medicare-survey-results.pdf

APA (American Psychological Association). (2010). *2008 Survey of psychology health services providers.* Retrieved from http://www.apa.org/workforce/publications/08-hsp/report.pdf

Baker, L., Wagner, T. H., Singer, S., & Bundorf, M. K. (2003). Use of the Internet and e-mail for health care information: Results form a national survey. *Journal of the American Medical Association, 289,* 2400–2406.

Bartels, S. J., Coakley, E. H., Zubritsky, C., Ware, J. H., Miles, K. M., Areán, P. A., & Levkoff, S. E. (2004). Improving access to geriatric mental health services: A randomized trial comparing treatment engagement with integrated versus enhanced referral care for depression, anxiety, and at-risk alcohol use. *American Journal of Psychiatry, 161,* 1455–1462.

Bean, J. F., Vora, A., & Frontera, W. R. (2004). Benefits of exercise for community-dwelling older adults. *Archives of Physical Medicine and Rehabilitation, 85,* S31–S42.

Ben-Sira, D., & Oliveira, J. M. F. (2007). Hypertension in aging: Physical activity as primary prevention. *European Review of Aging and Physical Activity, 4*(2), 85–89.

Blazer, D. (1996). The danger of reducing reimbursement for psychiatric disorders in late life. *American Journal of Psychiatry, 153*(7), 857–859.

Bower, P., & Gilbody, S. (2005). Stepped care in psychological therapies: Access, effectiveness and efficiency. *British Journal of Psychiatry, 186,* 11–17.

Boyer, C., Gaudinat, A., Baujard, V., & Geissbühler, A. (2007). Health on the net foundation: Assessing the quality of health Web pages all over the world. *Studies in Health Technologies and Informatics, 129*(2), 1017–1021.

Boyer, C., Selby, M., Scherrer, J. R., & Appel, R. D. (1998). The health on the net code of conduct for medical and health Web sites. *Computers in Biology and Medicine, 28*(5), 602–610.

Boyle, J. P., Honeycutt, A. A., Narayan, K. M., Hoerger, T. J., Geiss, L. S., Chen, H., & Thompson, T. J. (2001). Projection of diabetes burden through 2050: Impact of changing demography and disease prevalence in the U.S. *Diabetes Care, 24,* 1936–1940.

Bruce, M. L., Ten Have, T. R., Reynolds, C. F., III, Katz, I. I., Shulberg, H. C., Mulsant, B. H., & Alexopoulos, G. S. (2004). Reducing suicidal ideation and depressive symptoms in depressed older primary care patients: A randomized controlled trial. *Journal of the American Medical Association, 291*(9), 1081–1091.

Buchanan, J., & Fisher, J. (2002). Functional assessment and noncontingent reinforcement in the treatment of disruptive vocalization in elderly dementia patients. *Journal of Applied Behavior Analysis, 35*(1), 99–103.

Busse, E. W. (1969). Theories of aging. In E. W. Busse & E. Pfeiffer (Eds.), *Behavior and adaptation in later life* (pp. 11–32). Boston, MA: Little, Brown.

Byers, A. L., Yaffe, K., Covinsky, K. E., Friedman, M. B., & Bruce, M. L. (2010). High occurrence of mood and anxiety disorders among older adults: The national comorbidity survey replication. *Archives of General Psychiatry, 67*(5), 489–496.

Callahan, J. J. (1992). Aging in place. *Generations, 16,* 5–6.

Caracci, G., & Miller, N. (1991). Epidemiology and diagnosis of alcoholism in the elderly (a review). *International Journal of Geriatric Psychiatry, 6*(7), 511–515.

Carstensen, L. L. (1992). Social and emotional patterns in adulthood: Support for socioemotional selectivity theory. *Psychology and Aging, 7,* 331–338.

Cecile, M., Seux, V., Pauly, V., Tassy, S., Reynaud-Levy, O., Dalco, O., & Retornaz, F. (2009). Adverse drug events in hospitalized elderly patients in a geriatric medicine unit: study of prevalence and risk factors. *Revue de Medecine Interne, 30*(5), 393–400.

CDC (Centers for Disease Control and Prevention). (2003). Public health and aging: trends in aging—United States and worldwide. *Morbidity and Mortality Weekly Report, 52*(6), 101–106.

CDC (Centers for Disease Control and Prevention). (2005). National Center for Injury Prevention and Control. *Web-based injury statistics query and reporting system (WISQARS)*. Retrieved from www.cdc.gov/ncipc/wisqars

CDC (Centers for Disease Control and Prevention). (2006). Prevalence of doctor-diagnosed arthritis and arthritis-attributable activity limitation—United States, 2003–2005. *Morbidity and Mortality Weekly Report, 55*(40), 1089–1092.

CDC (Centers for Disease Control and Prevention). (2008). *National diabetes fact sheet: General information and national estimates on diabetes in the United States, 2007*. Retrieved from http://www.cdc.gov/diabetes/pubs/pdf/ndfs_2007.pdf

CDC (Centers for Disease Control and Prevention). (2009a). Prevalence and most common causes of disability among adults—United States, 2005. *Morbidity and Mortality Weekly Report, 58*(16), 421–426.

CDC (Centers for Disease Control and Prevention). (2009b). *Chronic disease overview*. Retrieved from http://www.cdc.gov/NCCdphp/overview.htm

Centers for Disease Control and Prevention and the Merck Company Foundation. (2007). *The state of aging and health in America 2007*. Retrieved from http://apps.nccd.cdc.gov/SAHA/Default/Default.aspx

Centers for Medicare & Medicaid Services. (2010). National health expenditures projections (2001–2019). Accessed at http://www.cms.gov/NationalHealthExpendData/downloads/proj2009.pdf

Charnock, D., Shepperd, S., Needham, G., & Gann, R. (1999). DISCERN: An instrument for judging the quality of written consumer health information on treatment choices. *Journal of Epidemiology and Community Health, 53*, 105–111.

Chiles, J. A., Lambert, M, J., & Hatch, A. L. (1999). The impact of psychological intervention on medical cost offset: A meta-analytic review. *Clinical Psychology: Science and Practice, 6*(2), 204–220.

Ciechanowski, P., Wagner, E., Schmaling, K., Schwartz, S., Williams, B., Diehr, P., et al. (2004). Community-integrated home-based depression treatment in older adults: A randomized controlled trial. *Journal of the American Medical Association, 291*(13), 1569–1577.

Cleary, M., Walter, G., & Matheson, S. (2008). What is the role of e-technology in mental health services and psychiatric research? *Journal of Psychosocial Nursing and Mental Health Services, 46*(4), 42–48.

Colliver, J. D., Compton, W. M., Gfroerer, J. C., & Condon, T. (2006). Projecting drug use among aging baby boomers in 2020. *Annals of Epidemiology, 16,* 257–265.

Conwell, Y., Duberstein, P. R., & Caine, E. D. (2002). Risk factors of suicide in later life. *Society of Biological Psychiatry, 52,* 193–204.

Crowther, M. R., Scogin, F., & Norton, M. J. (2010). Treating the aged in rural communities: The application of cognitive-behavioral therapy for depression. *Journal of Clinical Psychology: In Session, 66*(5), 502–512.

Dawson, P., Wells, D. L., & Kline, K. (1993). *Enhancing the abilities of persons with Alzheimer's and related dementias: A nursing perspective.* New York, NY: Springer.

Eastham, J. H., & Jeste, D. V. (1996). Differentiating behavioral disturbances of dementia from drug side effects. *International Psychogeriatrics, 8*(3), 429–434.

Eysenbach, G., Powell, J., Kuss, O., & Sa, E. R. (2002). Empirical studies assessing the quality of health information for consumers on the World Wide Web: A systematic review. *Journal of the American Medical Association, 287,* 2691–2700.

Fick, D., & Foreman, M. (2000). Consequences of not recognizing delirium superimposed on dementia in hospitalized elderly individuals. *Journal of Gerontological Nursing, 26*(1), 30–40.

Field, T. S., Gurwitz, J. H., Avorn, J., McCormick, D., Jain, S., Eckler, M.,...Bates, D. W. (2001). Risk factors for adverse drug events among nursing home residents. *Archives of Internal Medicine, 161*(13), 1629–1634.

Field, T. S., Mazor, K. M., Briesacher, B., Debellis, K. R., & Gurwitz, J. H. (2007). Adverse drug events resulting from patient errors in older adults. *Journal of the American Geriatric Society, 55*(2), 271–276.

Fisher, J. E., Drossel, C., Yury, C., & Cherup, S. (2007). A contextual model of restraint free care for persons with dementia. In P. Sturmey (Ed.), *The handbook of functional analysis and clinical psychology.* New York, NY: Elsevier.

Gallo, J., Zubritsky, C., Maxwell, J., Nazar, M., Bogner, H., Quijano, L., et al. (2004). Primary care clinicians evaluate integrated and referral models of behavioral health care for older adults: Results from a multisite effectiveness trial (PRISM-E). *Annals of Family Medicine, 2*(4), 305–309.

Garrison-Diehn, C. G., Rummel, C., Catlin, C., & Fisher, J. E. (2009). A training program to increase detection of excess disability in individuals with dementia. Poster session presented at the Association of Behavioral and Cognitive Therapies Annual Conference, November 2009.

Gatz, M., Kasl-Godley, J., & Karel, M. (1996). Aging and mental disorders. *Handbook of the psychology of aging* (4th ed.) (pp. 365–382). San Diego, CA: Academic Press.

German, P., Shapiro, S., & Skinner, E. (1985). Mental health of the elderly: Use of health and mental health services. *Journal of the American Geriatrics Society, 33*(4), 246–252.

Gfroerer, J. C., Penne, M. A., Pemberton, M. R., & Folsom, R. E. (2002). The aging baby boom cohort and future prevalence of substance abuse. In Substance Abuse and Mental Health Services Administration, Office of Applied Studies. *Substance use by older adults: Estimates of future impact on the treatment system.* OAS Analytic Series #A-21, DHHS publication no. (SMA) 03-3763, Rockville, MD. Retrieved from http://www.oas.samhsa.gov/aging/chap5.htm

Gurwitz, J. H., Field, T. S., Avorn, J., McCormick, D., Jain, S., Eckler, M.,...Bates, D. W. (2000). Incidence and preventability of adverse drug events in nursing homes. *American Journal of Medicine, 109*(2), 87–94.

Hebert, L. E., Beckett, L. A., Scherr, P. A., & Evans, D. A. (2001). Annual incidence of Alzheimer disease in the United States projected to the years 2000 through 2050. *Alzheimer Disease and Associated Disorders, 15,* 169–173.

Hegel, M. T., Imming, J., Cyr-Provost, M., Noel, P. H., Arean, P. A., & Unutzer, J. (2002). Role of behavioral health professionals in a collaborative stepped care treatment model for depression in primary care: Project IMPACT. *Families, Systems & Health, 20*(3), 265–277.

Hoffman, C., Rice, R., & Sung, H. (1996). Persons with chronic disease: Their prevalence and costs. *Journal of the American Medical Association, 276*(18), 1473–1479.

Hootman, J. M., & Helmick, C. G. (2006). Projections of U.S. prevalence of arthritis and associated activity limitations. *Arthritis and Rheumatism, 54*(1), 226–229.

Jeste, D. V., Alexopoulos, G. S., Bartels, S. J., Cummings, J. L., Gallo, J. J., Gottlieb, G. L., et al. (1999). Consensus statement on the upcoming crisis in geriatric mental health: Research agenda for the next two decades. *Archives of General Psychiatry, 56*, 848–853.

Kaur, S., Mitchell, G., Vitetta, L., & Roberts, M. S. (2009). Interventions that can reduce inappropriate prescribing in the elderly: A systematic review. *Drugs & Aging, 26*(12), 1013–1028.

Kertzman, S., Reznik, I., Hornik-Lurie, T., Weizman, A., Kotler, M., & Amital, D. (2010). Stroop performance in major depression: Selective attention impairment or psychomotor slowness? *Journal of Affective Disorders, 122*, 167–173.

Kessler, R., Berglund, P., Demler, O., Jin, R., Merikangas, K., & Walters, E. (2005). Lifetime prevalence and age-of-onset distributions of DSM-IV disorders in the national comorbidity survey replication. *Archives of General Psychiatry, 62*(6), 593–602.

Knight, B., Kaskie, B., Shurgot, G., & Dave, J. (2006). Improving the mental health of older adults. In *Handbook of the psychology of aging* (6th ed.) (pp. 407–424). Amsterdam, the Netherlands: Elsevier.

Kongkaew, C., Noyce, P. R., & Ashcroft, D. M. (2008). Hospital admissions associated with adverse drug reactions: A systematic review of prospective observational studies. *Annals of Pharmacotherapy, 42*(7), 1017–1025.

Koppel, R. (2002). *Alzheimer's disease: The costs to U.S. businesses in 2002.* Washington, DC: Alzheimer's Association.

Krahn, D. D., Bartels, S. J., Coakley, E., Oslin, D. W., Chgen, H., McIntyre, J.,...Levkoff, S. E. (2006). PRISM-E: Comparison of integrated care and enhanced specialty referral models in depression outcomes. *Psychiatric Services, 57*(7), 946–953.

Kravitz, R., Franks, P., Feldman, M., Meredith, L., Hinton, L., Franz, C.,...Epstein, R. (2006). What drives referral from primary care physicians to mental health specialists? A randomized trial using actors portraying depressive symptoms. *Journal of General Internal Medicine, 21*(6), 584–589.

Larson, E. B., Wang, L., Bowen, J. D., McCormick, W. C., Teri, L., Crane, P., & Kukull, W. (2006). Exercise is associated with reduced risk for incident dementia among persons 65 of age and older. *Annals of Internal Medicine, 144*(2), 73–81.

Levkoff, S., Chen, H., Coakley, E., Herr, E., Oslin, D., Katz, I., et al. (2004). Design and sample characteristics of the PRISM-E multisite randomized trial to improve behavioral health care for the elderly. *Journal of Aging and Health, 16*(1), 3–27.

Lewin Group. (2004). *Saving lives. Saving money: Dividends for Americans investing in Alzheimer research.* Washington, DC: Alzheimer's Association.

Liu-Ambrose, T., Nagamatsu, L. S., Graf, P., Beattie, L., Ashe, M. C., & Handy, T. C. (2010). Resistance training and executive functions. *Archives of Internal Medicine, 170*(2), 170–178.

Mackenzie, C., Scott, T., Mather, A., & Sareen, J. (2008). Older adults' help-seeking attitudes and treatment beliefs concerning mental health problems. *American Journal of Geriatric Psychiatry, 16*(12), 1010–1019.

Marek, K. D., Popejoy, L., Petroski, G., Mehr, D., & Rantz, M. (2005). Clinical outcomes of aging in place. *Nursing Research, 54*(3), 202–211.

MEDPAC (Medicare Payment Advisory Commission). (2008). Report to the Congress: reforming the delivery system. Washington, DC: Medical Payment Advisory Commission. Retrieved from http://www.medpac.gov/documents/Jun08_EntireReport.pdf

Monahan, G., & Colthurst, T. (2001). Internet-based information on alcohol, tobacco, and other drugs: Issues of ethics, quality, and accountability. *Substance Use and Misuse, 36*(14), 2171–2180.

Moore, T. J., Cohen, M. R., & Furberg, C. D. (2007). Serious adverse drug events reported to the Food and Drug Administration, 1998–2005. *Archives of Internal Medicine, 167*(16), 1752–1759.

National Advisory Committee on Rural Health and Human Services. (2004). *The 2004 report to the secretary: Rural health and human services issues,* 35–43.

National Institute of Mental Health. (2007). *Older adults: Depression and suicide facts (fact sheet).* Retrieved from http://www.nimh.nih.gov/health/publications/older-adults-depression-and-suicide-facts-fact-sheet/index.shtml#role

Oldenburg, B. (2002). Preventing chronic disease and improving health: Broadening the scope of behavioral medicine and research. *International Journal of Behavioral Medicine, 9*(1), 1–16.

Organization for Economic Cooperation and Development. (2009). *OECD health data 2009: How does the United States compare?* Retrieved from http://www.oecd.org/dataoecd/46/2/38980580.pdf

Oslin, D. W., Grantham, S., Coakley, E., Maxwell, J., Miles, K., Ware, J.,...Zubritsky, C. (2006). PRISM-E: Comparison of integrated care and enhanced specialty referral in managing at-risk alcohol use. *Psychiatric Services, 57*(7), 954–958.

Pew Internet and American Life Project (2009). *Internet, cell phone and broadband statistics.* Retrieved from http://www.authoring.pewinternet.org/Reports/2010/Internet-broadband-and-cell-phone-statistics.aspx?r=1

Pickard, J. G., & Tang, F. (2009). Older adults seeking mental health counseling in a NORC. *Research on Aging, 31*(6), 638–660.

Powell, J., & Clarke, A. (2002). The WWW of the World Wide Web: Who, what, and why? *Journal of Medical Internet Research, 4*(1), e4.

Qato, D., Alexander, G., Conti, R., Johnson, M., Schumm, P., & Lindau, S. (2008). Use of prescription and over-the-counter medications and dietary supplements among older adults in the United States. *Journal of the American Medical Association, 300*(24), 2867–2878.

Quinn, K., Laidlaw, K., & Murray, L. (2009). Older people's attitudes to mental illness. *Clinical Psychology & Psychotherapy, 16*(1), 33–45.

Regier, D., Boyd, J., Burke, J., & Rae, D. (1988). One-month prevalence of mental disorders in the United States: Based on five epidemiologic catchment area sites. *Archives of General Psychiatry, 45*(11), 977–986.

Ritchie, K., Touchon, J., & Ledésert, B. (1998). Progressive disability in senile dementia is accelerated in the presence of depression. *International Journal of Geriatric Psychiatry, 13*(7), 459–461.

Segal, D., Coolidge, F., Mincic, M., & O'Riley, A. (2005). Beliefs about mental illness and willingness to seek help: A cross-sectional study. *Aging & Mental Health, 9*(4), 363–367.

Seitz, D., Purandare, N., & Conn, D. (2010). Prevalence of psychiatric disorders among older adults in long-term-care homes: A systematic review. *International Psychogeriatrics, June 4,* 1–15.

Silberg, W. M., Lundberg, G. D., & Musacchio, R. A. (1997). Assessing, controlling, and assuring the quality of medical information on the Internet: Caveant lector et viewor. Let the reader and viewer beware. *Journal of the American Medical Association, 277*(15), 1244–1245.

Smith, T., Nealey, J., & Hamann, H. (2000). Health psychology. *Handbook of psychological change: Psychotherapy processes & practices for the 21st century* (pp. 562–590). Hoboken, NJ: John Wiley & Sons Inc.

Spector, W. D., Reschovsky, J. D., & Cohen, J. W. (1996). Appropriate placement of nursing-home residents in lower level care. *Milbank Quarterly, 74*(1), 139–160.

Speer, D. C., & Schneider, M. G. (2003). Metal health needs of older adults and primary care: Opportunity for interdisciplinary geriatric team practice. *Clinical Psychology Science and Practice, 10,* 85–101.

SAMHSA (Substance Abuse and Mental Health Services Administration), Office of Applied Studies. (2010). *The TEDS report: Changing substance abuse patterns among older admissions: 1992 and 2008.* Rockville, MD. Retrieved from http://www.oas.samhsa.gov/2k10/229/229OlderAdms2k10.htm

Unützer, J., Katon, W., Callahan, C. M., Williams, Jr., J. W., Hunkeler, E., Harpole, L.,...Langston, C. (2002). Collaborative care management of late-life depression in the primary care setting: A randomized controlled trial. *Journal of the American Medical Association, 288*(22), 2836–2845.

Unützer, J., Schoenbaum, M., Katon, W. J., Fan, M., Pincus, H. A. Hogan, D., & Taylor, J. (2009). Healthcare costs associated with depression in medically ill fee-for-service Medicare participants. *Journal of the American Geriatric Society, 57,* 506–510.

U.S. Administration on Aging. (2009). *A profile of older Americans: 2009.* Retrieved from http://www.aoa.gov/aoaroot/aging_statistics/Profile/2009/docs/2009profile_508.pdf

U.S. Department of Health and Human Services (1998). Treatment improvement protocol (TIP) series 26: Substance abuse among older adults. DHHS publication no. (SMA) 98-3179, Rockville, MD. Retrieved from http://www.ncbi.nlm.nih.gov/books/bv.fcgi?rid=hstat5.chapter.48302

U.S. Department of Health and Human Services. (2009). *National clearinghouse for long term care information.* Washington, DC: Author. Retrieved from www.longtermcare.gov/LTC/Main_Site/Paying_LTC/Costs_Of_Care/Costs_Of_Care.aspx#What

van't Veer-Tazelaar, P., Smit, F., van Hout, H., van Oppen, P., van der Horst, H., Beekman, A., & van Marwijk, H. (2010). Cost effectiveness of a stepped care intervention to prevent depression and anxiety in late life: Randomized trial. *British Journal of Psychiatry, 196,* 319–325.

Wang, P., Lane, M., Olfson, M., Pincus, H., Wells, K., & Kessler, R. (2005). Twelve-month use of mental health services in the United States: Results from the national comorbidity survey replication. *Archives of General Psychiatry, 62*(6), 629–640.

Webb, A., & Zhivan, N. (2010). *What is the distribution of lifetime health care costs from age 65?* Working paper 10-4. Chestnut Hill, MA: Center for Retirement Research at Boston College.

Xu, J., Kochanek, K. D., & Tejada-Vera, B. (2009). Deaths: Preliminary data for 2007. *National Vital Statistics Reports, 58*(1). Hyattsville, MD: National Center for Health Statistics.

Yury, C., & Fisher, J. (2007). Preventing excess disability in an elderly person with Alzheimer's disease. *Clinical Case Studies, 6*(4), 295–306.

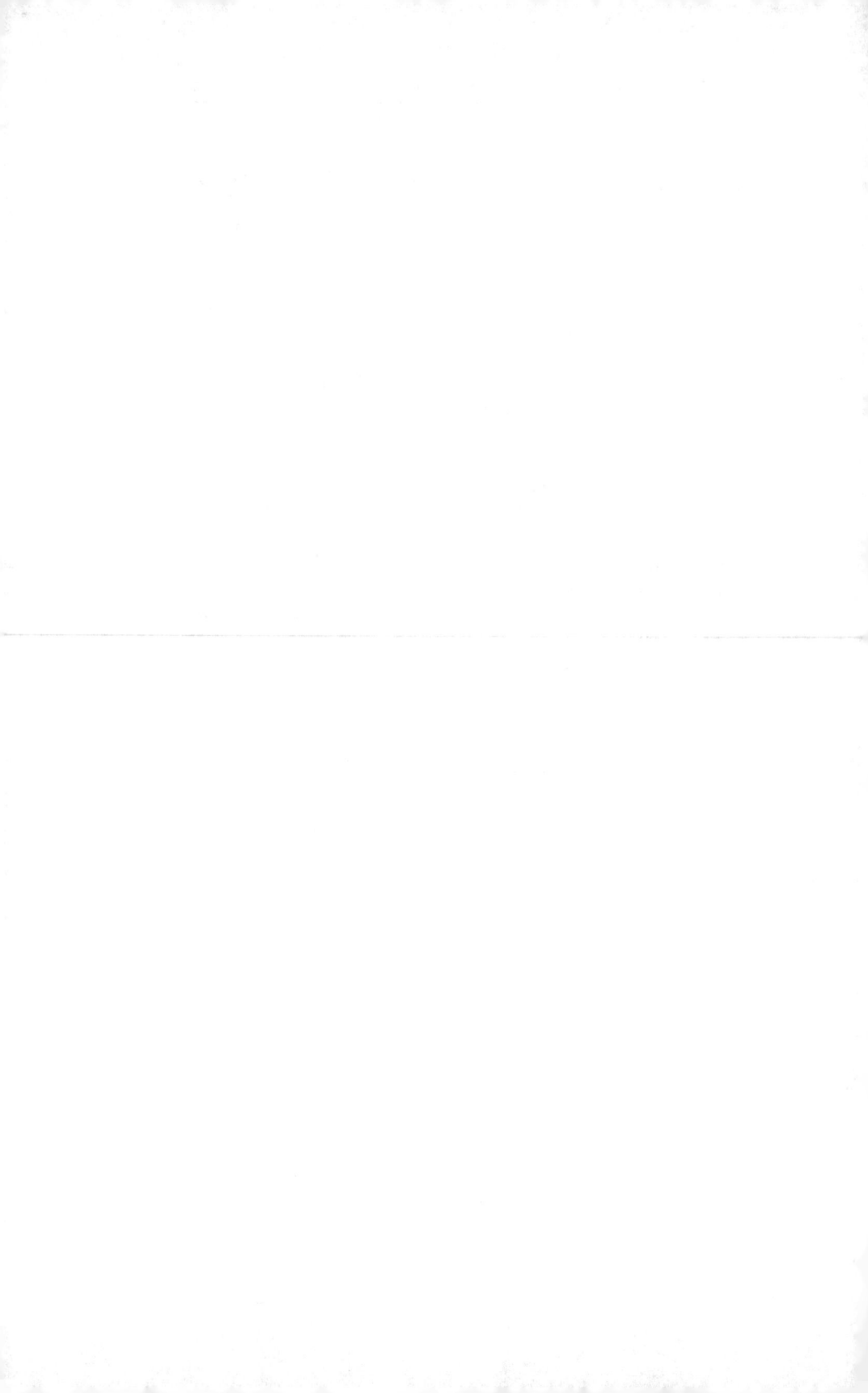

Fourteen

Failure to Serve
The Use of Medications as a First-Line Treatment and Misuse in Behavioral Interventions

JOHN L. CACCAVALE

WITH THE COLLABORATION OF JOSEPH CASCIANI,
NICHOLAS A. CUMMINGS, JERRY MORRIS,
DAVE REINHARDT, HOWARD RUBIN,
ELLE WALKER, AND JACK G. WIGGINS

Editor's note: This chapter is a summary of the extensive white paper, "A Failure to Serve," prepared by the National Alliance of Professional Psychology Providers (NAPPP), which is too lengthy to be included in its entirety. It has commanded considerable attention in both medical and psychological circles and addresses the need to restore psychotherapy as the first-line intervention in this era of health reform. The entire white paper on which this chapter is based, complete with references, may be obtained through http://www.nappp.org/White_paper.pdf. This summary chapter is published with the cooperation of the NAPPP.

INTRODUCTION: A STATEMENT OF CONCERN

There is a crisis in our nation's behavioral healthcare system. Many factors contribute to this crisis, including financial, regulatory, and cultural issues. One of the most glaring problems in this crisis is the corporate healthcare industry's practice of placing earnings and exorbitant profits above the public interest at the expense of quality services to those in need. There is another significant factor contributing to the poor quality of services provided to patients suffering from behavioral disorders: a significant shift of behavioral healthcare from specialists, such as psychologists and psychiatrists, to primary care physicians.

While well-meaning, the majority of primary care physicians are not trained or experienced enough to provide behavioral health treatment and diagnosis. These physicians have become naive distributors for drug manufacturers and collude with insurers in the face of solid research that shows that psychotropic medications are not effective or beneficial for an ever growing number of patients. NAPPP accepts that not every primary care physician is a puppet of drug companies or the insurance industry. Most are caring and hardworking professionals. However, as a profession, primary care physicians know, or should know, that psychotropic medications are mostly ineffective and potentially dangerous to patients. As such, most physicians who prescribe psychotropic medication do so to the detriment of their patients.

The full report upon which this chapter is based, "A Failure to Serve," addresses this crisis by providing a perspective of the problems encountered by patients who need behavioral healthcare but are not receiving it. The authors provide solid solutions based on sound, up-to-date research to support our assertions and conclusions about this crisis in behavioral healthcare. The problems of the present system, in which behavioral health is provided in primary care settings, will become even more pronounced as the new healthcare mandates take effect. NAPPP is concerned that healthcare reform will continue and even exacerbate the violation of patient care that is ubiquitous and characteristic of the present system.

We believe that the concerns and problems addressed in this report need to be taken seriously as a public policy issue and that this issue should be a matter of public interest. Consumers of behavioral healthcare must be protected and provided with positive and cost-effective treatments. Should the current practices of behavioral health treatment be continued by primary care physicians, NAPPP strongly believes that patients in desperate need of these services will suffer as drug companies, healthcare insurers, and physicians all gain at patients' and the public's expense.

Among the problems thoroughly documented and detailed in the full report are the following:

1. Medication as a first-line treatment for behavioral conditions is unsupported by the most recent outcome research.
2. Providing behavioral healthcare in a primary care setting without an appropriate evaluation by a doctoral level psychologist is ineffective, nonbeneficial, and costly, and it denies patients the standard of care required to treat behavioral disorders.
3. The growing incidence of adverse drug events can be directly tied to the lack of skills and training provided to physicians in medical school and practice. On-the-job training to prescribe medications must be preceded by solid educational preparation. Even the best medical schools provide only 90 hours of pharmacological education over a 4-year medical school curriculum. The vast majority of medical schools provide far less training.
4. There is a long-term shortage of psychiatrists that will not be resolved. Because of this shortage, primary care physicians have become the dominant prescribers of psychotropic medications. Seizing on physicians' lack of training, drug companies have deceived them and the public about the safety, effectiveness, and benefit of psychotropic medications. Consequently, patients have been put at risk and become guinea pigs for questionable medications such as antidepressants, antipsychotics, and other drugs marketed to treat behavioral disorders.
5. Children and the aged populations are at the most risk because they are receiving treatment from the least prepared physicians and are the targets of drug companies, which see children and the aged as "profit centers" in the ever increasing quest for market share. Off-label use of medications among these populations is promoted by drug companies simply to expand the profitability of their existing products.
6. Taxpayers are also victims of the healthcare industry. Healthcare reform will now require an additional 30+ million people to obtain healthcare insurance. For

those unable to afford insurance, their costs will be subsidized. NAPPP supports healthcare reform and universal coverage. We advocate and agree to extending care to everyone who needs it. What we are most concerned about, however, is having taxpayers subsidize drug companies, insurers, and providers whose products and services are not proven to work as advertised. Costs for medications will continue to increase to a projected $400 billion by the time the new reform takes effect. We have a right and responsibility to require physicians to work in the public interest—not as mere distributors for drug companies and in collusion with insurers who gladly reimburse for ineffective medications because they are cheaper than providing effective care.
7. Unlimited licensure of physicians contributes to a system in which patients are not being appropriately served and subjected to undue harm. Limited licensure can improve competence and treatment outcomes. It can greatly decrease the cost of healthcare while raising the standard of care provided to patients.

Patients suffering from behavioral disorders are among our most vulnerable citizens. We should not allow any profession or entity to hide behind selective science and the professional domination of healthcare to subject patients and the public to patently ineffective and nonbeneficial treatments. We do not argue that the healthcare industry and providers should be denied making a profit. Profit, however, must be balanced with the public good and must honestly and ethically be earned, be based on real need, and be based on sound theories and outcome research. Failure to hold physicians, providers, drug manufacturers, and insurers to these minimal standards will produce an even greater crisis in healthcare, aside from the misery afflicted on a trusting population at the mercy of a system concerned more with profit than results.

The NAPPP believes that we can all do better and that we should strive to do so.

For the purpose of this document, behavioral disorders are defined as any mental, emotional, or behavior disorder included in the *International Classification of Diseases, 9th Revision Clinical Modification* (ICD-9-CM) or the *Diagnostic and Statistical Manual* (DSM IV) diagnostic manuals.

SUMMARY OF THE DATA

Behavioral healthcare in America has largely been reassigned to primary care physicians as a result of the overall penetration in healthcare of for-profit managed care companies and insurers, the long-term campaign by drug manufacturers to replace effective behavioral interventions with medications, and a two-decades long shortage of psychiatrists. All of these factors have contributed to patients being denied effective treatments as the profits of these companies continue to increase. The healthcare reform bill recently signed by President Obama is unlikely to resolve any of the issues discussed in this report. In fact, the more likely outcome is that patients seeking and needing effective behavioral healthcare will not get it because the new healthcare bill further concentrates treatment and health decisions in primary care settings under the influence of insurance corporations and other third-party payers.

As gatekeepers for physical ailments, primary care physicians perform admirably under difficult circumstances. However, patients needing behavioral healthcare are not receiving and cannot receive effective treatment from primary care physicians, who generally are unskilled and lack training in evaluating, diagnosing, and treating behavioral disorders. This report discusses the problems and solutions associated with medications when they are used as a first-line treatment for behavioral disorders.

The Evidence Against Primary Care Physicians Providing Behavioral Healthcare

- The healthcare industry, composed of physician groups, insurers, large contract providers, medical device companies, and the pharmaceutical industry, has achieved total control of the healthcare system that routinely misleads and colludes with government regulators.
- The healthcare industry has embraced the myth that a behavioral disorder is a medical problem and implies that it is either genetically or neurohormonally caused, typically life long in duration and requiring treatment with medications.
- Primary care physicians providing behavioral healthcare overwhelmingly favor medications as first-line treatments for behavioral disorders despite the evidence that many of these drugs do not perform better than placebos.

- Renowned researchers have been writing voluminously for the need to require protocols that include psychosocial and behavioral treatments with medications and, in some cases, in place of medications.
- Primary care physicians routinely provide drugs without obtaining an evaluation or appropriate diagnosis from a doctoral level psychologist or psychiatrist.
- Patients treated in primary care settings for behavioral disorders receive less than 50% of the standard of care that is required by medical guidelines.
- Behavioral healthcare patients are exposed to undue risk and harm because primary care physicians account for more than 80% of the prescriptions written for psychotropic medications. In effect, physicians have become virtual distributors for drug companies despite the mounting evidence that many of these drugs are unwarranted and risky to patients.
- Visits to emergency rooms for the abuse of pain medications and sedatives are now equal to or exceed visits for heroin and other illegal drugs. This is a direct result of physicians writing too many prescriptions for these drugs.

Reducing Adverse Drug Events From Physician Error

- Physician errors attributed to prescribing medications account for many deaths and harm to patients. The Institute of Medicine (IOM) continues to report the risk to patients due to physician errors. While estimates may vary, the IOM believes that 100,000 deaths per year are caused by physician error. The IOM only counts deaths that occur in hospitals. There are no comparable data for harm occurring in outpatient settings because there is no formal reporting mechanism.
- Estimates of the annual cost due to increased harm from medication-related injuries range from a low of $72 billion to a high of $172 billion.
- Physician errors increase hospital costs on the average of $6,000 per patient.
- Annual nonfatal injuries from adverse drug events (ADEs) are estimated to be about 650,000.
- Many of the errors attributed to medications can be reduced or eliminated by better education and

training. However, few medical schools have developed a curriculum to confront this problem. At the best medical schools, physicians receive only 90 hours of training in pharmacology; most provide far less. Even fewer provide training to reduce adverse drug events.
- Medical psychologists are in the unique position of being a positive factor in reducing ADEs and they can provide behavioral health services effectively and efficiently. Primary care physicians and other nonpsychiatric physicians are not behavioral health specialists or psychopharmacologists.

Psychiatry in Crisis: Impacts on Primary Care, Patient Safety, and Public Healthcare Policy

- The number of medical students choosing psychiatry as a specialty has continued to decline over the past two decades. The shortage of psychiatrists has been very steep and there are no credible solutions that will impact the decline.
- As a result of this shortage, about 70% of primary care physicians have reported difficulty in obtaining high-quality outpatient behavioral health services.
- Psychiatrists, as a whole, have abandoned providing behavioral healthcare treatments outside medication. Few have sought or receive behavioral training. As a result, psychiatry no longer is a stakeholder in advancing effective patient care. Psychiatrists' economic survival is tied to drug companies, making their allegiance to patients highly questionable.
- Public safety has been compromised as psychiatry refuses to consider and implement alternative strategies to deal with its shortage. Public policy and public safety have been held hostage to economic factors as psychiatry continues to reject collaborative practice with psychologists.
- Despite the overwhelming evidence showing that some of the most successful outcomes in behavioral health treatment are a result of medications when appropriately diagnosed and used concurrently with behavioral therapy or psychotherapy alone, psychiatrists continue to subscribe to medication-only strategies.

Antidepressant Medications Are Ineffective and Claims Are Misleading

- Biologically based imbalance theories have long been posited as a basis for antidepressant medications. These theories, although largely unfounded, untested, and unproven, provide the foundation for medications sold by the millions of doses.
- There is no scientific substantiation or agreement that depression is caused by biological, chemical imbalances or defective genes or that it is remedied in any significant way by available medications.
- Antidepressant medications actually build negatively and impact the ability to function without the drug; over time, the condition becomes chronic. The data show that the longer that one stays on this type of drug, the higher the likelihood of relapse of depression.
- The side effects of these drugs include cardiac complications, withdrawal, akathisia and motor abnormalities, sexual side effects, drug-induced violence, and neuropsychiatric effects including insomnia, apathy, and mania. Physicians have responded to these side effects by prescribing additional medications, most of which are "off label" and not authorized by the FDA.
- Behavioral approaches for depression are now well established as effective first-line treatments for depression. They are just as effective and, in many cases, more effective than antidepressants and have no risk of side effects.
- The results of many clinical trials, meta-analyses, and reviews point to one inescapable conclusion: Behavioral therapy works for the treatment of depression, and the benefits are substantial.
- Antidepressants only dampen or partially control some symptoms of the disorder and that in a minority of patients; they therefore do not qualify as a "stand-alone" or a "first-line" treatment.
- The evidence is clear that antidepressant medications work no better than placebos in nearly all patients with depression. The use of these chemicals on 32 million people, when they simply do not work, presents a moral dilemma and should be a major public policy concern.
- Research shows that most people will respond positively to behavioral intervention. Typically, 13 sessions

of cognitive-behavioral intervention relieve symptoms and allow patients to resume work and family responsibilities and function well.
- Only a small number of patients, a minority of about 12–15%, respond solely to medications.

Physicians Often Do Not Provide Patients With Important Information When Prescribing Medications

Most physicians routinely do not provide important information to their patients when they prescribe a medication. Research shows that only 62% of the necessary information about a medication is communicated to patients. Only 35% of physicians advised patients of the adverse effects associated with a medication. In attempts to address this problem, it has become public policy to require dispensing pharmacists to provide the missing information that the physician is either too underinformed or too rushed to provide.

- Among the most profitable and growing segment of pharmaceuticals are psychotropic medications and their use by physicians for conditions for which they were not developed or approved by the FDA. Physicians continue to prescribe these medications with no research or data that can provide any clues to the side effects when prescribed for a condition that has not been studied.
- The Nonpartisan Center for Public Integrity reports that pharmaceutical companies spent more than $855 million for marketing, which is more than any other industry, between 1998 and 2006. Marketing comprises a significant portion of the cost of medications. These are at the low end of the estimates for drug company advertising. Advertising is unnecessary and many times violates FDA rules for marketing a drug.
- Even higher cost estimates for advertising by the Kaiser Foundation show manufacturer spending on advertising was almost twice as much in 2008 ($11.3 billion) as in 1998 ($5.9 billion). After increasing every year since 1996, the total amount manufacturers spent on advertising declined from 2004 to 2005 (from $12.1 billion to $11.7 billion), rose to $12.0 billion in 2006, and then fell to $11.8 billion in 2007 and $11.3 billion in 2008. The share directed toward consumers in 2008 through advertising on television, on radio, in magazines, and

in newspapers, as well as outdoor advertising, was more than three times that spent in 1998—$4.4 billion compared to $1.3 billion—though spending decreased 10% from 2007 to 2008 ($4.9 to $4.4 billion).
- The marketing strategy used by drug companies is similar to that employed by cereal makers, who line supermarket shelves with tens of boxes of the same sugar-laden cereals. Patients are being prescribed unnecessary medications and are not provided with important information; they are not receiving the appropriate treatment because psychologists are being kept out of the treatment mix and because drugs, in the short term, are cheaper than more appropriate and proven care.
- The use of medical psychologists—those trained in applying behavioral interventions to medical problems and clinical psychopharmacology—is an effective solution to control the unnecessary rise and subsequent costs for psychotropic medications while providing patients with the necessary information to make decisions.

Reducing Harm and Healthcare Costs: A Review of a Physician's Unlimited License to Practice

- Generally, physicians are licensed under what is termed an "unlimited" license. Underlying the intent of unlimited licensure is the expectation and requirement that physicians provide only those services for which they have received specific training and education. Unfortunately, there is no entity that can police or oversee that physicians adhere to the intent underlying the justification for unlimited licensure. As a result, unlimited licensure contributes to undue harm to patients and is a public policy issue that needs to be addressed and modified.
- Psychologists, nurses, nurse practitioners, and other healthcare professionals practice under what is termed a "limited" license. This means that these professionals can only practice what is stated in their scope of practice law. They can legally provide only those services for which they have specific training, education, and experience.
- State licensure boards establish procedures for granting initial licensure. However, in virtually all states,

it is possible for a physician to practice medicine for a lifetime without having to demonstrate to the state medical board that he or she has maintained an acceptable level of continuing qualifications or competence.
- The Federation of State Medical Boards (FSMB), raising the concern about ongoing physician competency and the consequences that lack of training and competence can have on patient care and outcomes, believes that leniency extended to physicians is no longer acceptable.
- The ongoing advances in science and technology and the knowledge that is required to digest and make use of this knowledge by physicians is at the core of why unlimited licensure is bad for patients and is a direct cause of excessive healthcare costs.
- The FSMB issued a report that raises concerns about the generally poor quality of medical school applicants, the small amount of time that physicians have to devote to patients, and the shortage of American-trained physicians and increased reliance on foreign-trained physicians with limited language skills.
- There needs to be a balance between professional autonomy and patient care. Unlimited licensure subverts treatment and ethical considerations because of economic issues or the interests of corporations such as drug manufacturers and insurers. It does not promote a balance. It sabotages professional ethics and the foundation for an effective and efficient healthcare system.

Medicating America's Children
- Prescriptions for antipsychotic medications to children aged 2–5 years doubled between the years 1999–2001 and 2007. The top-selling medicines in 2008 were antipsychotics for schizophrenia and bipolar disorder, with $14.6 billion in sales.
- The age of children being medicated with psychotropic drugs is getting younger, and the number of children given prescriptions is increasing every year. Yet, there is compelling research demonstrating the effectiveness of behavioral treatment to stabilize attention deficit disorder (ADD) and attention deficit hyperactivity disorder (ADHD) symptoms rapidly and without medication.
- There appears to be little evidence, if any, that these drugs are efficacious with this population of patients;

yet, physicians continue to prescribe drugs to children "off label" and at doses developed for adults.
- Drug manufacturers have been charged with hiding, obscuring, and falsifying the results of clinical trials. The efficacy of Prozac, for example, could not be distinguished from placebo in 6 out of 10 clinical trials. The FDA, nevertheless, allowed Prozac to be prescribed to millions of patients, including children.
- It is clear that bipolar disorder is being overdiagnosed in children and adolescents. Many of these patients are being treated in primary care settings. This is wrong, ill advised, and potentially dangerous to the patient. Patients diagnosed with bipolar disorder need to be evaluated and diagnosed by a doctoral psychologist or psychiatrist and regularly followed by both during the course of treatment.
- Many children are prescribed psychostimulants for attention-deficit problems. To date, not a solitary cause has yet been identified for ADHD. The National Institutes of Health Consensus Development Conference and the American Academy of Pediatrics agree that there is no known biological basis for ADHD. These drugs are top sellers for manufacturers.
- Large-scale research shows that children who are prescribed psychostimulants and are provided behavioral intervention have less need for these medications and experience rapid stabilization of their symptoms.
- Children are at great risk when taking psychostimulant drugs. In 2007, the FDA issued an administrative order that requires that all makers of ADHD medications develop and provide patients with medication guides. The FDA took this action because of complaints and the increasing data that concluded ADHD patients with heart conditions had a higher risk of strokes, heart attacks, and sudden death when using these medications.
- The psychological symptoms associated with these drugs include hearing voices, experiencing hallucinations, becoming suspicious for no reason, or becoming manic.
- Strattera, a psychostimulant prescribed to children and teenagers, is more likely to produce suicidal

thoughts in children and teenagers than in those who do not use this medication. Children who use Strattera must be supervised and their behavior carefully monitored because they may suddenly develop symptoms that are a serious threat to the child.
- ADD and ADHD are not the only conditions for which children are being prescribed potentially dangerous medications. Increasingly, children as young as 5 years old are being diagnosed with bipolar disorder by physicians, without an evaluation by a psychologist.
- Antidepressant medications are commonly prescribed for pregnant women. The use of these drugs during pregnancy is based upon the false assumption that they are safe to the fetus and the mother. They are not and they can cause serious medical impairments for newborns.

Patients Deserve to Be Evaluated and Treated by Real Doctors

- Since the penetration of managed care as the gatekeeper to healthcare, behavioral health services have been the most negatively impacted.
- As managed care became the gatekeeper for behavioral health services, costs dropped 40% as a result of delaying services, denying claims, arduous utilization review procedures, phantom panels, and the use of non-doctoral-level providers.
- The U.S. surgeon general, in a report on mental health, admitted that private health insurance is generally more restrictive in coverage of mental illness than in coverage for somatic illness.
- Mental health parity legislation has not remedied the disparity in treatment for behavioral health patients. Insurers and managed care companies employ sophisticated utilization review procedures to delay and deny treatment.
- Insurers state that they need these procedures to contain costs. Studies by health economists have concluded that unlimited mental health benefits under managed care cost virtually the same as capped benefits: The average increase was about $1 per employee compared with costs under a $25,000 cap, which is a typical limit under cost-containment plans.

The Treatment of the Aged in Long-Term Care

- The services psychologists provide patients in long-term care result in benefits to patients and the healthcare system. However, the underutilization of psychologists in these facilities remains a significant problem.
- The shift from a custodial care model to a functional capacity model that utilizes psychologists and other healthcare providers has increased the quality of care provided to nursing home patients.
- According to the American Geriatric Society, there are 1.5 million older adults in nursing homes. Anywhere from 65 to 91% have symptoms of a psychiatric disorder. Beyond these primary psychiatric diagnoses, many of the medical conditions presented on admission have underlying psychological factors that contribute to or exacerbate the conditions.
- Many research studies have repeatedly shown that higher costs and reduced quality of life for medically ill individuals are associated with depression, stress, and negative future outlook.
- The Institute of Medicine in a recent report projects significant shortages of all health professionals with specialized training in geriatrics and aging.
- Despite this prevalence of psychological disorders in nursing homes, psychological services, as elsewhere, have been negatively impacted by the medicalization of behavioral health. Elderly patients in nursing homes continue to be overmedicated and not provided the level of behavioral interventions that is needed.
- The Department of Health and Human Services published a report saying that 7 out of the 10 leading health and illness indicators are psychological, such as inactivity, obesity, smoking, substance abuse, behavioral illness, irresponsible sexual behavior, and violence. Many elderly patients never receive the appropriate treatment for these symptoms and are instead treated with ineffective drugs.
- Numerous studies looking at the effect of psychological interventions on medical utilization found that 90% of these studies showed reduced medical utilization following some psychological intervention and a corresponding reduction in cost.

- Studies show that there is an over-reliance on drugs in nursing home settings. These studies show that it is not uncommon for patients in nursing homes to be prescribed between 5 and 13 medications. The adverse drug events from this practice cause deaths and other harm to elderly patients.
- The increasing costs for medications clearly can be reduced if physicians, more often than not, would include behavioral interventions in the treatment plan.

CONCLUSION

In conclusion, the extent and magnitude of these proffered findings compel that the reader avail himself or herself of the comprehensive list of corroborating references through http://www.nappp.org/white-paper.pdf.

Fifteen

Reforms in Treating Children and Families

JAMES H. BRAY

INTRODUCTION

In the United States, the future directions of healthcare were dramatically changed during 2009 and 2010 as the federal government engaged in a major process to reform healthcare systems to meet the health needs of the population for the twenty-first century. This process resulted in the passage of the Patient Protection and Affordable Care Act, H.R.3590 (PPACA), which was signed into law by President Barack Obama on March 23, 2010 (P.L 111-148). This was followed by a package of key amendments, the Health Care and Education Reconciliation Act of 2010 (P.L. 111-152).

Major reform actually began in 2008 with the passage of the Mental Parity and Addiction Equity Act, H.R. 6983. Mental health parity was implemented and strengthened in the 2010 healthcare reform bill. This law specifies that services for mental and behavioral health problems will be treated and reimbursed with parity to other health problems. Specific aspects of parity and other changes are discussed later in this chapter and in Chapter 3 of this volume. The specifics of the parity regulations are being developed and will be gradually phased in through 2014. The implementation of the parity and healthcare reform bills may end mental health carve-outs, in which people with mental and behavioral health problems are treated differently and in separate systems of care than those with other health problems. The elimination of mental health carve-outs is essential for integrated healthcare to become a reality.

The focus of healthcare reform included four major areas: (1) increasing access to healthcare for uninsured and underinsured people, (2) creating a twenty-first century healthcare system that is supposed to be more efficient and effective, (3) revitalizing primary care, and (4) using comparative effectiveness research to inform practice (Clancy, 2009). However, the real driver of reform was economics and the escalating costs of healthcare. President Obama stated that the economy was in danger until healthcare costs were brought under control. Managed care and other healthcare systems have clearly failed in these efforts.

The PPACA creates new opportunities for the practice of psychology and behavioral health. The advocacy efforts by the American Psychological Association and its members and recommendations from the 2009 APA Presidential Task Force and Summit on the Future of Psychology Practice (Bray et al., 2009) were important factors in the reforms that impact the practice of psychology. These reforms build on the long-standing work by many who have demonstrated that behavioral health is cost effective in healthcare settings and who have called for psychologists to work in primary and integrated healthcare settings and to transform psychology from a mental health profession to a health profession (Bray, 1996; Cummings & Follette, 1968; Follette & Cummings, 1967; Hemmings, 2000; Newman & Rozensky, 1995; O'Donohue, Byrd, Cummings, & Henderson, 2005; Routh, Schroeder, & Koocher, 1983; Wright & Burns, 1986).

However, to take advantage of these opportunities requires that we *change where and how we practice* (Bray, 2010). Current models of practice are often not acceptable in the existing environments. We can move forward through collaboration with other disciplines and the integration of scientific and technological advances in our work.

The major reforms include many changes that will impact the care of children and families. The focus of this chapter will be to highlight some of these changes and discuss how psychology practice and behavioral healthcare can take advantage of these reforms. In this chapter, references to specific aspects of the PPACA are based on language and work reflected in the APA healthcare reform documents (APA, 2010). Before I discuss the child and family reforms, it is important to understand the current healthcare context and broader changes that will result from the implementation of the PPACA (Bray, 2010).

OVERVIEW OF ISSUES IN HEALTHCARE

Where does behavioral health fit within the current healthcare system? Saultz (2008) describes the healthcare system as a pyramid (see Figure 15.1). At the base of the system are primary care, mental health, and public health. Hospital care, speciality care, and tertiary care sit on this base. As one goes above the base, costs, specialization, and funding increase. Most people and many healthcare professionals think of behavioral health as solely or mainly within the specialized mental health realm. However, behavioral health issues are part of each area, and practices in all of these areas outside mental health are sources of future growth.

One of the major shifts in healthcare reform is to move more of the resources into the base of the pyramid—especially into primary care. The U.S. healthcare system spends significantly more on specialty medical care than primary care and this is one of the economic drivers of escalating healthcare costs (Clancy, 2009). The Obama administration and the PPACA have redirected some federal funds from specialty healthcare to primary care and prevention services to recognize the importance of these areas for the health of the nation. The concept is that if prevention services are provided and paid for within primary care, the incidence of chronic health problems will be reduced and will be less costly to treat.

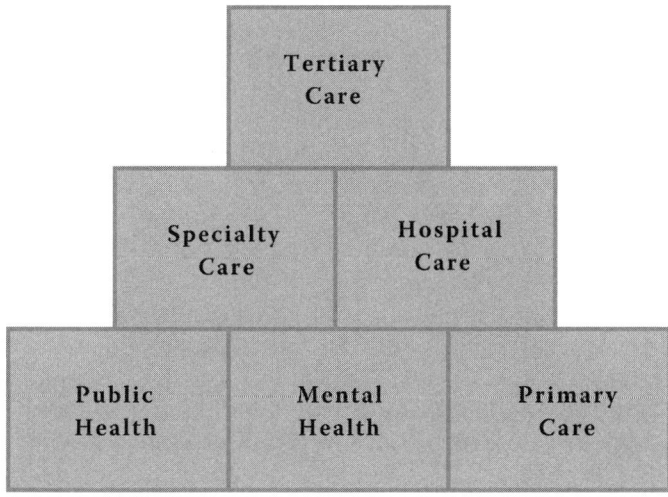

Figure 15.1 Healthcare pyramid. (Adapted from Saultz, J. 2008. http://www.fmdrl.org/index.cfm/saultz#17)

Over the past 30 years, there has also been a shift in the types of services provided for mental and behavioral health problems and the practitioners who provide the services (Frank, 2009; Kessler et al., 2005; Wang et al., 2006). General medical practitioners provide more mental health services than mental and behavioral health providers. In addition, in the last few decades there has been a tremendous increase in the use of psychotropic medications, mainly by general medical providers, and a decline in the use of psychotherapy to treat behavioral health problems (Frank, 2009; Medical Expenditure Panel Survey, 2009). This is an important reason for psychologists to obtain prescriptive authority: both to be able to prescribe medications (or take people off medications) and to use behavioral interventions.

Primary Care

Revitalization of primary care is a major part of healthcare reform; in addition, there is a move to more integrated systems of care. Many psychologists have called for the full integration of psychology and behavioral health into the general medical system for decades (Bray, 1996; Cummings, Cummings, & Johnson, 1997; Cummings & Follette, 1968; Follette & Cummings, 1967; Newman & Rozensky, 1995; O'Donohue et al., 2005; Routh et al., 1983). Cummings and Follette (1968), Follette and Cummings (1967), and Hemmings (2000) demonstrated that integrating behavioral health into healthcare settings is cost effective and decreases costs for general medical care. However, as noted by Cummings et al. (1997), partial or incomplete attempts at integrated care do not result in significant benefits.

The major model in the PPACA for primary care is called the patient-centered medical home (PCMH; PCMH Collaborative, 2007). The PCMH is designed to provide comprehensive primary care for children, youth, and adults that facilitates partnerships between individual patients and their personal physicians and, when appropriate, the patient's family. The twenty-first century healthcare medical homes should include interdisciplinary teams and care management and care coordination programs. There is an emphasis on quality assurance mechanisms and health information technology systems that are supposed to lead to improved quality and better access. These changes are designed to contain and reduce costs (Clancy, 2009; PCMHC, 2007).

There have been a number of PCMH pilot and demonstration projects that examined how to implement the model in integrated care systems, chronic care practices, and private medical practices with promising initial results for cost savings and access to care (Crabtree et al., 2010; Patient-Center Primary Care Collaborative, 2010). Most of the projects have been regional or healthcare system specific. The National Demonstration Project on the Patient-Centered Medical Home (Crabtree et al., 2010; Stange et al., 2010), sponsored by the National Academy of Family Physicians, began in 2006 and compared facilitated and self-directed implementation approaches in a group randomized clinical trial of the PCMH in 36 family practices. The preliminary results showed that implementation of the model improved access and prevention efforts and improved chronic disease care, but did not demonstrate improved patient-rated outcomes or health status. The authors concluded that more time is needed to examine these changes and that other parts of the healthcare system may need to be integrated in order to see the full positive benefits of the PCMH.

The initial proposals for PCMHs did not explicitly include the integration of behavioral health. However, strong outcries from primary care physicians and behavioral health professionals convinced the government and the PCMH leaders to include behavioral health explicitly (APA, 2010; Petterson et al., 2008). Because the authors do not report in their published papers, it is unclear whether any of the PCMH projects included behavioral health as a part of the implementation of the model. Inclusion of behavioral health as an essential component of integrated care and PCMHs in the PPACA will facilitate changes in future efforts to implement the PCMH.

There are compelling data why psychologists and behavioral health need to be key components of any healthcare reform system. Research indicates that behavioral factors, such as diet, stress management, exercise, and lifestyle, account for the largest proportion of variance in health; over 50% of visits to primary care providers are for psychosocial problems and not due to biomedical problems (Blount et al., 2007; CDC, 2003; Farley, 2009). The epidemic rise in obesity in children and adults and subsequent increase in chronic diseases, such as diabetes and hypertension, is just one example of this problem (O'Donohue, Moore, & Scott, 2007).

In many cases, increasing healthy behaviors and behavioral change to promote medical compliance are the most critical factors in health promotion and disease prevention. Whether the focus is on prevention or chronic disease management, it takes health behavior change to improve health. This is why psychologists need to be more involved in the primary care health system and patient-centered medical homes (Bray, 1996, 2010; Frank, McDaniel, Bray, & Heldring, 2004; McDaniel & Fogarty, 2009).

Evidence-Based Practice Through Comparative Effectiveness Research

Healthcare reforms emphasize the need to use evidence-based practice (EBP). The PPACA places greater emphasis on finding out which treatments are most effective and paying only for those treatments. The system for determining effective treatments is called *comparative effectiveness research* (CER) and it is designed to inform healthcare decisions at both individual and population levels by providing evidence on the effectiveness, benefits, and harms of different treatment options. CER is research designed to compare the effectiveness of different treatments for the same problem and determine which treatment works best, for whom, and under what circumstances.

Through testimony at the Institute of Medicine (Bray, 2009), APA proposed a number of areas for CER behavioral research—for example, determining (1) the most cost-effective treatment of school-based interventions in preventing and treating overweight and obesity in children and adolescents, or (2) the best treatment strategies (e.g., symptom management, cognitive behavior therapy, biofeedback, social skills, educator/teacher training, parent training, pharmacologic treatment) for attention deficit hyperactivity disorder (ADHD) in children. The results of these studies will be used to guide future practice and reimbursement policies for treatments (Institute of Medicine, 2009; PPACA, 2010). CER can utilize established evidenced-based programs for children, adolescents, and families (Effective Child Therapy, 2009; Kazdin & Weisz, 2003; SAMHSA, 2009; Yannacci & Rivard, 2006).

Expand the Focus of Traditional Behavioral Health Practice

While there will continue to be a demand and need for traditional mental health services in the future, the growth areas are in integrated healthcare, primary care, and preventive care (Bray, 2010). These are all areas that are authorized and expanded within the PPACA. In addition, with increased competition from master's level providers for providing psychotherapy, it is important that doctorally trained psychologists become clinical leaders and use their expertise in research and evaluation to develop and implement evidence-based psychological services and programmatic changes in health service delivery systems.

Integrated Healthcare Within Patient-Centered Medical Homes

To participate fully in PCMHs, behavioral health providers need to be full partners in the healthcare system and identify as *healthcare providers, not just mental health providers* (Bray, 1996; Cummings et al., 2003; Frank et al., 2004; O'Donohue et al., 2005). Most behavioral health providers are not trained in biomedicine and the lack of understanding can interfere with their participation in healthcare systems. Every medical exam room needs a psychologist and behavioral health provider (Farley, 2009); primary care providers treat over 70% of mental health problems without assistance from psychologists or any other behavioral health providers (Blount et al., 2007).

The PPACA authorizes grants to establish community-based, interdisciplinary, interprofessional health teams to support primary care practices. Health teams may include behavioral health providers. One requirement of health teams receiving grants includes establishing a coordinated system of early identification and referral (such as through the use of health information technology) for children at risk for developmental or behavioral problems.

In addition, the PPACA authorizes the development of coordinated and integrated services in community-based mental health settings. This includes the colocation of primary care in community mental and behavioral health settings. This program is to provide comprehensive care for adults and children with mental illnesses who have co-occurring health problems and chronic disease to receive services in mental health clinics. Thus, whether one practices in a traditional mental health system or in an integrated health system, the government is promoting collaborative care among providers. There is an intentional shift to reduce the mind/body split and treat the whole person in healthcare. This will require practicing differently than in traditional mental health models.

Primary care psychology is the provision of health and mental health services that involves the prevention and treatment of health problems and the promotion of healthy behaviors in individuals, families, and communities (Bray, Frank, McDaniel, & Heldring, 2004). To practice in primary care, a behavioral health professional needs to understand the common biomedical conditions seen within primary care, the medical and pharmacological treatments of those conditions and how they interact with and impact the psychosocial functioning of patients and their families and communities. In addition, it is essential to understand how mental health problems show up in primary care because patients often present with somatic complaints and have subthreshold levels of anxiety and depression, yet they benefit from treatment of these conditions (Petterson et al., 2008).

Integrated primary care practice is different from usual mental health settings (Bray & Rogers, 1995; Cummings et al., 2003; O'Donohue et al., 2005; Robinson & Reiter, 2007). Rather than the weekly 50-minute psychotherapy hour, patients are often seen more quickly in varying time frames—from brief consults to 15- to 20-minute sessions to longer sessions. Psychotherapy focuses on symptom resolution using brief interventions. This requires specialized training and experience in these settings (Bray, 2004; McDaniel, Belar, Schroeder, Hargrove, & Freeman, 2002; O'Donohue et al., 2005; Robinson & Reiter, 2007).

For behavioral health practice, we need to adopt some of the language of medicine and public health. This includes the use of medical diagnostic systems. In most of medicine, the World Health Organization's *International Classification of Disease* (ICD) is used for diagnosis, rather than the American Psychiatric Association's *Diagnostic and Statistical Manual* (DSM). Primary care providers do not generally use the DSM. The APA is sponsoring a psychologist to work on the next revision of the ICD system, which is due out in 2012.

Integrating Technology Into Practice

Through the HITECH (Health Information Technology for Economic and Clinical Health) Act (2009) and the PPACA, Congress provides billions of dollars for the implementation of electronic health records (EHRs) technology. To participate in these changes and, more specifically, in integrated healthcare systems, psychologists and behavioral health providers will be required to use EHRs and other technological advances. Providing services via the Internet (e.g., Skype) and other electronic means of telehealth is also likely to be part of the future of practice. Children and adolescents are more tech savvy and psychologists and behavioral health providers need to update their assessments and interventions to include technology in order to have greater access and to meet clients' expectations, which often include high-tech access and solutions.

REFORMS SPECIFIC TO CHILDREN AND FAMILIES

This section focuses on three major changes of healthcare reform that are specific to children and families. First, as previously discussed, PPACA provides increased access to behavioral healthcare through a variety of programs. Second, prevention efforts are now authorized and covered for many services. Third, there is an emphasis on understanding and decreasing health disparities across all aspects of health services.

Access to Care for Children and Families

The PPACA authorized increased access to healthcare for millions of Americans who are currently uninsured or underinsured. Mental, behavioral health and substance abuse services are considered part of the essential benefits package mandated by the Congress in the PPACA. The combination of increased access, mental health parity act, and the provisions that end discrimination against individuals with preexisting conditions means that more children and families will have greater access to behavioral healthcare. Private insurers can no longer deny coverage for people because of any of the following: health status; medical condition, including both physical and mental illness; claims experience; receipt of healthcare; medical history; genetic information; evidence of insurability (including conditions arising out of acts of domestic violence); or disability (APA, 2010). Further, children are eligible to stay on a parent's insurance plan through age 26. These provisions apply to both private and public insurers and health systems.

Extended coverage is also provided for former foster care children. This change makes mandatory the current state option to extend Medicaid coverage up to age 26 to foster children who have aged out of the foster care system. This provision becomes effective in 2014.

From CHIP to CHIPRA

The reauthorization of the Children's Health Insurance Program (CHIP) with the Children's Health Insurance Program Reauthorization Act of 2009 (CHIPRA) continues health coverage for poor children and families who do not qualify for Medicaid. PPACA extended this program through September 30, 2015. CHIPRA called for new measures of child healthcare quality, quality improvement, and information technology demonstration grants that include the development of a model electronic health record format for children enrolled in CHIP and Medicaid.

Implications of these changes are far reaching: Parents can be less concerned that a child with a mental health problem will be unable to secure health insurance in the future and as an adult. Lifetime and other limits for coverage are lifted as children and families are guaranteed coverage by either private or government-sponsored programs. It is hoped that these changes will persuade parents to seek help for their children's mental and behavioral health problems earlier rather than later—before they develop into more serious conditions.

School-Based Health Centers

The PPACA authorizes grants for the establishment and operation of school-based health centers (SBHCs), which provide comprehensive primary health services, including mental and behavioral health. Preference will be given to

- centers that serve a large population of children eligible for Medicaid
- schools that serve communities with evidenced barriers to primary healthcare and mental health and substance use disorder prevention services for children and adolescents
- communities with high per-capita numbers of children and adolescents who are uninsured, underinsured, or enrolled in public health insurance programs
- populations of children and adolescents who have historically demonstrated difficulty in accessing health and mental health and substance use disorder preventive services

Grantees are required to offer comprehensive mental health services that include mental health and substance use disorder assessments, crisis intervention, counseling, treatment, and referral to a continuum of services including emergency psychiatric care, community support programs, inpatient care, and outpatient programs (APA, 2010).

Women With Postpartum Conditions and Their Families

The PPACA authorizes the secretary of the Department of Health and Human Services to expand the understanding of the causes of and treatments for postpartum conditions. Behavioral health providers can help with the development of improved screening and diagnostic techniques, development and evaluation of new treatments, and development and implementation of education programs for healthcare professionals and the public. New funds will be available for the establishment, operation, and coordination of effective and cost-efficient systems for the delivery of essential services to individuals with or at risk for a postpartum condition and their families.

Pregnant Women

The PPACA requires Medicaid to provide coverage for counseling and pharmacotherapy for cessation of tobacco use for pregnant women. This change also eliminates copayments for these services. Psychological approaches to smoking cessation are well established and successful (Science of Behavior Change Report, 2009).

Preventive Services for Children and Families

Community Prevention Efforts

The PPACA authorizes funding for the implementation, evaluation, and dissemination of evidence-based community preventive health activities to reduce chronic disease rates and address health disparities. These include many areas in which behavioral health providers can contribute: (1) creating healthier school environments; (2) creating programs to increase access to smoking cessation, to improve social and emotional wellness, and to prevent chronic health and mental health problems for children and families; and (3) addressing the needs of special populations with mental and physical disabilities. Behavioral health professionals can contribute to these efforts by providing services, designing programs, and evaluating the effectiveness of the programs.

There are established prevention and intervention programs that can be implemented in these school-based centers (Effective Child Therapy, 2009; Kazdin & Weisz, 2003; SAMHSA, 2009; Yannacci & Rivard, 2006). For example, Dishion developed several programs for use in middle schools that provide evidence-based parenting interventions that address behavior problems and increase social and emotional wellness (Dishion & Stormshak, 2009). Demonstrated outcomes include reductions in substance use and in deviant peer involvement. In addition, there are evidence-based programs to prevent HIV/AIDS, early sexual initiation, and substance use (Pequegnat, 2009).

Coverage of Preventive Health Services

Insurers are now required to provide coverage, without cost sharing or coinsurance payments, for evidence-based services that have a rating of "A" or "B" in the current recommendations of the U.S. Preventive Services Task Force, as well as preventive care and screenings for infants, children, adolescents, and women as provided for in the comprehensive guidelines supported by the Health Resources and Services Administration (HRSA). In addition, coverage for annual wellness visits to provide a personalized prevention plan are now required in Medicare and Medicaid. The law specifically authorizes screening for detection of any cognitive impairment. There are incentives for grants to develop programs within Medicaid to address causes of chronic health problems such as ceasing use of tobacco products, controlling or reducing weight, and addressing comorbidities such as depression that are related to the cause and effects of chronic disease.

Maternal, Infant, and Early Childhood Home Visiting Programs

Services are authorized to provide home visits to promote improvements in maternal and prenatal health, infant health, child health and development, parenting related to child development outcomes, school readiness, and reductions in child abuse, neglect, and injuries. Families who have a history of child abuse or neglect and substance abuse or the need for substance abuse treatment; families who have users of tobacco products in the home; and families who have children with low school achievement, developmental delays, or disabilities receive top priority for these services.

Behavioral health providers can implement many well-established evidence-based programs, such as the multisystemic therapy (Henggeler, Sheidow, & Lee, 2009), within home visiting programs. Multisystemic therapy is an intensive evidence-, family-, and community-based treatment program that focuses on the entire world of chronic and violent juvenile offenders. The therapy is offered in their homes and includes work with schools and teachers, in their neighborhoods, and with their friends.

The emphasis on payment for prevention services may provide new behavioral health opportunities. For example, research on marriage and parenting allows identification of early markers and predictors of couple and family conflict, divorce, and parenting problems that lead to childhood behavior problems and divorce (Dishion & Stormshak, 2009; Gottman, 1994; Ragan, Einhorn, Rhoades, Markman, & Stanley, 2009). Prevention and intervention programs have demonstrated evidence to address these issues. However, the U.S. Preventive Services Task Force does not yet recognize these programs. Thus, additional policy work will be required to have them recognized.

Health Disparities

While many are fortunate to have access to healthcare through private or government-sponsored programs, many people have no health insurance or regular access to healthcare. The implementation of the PPACA should increase access to care. However, even when access is available, there are clear health disparities for ethnic minorities, the poor, and homeless people (Agency for Healthcare Research and Quality, 2010; Institute of Medicine, 2003). Ethnic minorities receive less effective care for chronic health problems, including mental health and substance abuse problems, and this results in increased morbidity and mortality (AHRQ, 2010; see Chapter 16 in this volume). The reasons for this are complex and need further study.

Because many providers do not accept Medicare or Medicaid, even when people have insurance (especially Medicaid), people often resort to emergency rooms and community health centers for their care—places where psychologists and behavioral health providers frequently do not practice. The PPACA has a major emphasis on decreasing and eliminating health disparities. This includes the development of standards and measures for the evaluation of health disparities. Other areas to improve health disparities include providing incentives and rewarding quality for the implementation of activities that reduce healthcare disparities through the use of cultural competency training. Behavioral health providers need to ensure, through multicultural education and policy changes, that they are properly trained to work with diverse populations and that their services are included in funding designed to reduce health disparities (Bray, 2010).

PAYMENT ISSUES

A challenge in these reforms is that most of the increased access to health services is through Medicaid, CHIP, and Medicare. Many private practitioners do not provide services to people with this form of insurance because of the low reimbursement rates and difficult regulations in many states. Reimbursement rates vary by state and region; some provide reimbursement levels similar to private insurance rates (e.g., West Virginia), while others are significantly lower (e.g., Texas) than private rates and make it difficult for providers to make a reasonable living. In addition, many of these services are provided in community health centers, which frequently do not employ psychologists or behavioral health specialists.

The federal government is developing treatment models that move away from fee for service and into more organized systems of care, such as community health systems and integrated care systems in which healthcare providers are likely to be paid salaries and/or flat rates for providing care. While the public may continue to value psychological services and pay out of pocket for them, psychologists who choose to practice in traditional independent practices will face increasing pressures from the federal government to join organized systems of care, such as PCMHs, as well as additional competition from master's level providers who will provide similar services for reduced costs. There appears to be pressure for private insurers to lower their rates to Medicare standards for payment as a method of reducing healthcare costs.

TRAINING OPPORTUNITIES

The PPACA provides funds for investment in a future pediatric healthcare workforce. A loan repayment program for qualified health professionals, including psychologists, who agree to be employed full-time for no less than 2 years providing pediatric care (including mental and behavioral healthcare) was authorized. Priority will be given to providers who have familiarity with evidence-based methods and cultural and linguistic competence in healthcare services.

In addition, the graduate psychology education (GPE) grant program provides funding to train master's, doctoral, and postdoctoral trainees. GPE is a grant program that provides funds to interdisciplinary programs that train psychologists to work with poor, underserved children, families, and adults. In order to be eligible for these funds, psychologists have to partner with at least two other disciplines in their training program. Authorization for funding the GPE program increased in the PPACA.

Traditional psychology and mental health training programs need to change their programs radically for the new realities created with healthcare reform, the move to integrated healthcare systems, and emphasis on primary care (Bray, 2010). While there will continue to be a need for traditional and specialty mental health services, the future opportunities are in providing behavioral healthcare to people with chronic disease and the elderly. People with these conditions or in these situations are the economic drivers of healthcare. As demonstrated by Cummings and colleagues (1967, 1968, 2003), when full integration of behavioral health occurs in medical systems, it is efficacious and cost effective and saves money.

EVIDENCE-BASED PRACTICE FOR CHILDREN, ADOLESCENTS, AND FAMILIES

There are many established evidence-based therapies to treat children, adolescents, and families (Bray & Stanton, 2009; Effective Child Therapy, 2009; Kazdin & Weisz, 2003; SAMHSA, 2009; Yannacci & Rivard, 2006). It is beyond the scope of this chapter to review the many effective treatments that are currently available. Several resources provide practitioners with reviews of currently available treatments and interventions. Overviews of EBP family interventions are found in Bray and Stanton (2009) and Fisher and O'Donohue (2006).

The Effective Child Therapy (2009) Web site developed by the APA Society of Clinical Child and Adolescent Psychology (Division 54) and the Association for Behavioral and Cognitive Therapies provides information and reviews of EBP programs. Therapies are organized for the public by problems (e.g., sadness, worry, rule breaking) and for professionals by disorder and diagnosis (e.g., conduct disorder, OCD). This Web site is regularly maintained and updated to provide both professionals and the public with information about effective treatments.

SAMHSA has developed several Web sites that provide information about EBP. The Systems of Care (SOC, 2009) Web site provides information on programs and resources for transforming the mental health of America's children. Yannacci and Rivard (2006) reviewed the literature on EBP for children for SAMHSA. Their report and matrix of interventions provides a quick and user-friendly resource for locating peer-reviewed programs. This report can be downloaded from the SOC Web site. The National Registry of Evidence-Based Programs and Practices (NREPP, 2009) is a searchable database of interventions for the prevention and treatment of mental and substance use disorders. SAMHSA developed this resource to help the public, agencies, and organizations implement programs and practices in their communities. Both Web sites include information directed at the public and professionals and are regularly updated based on new research findings. The SAMHSA Web sites are broader than that of Effective Child Therapy and include information about community programs and populations targeted by SAMHSA, such as minorities, the underserved, and the poor.

FUTURE CHILD AND FAMILY PRACTICE OPPORTUNITIES

While there will continue to be a need for specialty and traditional mental health services, the clear growth areas are in the broader healthcare arena and in other areas outside mental healthcare. The growth areas for practice are in all of the sectors of healthcare (see Figure 15.1), especially in primary care, patient-centered medical homes, and public health and clinical and team leadership (Bray, 2010; Bray et al., 2009).

However, many other areas are also open and in need of behavioral health services, and these services are not necessarily for psychotherapy and traditional mental health. Future practice opportunities include the application of the evidence-based behavior change strategies for a wide variety of health problems that range from compliance with medical regimes to the promotion of lifestyle changes that may prevent chronic disease to helping children and families adapt to health problems (Science of Behavior Change Report, 2009). With the development of the health and behavior CPT (current procedural terminology) codes, behavioral health professionals can be reimbursed for treating children with medical problems that do not have a mental health diagnosis (APA Practice Organization, 2004). The use of these codes is for behavioral assessment and treatment of medical conditions that have been diagnosed by a physician.

For example, a child with diabetes and no mental health problems can be assessed and treated for the behavioral aspects of the impact of diabetes on children and to help families cope with their diabetic child (Johnson, 2006). In addition, using behavior change strategies and interventions, behavioral health professionals can help children and families be compliant with medical regimes and help them develop healthier lifestyles that decrease morbidity from the disease.

Currently, most psychologists and behavioral health providers practice in independent settings in solo or small-group practices. Some have multidisciplinary practices, but usually they are with other mental health specialists. They provide traditional mental health services, usually seeing their clients or patients in isolation from the general healthcare system. This system of care is supported by mental health carve-outs and confidentiality standards that keep mental health separate from general healthcare. However, there are multiple examples of independent practices that collaborate closely with pediatricians and family physicians to provide behavioral health services for children and families (Bray, 2004; Driscoll & McCabe, 2004). The models of care range from separate practices with close referrals to colocation of practices within the same locations to fully integrated systems of care (Bray & Rogers, 1995).

The PPACA promotes the move to integrated healthcare with a greater emphasis on primary care through the PCMH. Behavioral health is part of this new model and it is up to psychologists and other behavioral health providers to take advantage of these opportunities because many of the authorized programs include but *do not require* behavioral health providers to participate. If we do not step up and participate, other professionals, such as nurses, health educators, and social workers, will fill these roles. With the implementation of healthcare reform, we have many new and exciting opportunities to help children and families who have not had adequate access to our services. However, to take full advantage of these opportunities, we will need to practice in different ways, with different methods, and in different settings.

The PPACA creates many new opportunities for psychologists and other behavioral health providers, yet there are areas that need further work and advocacy. For example, the reliance on the USPS prevention guidelines does not explicitly include prevention programs developed by psychologists for problems such as childhood behavior problems, obesity, and other chronic diseases. Further, most psychologists and behavioral health specialists are not trained to work in integrated health or primary care systems. Inclusion of psychologists in the U.S. workforce analysis plans authorized in the PPACA may demonstrate a shortage, and justify increases in federal training dollars that are dedicated to producing more psychologists who work in primary and integrated care systems.

These types of changes require that we not only change our profession and educational systems, but that we also increase our engagement in public policy advocacy efforts (Bray, 2010). To truly realize the potential of full behavioral health integration, we need federal and state policy makers to recognize and increase our participation in healthcare legislation and programs. I previously called for the creation of a new department of behavioral health and senior director of the department within the federal government (Bray, 2010). The data on behavioral and psychosocial factors support this need. It is time to recognize this reality with a high-level department within our government, similar to what has been done with the undersecretary of the Office for Minority Health within DHHS. This type of investment will help ensure that our nation's children and adolescents receive the kind of care that they need to be productive citizens in the generations to come.

REFERENCES

AHRQ (Agency for Healthcare Research and Quality). (2010). National healthcare disparities report: 2009. AHRQ report publication no. 10-0004. Rockville, MD. Retrieved from www.ahrq.gov/qual/qrdr09.htm

APA (American Psychological Association). (2010). *Healthcare reform*. Washington, DC: APA. Retrieved from http://www.apa.org/health-reform/

APA (American Psychological Association) Practice Organization. (2004). Health and behavior CPT codes. Washington, DC: APA. Retrieved from http://www.apapracticecentral.org/reimbursement/billing/secure/new-codes.aspx

Blount, A., Schoenbaum, M., Kathol, R., Rollman, B. L., Thomas, M., O'Donohue, W., & Peek, C. J. (2007). The economics of behavioral health services in medical settings: A summary of the evidence. *Professional Psychology: Research and Practice, 38*, 290–297.

Bray, J. H. (1996). Psychologists as primary care practitioners. In R. J. Resnick & R. H. Rozensky (Eds.), *To your health: Psychology across the life span* (pp. 89–100). Washington, DC: American Psychological Association.

Bray, J. H. (2004). Training primary care psychologists. *Journal of Clinical Psychology in Medical Settings, 11,* 101–107.

Bray, J. H. (2009). Behavioral research in comparative effectiveness research. Testimony to Institute of Medicine Committee on Comparative Effectiveness Research Priorities, March 20, Washington, DC. Retrieved from www.apa.org/news/press/releases/IOM-Bray.pdf

Bray, J. H. (2010). The future of psychology practice and science. *American Psychologist, 65,* 355–369.

Bray, J. H., Frank, R. G., McDaniel, S. H., & Heldring, M. (2004). Education, practice and research opportunities for psychologists in primary care. In R. G. Frank, S. H. McDaniel, J. H. Bray, & M. Heldring (Eds.), *Primary care psychology* (pp. 3–21). Washington, DC: American Psychological Association.

Bray, J. H., Goodheart, C., Heldring, M., Brannick, J., Gresen, R., Hawley, G.,...Strickland, W. (2009). *Task Force on the Future of Psychology Practice Final Report.* Washington, DC: American Psychological Association.

Bray, J. H., & Rogers, J. C. (1995). Linking psychologists and family physicians for collaborative practice. *Professional Psychology: Research and Practice, 26,* 132–138.

Bray, J. H., & Stanton, M. (Eds.). (2009). *Handbook of family psychology.* London, England: Wiley-Blackwell.

CDC (Centers for Disease Control and Prevention). (2003). *Health, United States, 2003 with chartbook on trends in the health of Americans.* Washington, DC: Department of Health and Human Services.

Clancy, C. M. (July, 2009). Federal perspective on health care reform: Agency for Health Research and Quality. Paper presented at the Patient Center Medical Home Stakeholders meeting, Washington, DC.

Crabtree, B. F., Nutting, P. A., Miller, W. L., Stange, K. C., Stewart, E. E., & Jaén, C. R. (2010). Summary of the National Demonstration Project and recommendations for the patient-centered medical home. *Annals of Family Medicine, 8*(Suppl 1), s80–s90.

Cummings, N. A., Cummings, J. L, & Johnson, J. N. (1997). *Behavioral health in primary care: A guide for clinical integration.* Madison, WI: Psychosocial Press.

Cummings, N. A., & Follette, W. T. (1968). Psychiatric services and medical utilization in a prepaid health plan setting: Part 2. *Medical Care, 6,* 31–41.

Dishion, T. J., & Stormshak, E. (2009). A family-centered intervention strategy for public middle schools. In J. H. Bray & M. Stanton (Eds.), *Handbook of family psychology* (pp. 499–514). London, England: Wiley-Blackwell.

Driscoll, W. D., & McCabe, E. P. (2004). Primary care psychology in independent practice. In R. G. Frank, S. H. McDaniel, J. H. Bray, & M. Heldring (Eds.). *Primary care psychology* (pp. 133–148). Washington, DC: American Psychological Association.

Effective Child Therapy. (2009). Evidence-based mental health treatments for children and adolescents. Society of Clinical Child and Adolescent Psychology and Association of Cognitive and Behavioral Therapies. Retrieved from http://www.effectivechildtherapy.com/

Farley, T. (May, 2009). Extreme collaboration: Total integration of behavioral clinicians into primary care practice. Presentation at the 2009 Presidential Summit on the Future of Psychology Practice. American Psychological Association, San Antonio, TX. Retrieved from http://www.apa.org/practice/resources/summit/index.aspx

Fisher, J. E., & O'Donohue, W. T. (2006). *Practitioner's guide to evidence-based psychotherapy.* New York, NY: Springer.

Follette, W. T., & Cummings, N. A. (1967). Psychiatric services and medical utilization in a prepaid health plan setting. *Medical Care, 5,* 25–35.

Frank, R. (May, 2009). Mental health economics. Presentation at the 2009 Presidential Summit on the Future of Psychology Practice. American Psychological Association, San Antonio, TX. Retrieved from http://www.apa.org/practice/resources/summit/index.aspx

Frank, R. G., McDaniel, S. H., Bray, J. H., & Heldring, M. (Eds.). (2004). *Primary care psychology.* Washington, DC: American Psychological Association.

Gottman, J. M. (1994). *What predicts divorce? The relationship between marital processes and marital outcomes.* Hillsdale, NJ: Lawrence Erlbaum Associates.

Health Information Technology for Economic and Clinical Health (HITECH) Act. (2009). American Recovery and Reinvestment Act of 2009. U.S. Congress. Retrieved from http://www.opencongress.org/bill/111-h1/show and http://www.cms.hhs.gov/recovery/11_healthit.asp

Hemmings, A. (2000). A systematic review of the effectiveness of brief psychological therapies in primary health care. *Family, Systems and Health, 18,* 279–313.

Henggeler, S. W., Sheidow, A. J., & Lee, T. (2009). Multisystemic therapy. In J. H. Bray and M. Stanton (Eds.), *Handbook of family psychology* (pp. 370–387). London, England: Wiley-Blackwell.

Institute of Medicine. (2003). *Unequal treatment: Confronting racial and ethnic disparities in health care.* B. D. Smedley, A.Y. Stith, & A. R. Nelson (Eds.). Washington, DC: National Academies Press.

Institute of Medicine. (2009). *Initial national priorities for comparative effectiveness research.* Washington, DC: National Academies Press.

Johnson, S. B. (2006). Genetic screening for type 1 diabetes: Psychosocial impact on families. In S. M. Miller, S. H. McDaniel, J. S. Rolland, & S. L. Feetham (Eds.), *Individuals, families, and the new era of genetics: Biopsychosocial perspectives* (pp. 404–422). New York, NY: Norton & Co.

Kazdin, A. E., & Weisz, J. R. (2003). *Evidence-based psychotherapies for children and adolescents.* New York, NY: Guilford Press.

Kessler, R. C., Demler, O., Frank, R. G., Olfson, M., Pincus, H. A., Walters, E. E.,...Zaslavsky, A. M. (2005). Prevalence and treatment of mental disorders, 1990 to 2003. *New England Journal of Medicine, 352,* 2515–2523.

McDaniel, S. H., Belar, C. D., Schroeder, C., Hargrove, D. S., & Freeman, E. L. (2002). A training curriculum for professional psychologists in primary care. *Professional Psychology: Research and Practice, 33,* 65–72.

McDaniel, S. H., & Fogarty, C. T. (2009). What primary care psychology has to offer the patient-centered medical home. *Professional Psychology: Research and Practice, 40,* 483–492.

Medical Expenditure Panel Survey. (2009). Agency for Healthcare Research and Quality, Washington, DC: Department of Health and Human Services. Retrieved from http://www.meps.ahrq.gov/mepsweb

Miller, S. M., McDaniel, S. H., Rolland, J. S., & Feetham, S. L. (2006). *Individuals, families, and the new era of genetics: Biopsychosocial perspectives.* New York, NY: Norton & Co.

Newman, R., & Rozensky, R. (1995). Psychology and primary care: Evolving traditions. *Journal of Clinical Psychology in Medical Settings, 2,* 3–6.

O'Donohue, W. T., Byrd, M. R., Cummings, N. A., & Henderson, D. A. (2005). *Behavioral integrative care: Treatments that work in the primary care setting.* New York, NY: Brunner-Routledge.

O'Donohue, W. T., Moore, B., & Scott, B. (Eds.). (2007). *Handbook of pediatric and adolescent obesity treatment.* New York, NY: Routledge.

PCMHC (Patient Centered Medical Home Collaborative). (2007). Joint principles of the patient centered medical home. Washington, DC. Retrieved from http://www.pcpcc.net/content/joint-principles-patient-centered-medical-home

Patient-Center Primary Care Collaborative. (2010). Proof in practice: A compilation of patient-centered medical home pilot and demonstration projects. Washington, DC. Retrieved from http://www.pcpcc.net/content/lesson-learned

Petterson, S., Phillips, B., Bazemore, A., Dodoo, M., Zhang, X., & Green, L. A. (2008). Why there must be room for mental health in the medical home. *American Family Physician, 77,* 757.

Ragan, E. P., Einhorn, L. A., Rhoades, G. K., Markman, H. J., & Stanley, S. M. (2009). Relationship education programs: Current trends and future directions. In J. H. Bray & M. Stanton (Eds.), *Handbook of family psychology* (pp. 450–462). London, England: Wiley-Blackwell.

Robinson, P. J., & Reiter, J. T. (2007). *Behavioral consultation and primary care: A guide to integrating services.* New York, NY: Springer.

Routh, D. K., Schroeder, C. S., & Koocher, G. P. (1983). Psychology and primary health care for children. *American Psychologist, 38,* 95–98.

Saultz, J. (2008). Something you somehow haven't to deserve: A medical home for every American. Retrieved from http://www.fmdrl.org/index.cfm/saultz#17

Science of Behavior Change Report. (2009). National Institutes of Health. Washington, DC. Retrieved from http://www.nia.nih.gov/NR/rdonlyres/AF0997F6-0C16-4A76-96C0-D3780F00E6D4/13545/2009Jun_SOBCMeetingReport_final.pdf

Stange, K. C., Miller, W. L., Nutting, P. A., Crabtree, B. F., Stewart, E. E., & Jaén, C. R. (2010). Context for understanding the national demonstration project and the patient-centered medical home. *Annals of Family Medicine, 8*(Suppl 1), s2–s8.

SAMHSA (Substance Abuse and Mental Health Services Administration). (2009a). National registry of evidence-based programs and practices. Washington, DC. Retrieved from http://www.nrepp.samhsa.gov/

SAMHSA (Substance Abuse and Mental Health Services Administration). (2009b). Systems of care: Transforming children's mental health care in America. Washington, DC. Retrieved from http://systemsofcare.samhsa.gov/

U.S. Congress. (2008). H.R. 6983: Wellstone and Domenici Mental Parity and Addiction Equity Act. Washington, DC. Retrieved from http://www.govtrack.us/congress/bill.xpd?bill=h110-6983

U.S. Congress. (2010). H.R. 3590 Patient Protection and Affordable Care Act. Washington, DC. Retrieved from http://www.opencongress.org/bill/111-h3590/show

Wang, P. S., Demler, O., Olfson, M., Pincus, H. A., Wells, K. B., & Kessler, R. C. (2006). Changing profiles of service sectors used for mental health care in the United States. *American Journal of Psychiatry, 163,* 1187–1198.

Wright, L., & Burns, B. J. (1986). Primary mental health care: A "find" for psychology. *Professional Psychology: Research and Practice, 17,* 560–564.

Yannacci, J., & Rivard, J. C. (2006). Matrix of children's evidence-based interventions. NRI Center for Mental Health Quality and Accountability, Washington, DC. Retrieved from systemsofcare.samhsa.gov/headermenus/docsHM/MatrixFINAL1.pdf

Sixteen

Reforms for Ethnic Minorities and Women

LORRAINE BENUTO AND BRIAN D. LEANY

INTRODUCTION

Our general interest in the current healthcare reform lies in how it will impact the mental and behavioral healthcare system. Our specific interest lies in how these reforms will impact ethnic minorities and women. The healthcare reform bill specifically addresses 10 domains, 7 of which are relevant to our discussion here: quality, affordable healthcare for all Americans; the role of public programs; improving the quality and efficiency of healthcare; prevention of chronic disease and improving public health; the healthcare workforce; improving transparency and program integrity; and reauthorization of the Indian Health Care Improvement Act (www.whitehouse.gov/health-care-meeting/proposal).

Even though legislation was recently signed (U.S. Congress, 2010), it is still not clear how the reform will impact the mental and behavioral health industries and, even more, how it will affect ethnic minorities and women. It would seem that there would be some improvement in that converting the uninsured will allow many minorities and poor women to be insured. While the full details of this new legislation are still coming to light, this chapter examines how the reform might impact both behavioral and mental healthcare for ethnic minorities and women. Specifically, we explore problems with the conceptualization of cultural sensitivity, discuss the most prevalent issues faced by ethnic minorities and women, and examine considerations for maximizing the utilization of behavioral health services by these groups in an integrative healthcare setting.

PROBLEMS WITH THE CULTURAL SENSITIVITY MOVEMENT

The cultural sensitivity movement is not new. Scholars and researchers alike have been writing about ethnic differences and their relationship to mental health for decades (e.g., Cardemil, 2010; Chavez, Cornelius, & Jones, 1985; Conner, Koeske, & Brown, 2009; Falicov, 1996; Givens, Houston, Van Voorhees, Ford, & Cooper, 2007; Leaf, Bruce, & Tischler, 1986; Snowden, 1998). In fact, a search in the psycinfo database—which houses the vast majority of scholarly works in the area of psychology—yielded almost 2,000 results using the terms "ethnic minority" and "mental health"; the oldest result was from 1967. A cursory review of this vast literature indicated that a large portion of scholarly works have focused on discussing ethnic differences (in attitudes, use of healthcare, prevalence for certain disorders, etc.), identifying putative barriers to access, or discussing the problems associated with the lack of cultural sensitivity.

Thus, while a number of works have provided theoretical discussions of the hypothesized problems faced by ethnic minorities (unique to as well as not specific to ethnic minorities), few have offered or implemented practical solutions to these redundantly identified problems. Fewer still have systematically evaluated outcomes and proposed reforms to improve any of these putative problems. In fact, one might say that, as a field, we are experts in discussing how we should be culturally sensitive yet we do a poor job at even defining and discussing the construct of cultural sensitivity. This problematic trend was noted by O'Donohue (1995), who operationalized the construct of cultural sensitivity and proposed seven dimensions for it:

- Accurately identifying the culture to which the person belongs
- Accurately knowing actual regularities associated with the culture or cultures
- Knowing when these regularities are potentially relevant to the task with which the psychologist is concerned
- Making proper ethical judgments that acting on or respecting this cultural regularity is not ethically impermissible

- Knowing how to implement effectively any action in a culturally sensitive manner
- If cultural sensitivity is regarded as a global construct, all issues are nested by all relevant cultures and all possible permutations
- Awareness of what the psychologist's own cultural values, assumptions, and the like bring to the task at hand

Defining cultural sensitivity was an important first step because discussing and solving a problem requires defining key constructs related to the problem.

While examining specific ethnic differences can be useful (e.g., if we know that X ethnic group has a high prevalence rate of depression, we know that we need to have an efficacious treatment for depression for this group), to withhold services in the interest of studying ethnic differences exhaustively would not allow us to move forward at a desirable pace and has a tendency to prevent the attainment of the goals set out in the current healthcare plan (e.g., improving quality and efficiency of healthcare, prevention of chronic disease, and improving public healthcare as well as improving transparency and program integrity). For example, if it takes 1 year to collect data to determine all ethnic differences in, for example, sexual attitudes, that year might be better spent examining the efficacy and effectiveness of an established treatment for a specific ethnic group, especially because leaders in the field have recommended that we not assume that an evidence-based treatment is generalizable to other ethnic groups until it is proven to be.

Thus, a second step that has not been taken is moving out of "discussing" and into "doing" and evaluating. Our first recommendation is that researchers begin conducting outcome studies to establish which treatments work with ethnic minorities and women and in the meantime use evidence-based treatments when working with cultural minorities.

BARRIERS: A REDUNDANT DISCUSSION

As mentioned previously, the literature is replete with works that discuss the barriers faced by ethnic minorities (e.g., Barrett et al., 1998; Conner et al., 2009; Garrett, Treichel, & Ohmans, 1998; Harrell & Carrasquillo, 2003; Hubbell, Waitzkin, Mishra, Dombrink, & Chavez, 1991; Jenkins, Le, McPhee, Stewart, & Ha, 1996; Jones, Cason, & Bond, 2002; Scheppers, van Dongen, Dekker, Geertzen, & Dekker, 2006; Smith, Kreutzer, Goldman,

Casey-Paal, & Kizer, 1996). This particular discussion will be brief, although certainly not unique.

We are well aware of the issues faced by ethnic minorities, although many of these issues seem not to be ethnic specific but rather appear to be related more to issues of socioeconomic status (SES). In fact, lower socioeconomic status, simply conceptualized as an amalgam of economic, educational, racial, cultural, and/or ethnic variables, can also act as a barrier to healthcare. This can be seen in the poor efficacy of healthcare advertising targeted at specific ethnic groups, which would most likely be more efficacious if it were instead more broadly targeted at lower SES groups (Garrett et al., 1998; Jenkins et al., 1996; Jones et al., 2002). Even more commonly, these issues seem to relate to a communication breakdown due to the disparity of socioeconomic status between the ethnic minority patient and his or her care provider (Flores & Vega, 1998; Smith et al., 1996).

Furthermore, these problems have the potential to have a negative impact on the patient's perceptions and use of healthcare services (Jones et al., 2002). Any reform that can improve the understanding of these difficulties for healthcare providers and those who are tasked with creating, administering, maintaining, and revising public health programs would meet the goals of healthcare reform legislation and provide a better service to ethnic minorities and women, as well as those who share similar socioeconomic status.

From a more practical perspective (and, again, certainly not specific to ethnic minorities), research has indicated that families perceive lack of transportation, long waits, inflexible hours, and distance between home and the treatment location as barriers to treatment (Leaf et al., 1986; Trupin, Forsyth-Stephens, & Low, 1991). Lack of health insurance has also been cited as a barrier to healthcare and has been reported to prevail among Latinos (Bolen, Rhodes, Powell-Griner, Bland, & Holtzman, 2000); an alarming 32.4% of Latinos residing in the United States lack health insurance coverage, although this should change dramatically with recent federal legislation. African Americans and Asian Americans also constitute high numbers of individuals who lack coverage, with 19.9 and 18% lacking coverage, respectively (U.S. Census, 2002).

Cost has been cited as a barrier to healthcare among certain ethnic groups (e.g., Latinos; Bolen et al., 2000) and lower socioeconomic status is associated with greater barriers to receiving services for mental health conditions (Eiraldi, Mazzuca, Clarke, & Power, 2006). Considering that we live in a multicultural society replete with many different languages, it is not surprising that linguistic limitations have been cited as a constraint in the current healthcare system (e.g., Barrett et al., 1998). The barriers discussed earlier are compounded for ethnic minorities, given the high number who are establishing residence in rural communities (Yellowlees, Marks, Hilty, & Shore, 2008). The U.S. Department of Agriculture has indicated that the Hispanic/Latino population in rural and frontier America has increased from 1.4 to 2.7 million (Hamrick, 2005).

Researchers have indicated that stigma surrounding the use of mental health services is prevalent among ethnic minority groups in the United States (Akutsu, Snowden, & Organista, 1996; Alvidrez & Azocar, 1999b), perhaps creating an additional barrier to the attainment of behavioral healthcare services. The issue of access has been cited as being worse for undocumented immigrants (Harrell & Carrasquillo, 2003); for example, 64% of the approximately 6.6 million undocumented Latinos do not have health insurance (Passel & Cohn, 2009). However, this is a number that over the last decade has increased numerically, but decreased proportionately, as past estimates suggested that 75% of undocumented immigrants were uninsured, for a total of 3.3 million (Quinn, 2000). Considering that the vast majority of social services require proof of legal residency, a majority of noncitizens cannot use this avenue to obtain behavioral health services. Additionally, individuals who are undocumented may be afraid to seek out behavioral health services out of fear of arrest, deportation, etc.

Our second recommendation is that, as a field, we become more proactive and identify and implement solutions to the problems we have been discussing for decades. This recommendation is related to healthcare reform's goals as they relate to the domains of healthcare workforce and the role of public programs. The number of healthcare providers will be augmented and additional funding can be used to facilitate patient transportation to service centers, decrease long waits, and establish more flexible treatment hours by increasing practitioner availability and decreasing the distance between patient homes and service centers. This can be accomplished by creating new treatment centers staffed with providers who benefit from programs such as student loan repayment, etc.

SOME CULTURAL FACTORS ARE TWO-FACED

While anybody would be hard-pressed to argue that the barriers discussed earlier can facilitate the treatment process or contribute to improved mental health, some cultural factors appear to be two-faced; that is, in certain instances they can act as a barrier to services, but in others they may facilitate ethnic minority mental health. For example, family support can be advantageous in providing emotional support to the ethnic minority patient (Lipton, Losey, Giachello, Mendez, & Girotti, 1998) and kinship may furnish assistance, companionship, and stability (Morgan, 1996). However, family support can also be viewed in an unconstructive way when collective family responsibilities take precedent over individual needs (El-Kebbi et al., 1996; Lipton et al., 1998). Therefore, family and social support can act as a facilitator to healthcare while over-reliance on family members can act as a barrier to mental healthcare services.

A similar issue has been observed in cultures where there is a large premium on religion. Research has suggested that ethnic minorities may have a preference for religious practices (e.g., U.S. Department of Health and Human Services, 2001) and tend to reject antidepressant medications (Givens et al., 2007)—both of which may create barriers to effective mental and behavioral healthcare treatments. However, there is also good evidence that religion can be a buffer to forming a mental disorder as well as a good resource for improving any conditions that do develop (for a review of the influence of spirituality as a buffer to mental health, see Koenig, 2010). Additionally, the presenting problem can also determine whether or not certain cultural factors may act as a barrier or a facilitator.

For example, if a Catholic male (ethnic minority or not) loses his wife, it may in fact be helpful for him to rely on a priest and/or his family as he is working through his grief over her death. However, if a Catholic mother (ethnic minority or not) has a 4-year-old with enuresis and she goes to her priest for help, the priest may be able to lend a listening and empathic ear (which could result in her feeling better—considering the literature on common factors), but she is likely to be equally frustrated the next day when her child continues to urinate in his or her pants because the priest is not likely to have the knowledge and background necessary to help her effectively treat the enuresis. In this instance, the better course of action would be the use of a urine alarm system (Friman, 1986), which she could learn about from a behavioral healthcare specialist.

Finally, it is important to keep in mind that in some instances cultural factors are simply not relevant to treatment. This may also be related to the presenting problem; in our previous enuresis example, cultural factors may have a limited place because the treatment for enuresis is largely behavioral and the principles of learning are easily translated cross culturally. Thus, our third recommendation is that behavioral healthcare specialists recognize and make use of cultural factors that may act as facilitators in the treatment of cultural minorities and be mindful that not all treatments require cultural modifications.

WILL THE REAL CULTURAL MINORITY PLEASE STAND UP?

An additional problem that we need to consider (especially when we discuss the efficacy of evidence-based treatments) is what determines cultural minority status. Determinations could be made by ethnicity, gender, sexual orientation, age, religion, etc. O'Donohue and Benuto (2010) discuss how Betancourt and Lopez's (1993) definition of culture is typically used—that is, "culture refers to a shared set of social norms, beliefs and values that particular groups hold and transmit across generations" (p. 8)—but seems to exclude some groups that are typically included in the culturally sensitive movement (e.g., gay, lesbian, bisexual, and transgender; GLBT) while simultaneously seems too inclusive for the cultural sensitivity movement (i.e., includes groups traditionally thought to be outside the cultural sensitivity movement tent, such as Jewish Americans or Irish Catholics).

Considering that leaders in the cultural sensitivity movement are recommending that treatments not be considered generalizable until proven to be so, we need to establish what determines how exhaustive we need to be when considering the range of possible cultural group permutations. If we know cognitive behavioral therapy (CBT) is effective for treating depression, to whom does this effectiveness generalize? If this hypothetical study were conducted with Irish Catholic males, do we assume that CBT is effective only with Irish Catholic males? What about Irish females? Catholic females? Non-Irish males? Non-Catholic males?

Thus, our fourth recommendation is that as a field we establish parameters to guide how exhaustive we need to be when considering the range of possible cultural group permutations and, in the meantime, behavioral healthcare specialists use evidence-based treatments when working with cultural minorities. We further recommend that treatments be considered generalizable unless there is a cultural factor that directly contradicts a treatment component; as discussed previously, not all treatments require a cultural modification. We need to develop better heuristics for this judgment.

HOW IS THIS CHAPTER DIFFERENT?

So far, we have provided limited innovative content. We have discussed the problems with the idea of cultural sensitivity, engaged in a redundant discussion of the literature on cultural sensitivity, and offered approximately four recommendations. In the remainder of this chapter, we will provide additional simple recommendations to the problems identified in the literature and emphasize how, in the context of what we understand to be the goals of healthcare reform, integrated care is perfectly positioned to address many of these issues.

EVIDENCE-BASED TREATMENTS AND THE CULTURAL SENSITIVITY MOVEMENT

As a field, the majority of training programs for behavioral healthcare specialists emphasize the use of science in establishing and selecting treatments; however, when it comes to selecting evidence-based treatments for individuals from different cultural backgrounds, we are left poorly trained. This may be due in part to the current position of the cultural sensitivity movement. As discussed previously, we have only recently begun to define cultural sensitivity and at present it is not clear who should be considered a cultural minority. Unfortunately, as a field, it seems that we have remained stagnant and have not managed to be solution focused. Instead, we have become experts at identifying and discussing barriers, discussing how things should be culturally sensitive, etc.

While identifying barriers is certainly an important first step in meeting the goals of healthcare reform, what is even more important is figuring out how to reduce and/or overcome them; this will be discussed momentarily. We absolutely maintain that cultural considerations are important but fear that our well-intended desire to be culturally sensitive has caused a disservice to those we are desperately trying to serve. We believe that it is crucial that we not detour from using evidence-based treatments on the premise that our clients' cultural characteristics justify deviating from gold standards of treatment. Selecting treatments that have little or no scientific basis acts as a disservice to cultural minorities seeking behavioral healthcare services.

For example, Garrett and Carroll (2000) discuss the value of the circle (among other cultural factors) in Native American culture and its potential use in the treatment of alcohol abuse and/or dependence. While they do not specifically recommend the explicit use of the "sacred circle" to treat this population, their article sheds light on the idea that seems to prevail among clinicians: that certain cultural factors should be incorporated into treatment (despite such incorporations having little or no scientific basis). A search of the psycinfo database using the terms "American Indians," "circle," and "therapy" yielded seven publications in peer-reviewed journals. Of these, only two (Heilbron & Guttman, 2000; Moody, 1995) consisted of outcome studies. The other five (BigFoot & Schmidt, 2010; Garrett, Garrett, & Brotherton, 2001; Garrett & Osborne, 1995; Rhinehart & Engelhorn, 1984; Tafoya, 1989) provided recommendations for the incorporation of certain cultural phenomena related to American Indians (e.g., the use of color, circles, the sweat lodge).

Using interventions that have no scientific basis (e.g., "drum circle therapy" to treat depression) when we have established which treatments work (e.g., cognitive behavioral therapy to treat depression) is akin to using herbs to treat cancer simply because herbs are a part of a specific group's culture when, in fact, we know that cancer is best treated using chemotherapy, radiation, etc.

As discussed earlier, leaders in the cultural sensitivity movement (e.g., Cardemil, 2010) suggest that therapies should be considered nongeneralizable to a particular group until they are shown to be so. This could involve an infinite number of outcome studies to establish the efficacy of many different treatments for each minority group (e.g., Gay Aleutian Islanders) (O'Donohue & Benuto, 2010), which is simply not feasible. Nonetheless, it seems unjust to provide non-evidence-based treatment to cultural minorities.

We propose that while it is certainly appropriate to consider the psychosocial backgrounds, language (including variations in description of symptoms), traditions, customs, beliefs, etc. of the racial and ethnic groups we are serving (U.S. Department of Health and Human Services, 2001; Yellowlees et al., 2008), treatments should ultimately be selected based on the extent to which they have established efficacy. For example, an evidence-based treatment should be the treatment of choice even if there is not a single published study on the specific cultural group with which a behavioral health specialist is working. For example, if prolonged exposure therapy is the gold standard treatment for PTSD (Foa, Hembree, & Rothbaum, 2007) but we do not know the efficacy with X cultural group, we should not justify doing hypnotherapy or utilizing a drum circle with a client who has PTSD simply on the basis of cultural sensitivity if hypnotherapy or drum circles are not considered evidenced-based treatments.

The medical world has long been practicing from an evidence-based perspective, tracing it as far back as the ancient Greeks and Chinese (Sackett, Straus, Richardson, Rosenberg, & Haynes, 2000). The social sciences that provide treatment have recently been employing this process. While outcome research specifically designed for use with specific cultural minorities may be lacking, we must also begin to test treatments (when it seems appropriate to do so) that have established efficacy with different cultural groups and, in the meantime, use rather than avoid evidence-based practices (even in the absence of specific studies for these populations). As the two groups (i.e., medical and social science) converge in their style of process, this is likely to produce a confluence in the literature of *best practices* that would identify when best to refer to the appropriate provider (e.g., primary care provider, psychologist, dietician, etc.), based upon outcome measures. This process is likely to be the most effective in an integrated care setting and improve the access of ethnic minorities to innovative treatment.

TECHNOLOGY: ADDRESSING ISSUES FACED BY ETHNIC MINORITIES AND WOMEN

E-health and Telehealth as Alternatives for Reducing Barriers to Access

Considering the detrimental effects of untreated mental illness and the fact that access difficulties seem to be the most often cited barrier to obtaining mental health services for ethnic minorities, women, and individuals of low socioeconomic status, it seems necessary that healthcare reform specifically incorporate means for providing access to effective behavioral healthcare services. Access to services for those who are at risk for chronic illness increases both the efficiency and cost effectiveness of treatments. This is particularly relevant to underserved, ethnically diverse, and socioeconomically disadvantaged groups because they often face additional access difficulties and are at greater risk for chronic, high-cost diseases such as diabetes and hypertension.

Internet healthcare delivery seems to be a viable option for reducing barriers to access because it has many benefits, including improving the quality of services, increasing access to treatment, and controlling the rapidly increasing costs of healthcare delivery. With the growing interest and use of electronic mental health options, we must consider how to expand our delivery of mental and behavioral health interventions in a culturally appropriate manner using technology.

Access to the Internet

The Internet can aid in reducing barriers of access for both rural and metropolitan communities. It is likely the most effective and efficient means of reducing or overcoming barriers, improving access, and meeting the overarching goals of quality affordable healthcare, improved quality and efficiency of healthcare access, and improved access to innovative therapies—all at an acceptable level of quality and affordability (all of which are stated goals of healthcare reform). However, the use of technology as a medium for dissemination presents its own set of barriers.

To address these barriers, it is important that culturally appropriate electronic mental health programs consider patient attitudes toward technology and patient socioeconomic status (Yellowlees et al., 2008). Despite the fact that ethnic minorities have less access to technology than Euro-Americans (Mossberger, Tollbert, & Gilbert, 2006), statistics show that high numbers of ethnic minorities are connected to the Internet. According to NAS (2009), nearly 73% of the American population has access to the Internet; this includes comparable numbers of men and women and a broad range of age groups. In fact, even children are online at very high rates (over 70% of children have home access to the Internet; DeBell & Chapman, 2003). These data include families from ethnically, geographically, and socioeconomically diverse settings. Furthermore, America is online at high speeds; 79% of Internet users have a broadband connection compared to the 15% who use dial-up (NAS, 2009).

With regard to ethnic minority use of the Internet, Hispanics make up the largest minority group; over 23 million

Hispanics use the Internet, constituting 12% of all Internet users. African Americans are close behind Hispanics, making up 11% of American Internet users. Finally, an estimated 83% of Asian Americans have Internet access in their homes (NAS, 2009). Specific to healthcare, data have suggested that 50–80% of families use the Web to access healthcare information (Fox & Fallows, 2003) and interactive, Web-based, behavioral interventions have shown proven efficacy for an array of conditions (i.e., headaches: Sciamanna et al., 2006; anxiety disorders: Klein & Richards, 2001; trichotillomania: www.stoppulling.com; smoking cessation: www.committedquitters.com). Moreover, large, randomized controlled trials have demonstrated equivalence in efficacy to both adjunctive (Strecher, Shiffman, & West, 2005) and face-to-face (Mouton-Odum, Keuthen, Wagener, Stanley, & DeBakey, 2006) care.

While a perfect intervention would certainly include a medium that is accessible by all, it is important to note that 100% accessibility is nearly impossible (clinics constructed of bricks and mortar do not meet this standard either and never will). This expectation may stall the advancement of viable interventions. Thus, while recommendations for using Internet and telehealth technology for reducing access barriers will not completely close the gap of access to treatment, we believe that it will be accessible to many ethnic minorities (and women) and therefore reduce the number of barriers to behavioral healthcare. Web-based care should therefore improve mental health for many because these treatment modalities are low cost and reduce many barriers to treatment (i.e., can be accessed from home, a public library, etc.).

Thus, we recommend the use of Web-based care for ethnic minorities and women. In light of this recommendation, it is important to consider a stepped-care system. Bower and Gilbody (2005) discuss how, in a stepped-care system (specific to psychological therapies), less intensive treatments are administered first and may consist of brief therapies, group treatments, self-help approaches (i.e., bibliotherapy), and computerized treatments. After such treatments are administered, the patient is assessed and it is determined whether a significant health gain has been attained or improvement has occurred. Based on this assessment it is determined whether "stepping up" (i.e., beginning a more intense treatment such as individual therapy) is necessary.

This certainly provides increased access to treatments that are less intensive but likely to yield improvement and significant health gains. The allocation of federal funding for "less intensive treatments" (either the development or actual implementation of such treatments) would increase access to general services and decrease barriers associated with access—not to mention reduce the sequelae of untreated mental health conditions. Thus, we recommend funding be directed at the development of less intensive treatments for ethnic minorities and women.

Cultural Sensitivity and Technology as a Medium for Treatment Delivery

While high-tech advances are likely to provide a simple solution to many of the barriers associated with access, it is crucial that we consider and address the additional barriers that technology may bring. Yellowlees et al. (2008) discuss how differences in affinity for using technology may have a number of different sources, including access, training, and socioeconomic variables that are not necessarily directly tied to an individual's cultural background. They thus suggest a degree of variability among and within cultural groups for attitudes toward as well as their familiarity with technology. They further identify poverty as the most significant barrier to receiving culturally appropriate mental healthcare (including healthcare delivered via telecommunications).

Poverty can affect (1) technology experience (i.e., it may limit easy access or access only via outdated technologies), (2) capacity to change healthcare outcomes, (3) education level, and (4) socioeconomic status—all of which may be related to decreased use of appropriate mental health services. Finally, previous exposure to technology can impact comfort and openness to engage in electronic mental healthcare. In light of this, Yellowlees and colleagues (2008) have posed questions that are extremely relevant to the healthcare reforms that are currently taking place. They explore how we might

- Assess for the provision of services that are culturally appropriate
- Distinguish between cultural, socioeconomic, and geographic barriers
- Use technology to overcome access barriers while avoiding confounds (e.g., socioeconomic and geographic barriers)
- Attempt to overcome culturally linguistic barriers through electronic means

This is also generational in that most kids in school get a good dose of computers and the Web.

Yellowlees et al. (2008) have looked at similar questions from a perspective of policy making by exploring where best to spend money (e.g., if we identify more barriers related to socioeconomic status, would money be best allocated targeting low-income groups rather than a specific cultural or linguistic group?). This examination from a cost-benefit perspective proposes evaluating new technologies and innovations to improve access while reducing or minimizing costs and providing maximal benefit to traditionally underserved groups.

In terms of how technology acting as a medium for treatment delivery relates to the cultural sensitivity movement, Shore, Savin, Novins, and Manson (2006) conducted a review of the impact of culture on telepsychiatry and identified two components that are particularly relevant in telepsychiatry:

- How a patient's cultural background (the cultural identity of the individual) influenced his or her comfort level with technology
- The impact of cultural differences on the patient–provider relationship (i.e., the need for the psychiatrist to attend to how culture-specific communication styles may impact the videoconferencing session)

Thus, if video-conferencing is being used as a medium to deliver treatment, it may be effective simply to increase comfort level with technology while making special efforts to attend to nonverbal cues. It is important this be compared to a practical alternative, which in many instances would be no access to care or access to low quality care.

Certainly the ethnic minority population will continue to grow along with a corresponding higher need for easily accessible, widely disseminated, culturally appropriate interventions. It seems that the Internet is a viable option for providing these behavioral health interventions. We agree with Yellowlees et al. (2008) that part of healthcare should include increased funding from both federal and state levels and private payers so that scientific and behavioral healthcare specialists can focus on developing these much needed interventions. We also believe that funding geared at computer literacy can help address issues of comfort with technology as well as close the literacy gap attributable to SES.

ACCESS PROBLEMS

Lack of Health Insurance Coverage and Cost of Healthcare

Given the skyrocketing costs associated with healthcare, it is no wonder that lack of health insurance coverage is cited as a major access barrier. A large portion of the current healthcare reform is directed at how to get insurance and hence care to the uninsured (quality, affordable healthcare). Generally speaking, lack of health insurance coverage is likely to decrease care-seeking behavior (contrary to the goal of prevention of chronic disease and improving public health); however, this decrease in care-seeking behavior is even more likely to be associated with specialty services (e.g., mental and behavioral health services). The use of the integrated care model (Cummings, O'Donohue, & Cummings, 2009) may help to increase access to specialty services at a reduced cost because individuals seeking general services will have greater access to mental/behavioral health specialists.

Ethnic Minorities in Rural Communities

When access is limited, individuals are most likely to receive care for medical conditions and least likely to receive specialized care. This may be especially true in rural communities because it is hardly a surprise that psychologists, social workers, counselors, etc. are often simply not available. The use of an integrated care system would help improve access in rural communities because behavioral healthcare specialists would be located in settings where medical care is available. These specialists might be physically accessible or accessible via electronic media.

Language Barriers

Language barriers frequently complicate access to services. While an integrated care model may not directly solve such issues, the increased utilization of electronically administered assessments (that are easily translatable to different languages) utilized in integrative care systems should decrease the barrier of language. Additionally, Internet tools, such as "Google Language Tools," can translate the content of Web sites, increasing the probability that resources available in English will also be accessible in other languages.

Stigma and Cultural Attitudes

Because stigma and cultural attitudes are an often cited reason why ethnic minority individuals do not seek mental health services, integrated care is perfectly positioned to address this barrier. If an ethnic minority individual is being seen for a medical concern (perhaps medical concerns produce less stigma) and the primary care physician notes a potential behavioral or mental health condition, a behavioral health specialist can be quickly located.

Other Barriers

The implementation of an integrative care system can greatly reduce other barriers (relevant to both ethnic minorities and women), such as long waits and long periods of time between initial contact and appointment, through increased efficiency. Consider the example of Dr. Arrendando, a family practice physician, who has a very busy schedule ahead of him. His first patient bursts into tears in his office during a routine physical, putting Dr. Arrendando behind schedule and leaving many frustrated patients to wait in the waiting room.

In an integrated care system, a behavioral healthcare specialist is easily accessible when patients become tearful or express symptoms that may represent a mental health problem. An integrated care system would have provided Dr. Arrendando with immediate access to a behavioral healthcare specialist. When the patient burst into tears, the specialist could have completed an assessment and provided treatment recommendations for the patient, thus allowing Dr. Arrendando to move on with his next patient, increasing efficiency, and reducing barriers such as long waits.

Immigration Status

Will Undocumented Immigrants Be Covered?

With regard to undocumented immigrants, the question is, naturally, whether undocumented immigrants are covered under healthcare reform. While the sound bites and the speeches in the political town hall meetings to support the president's healthcare plan denied it would cover undocumented immigrants, the language of the legislation is unclear. The resulting arguments are easily dichotomized. Most problematic is the fact that any additional costs or benefits are dependent upon variables whose true numbers will only come to light once the legislation is implemented. The following section will explore potential outcomes of this reform with regard to undocumented immigrants.

Determining Eligibility

The first and probably largest logistical question is how we determine who is eligible for services. Is eligibility a birthright? Will eligibility be determined by contribution into the system? Emergency rooms across the country already provide services to those who are uninsured. Can we begin patently to deny those who may be in the country illegally and who cannot show proof of insurance? Will people be asked to present passports or proof of residency? More important may be the question of who will make the determination (e.g., clerk, triage nurse, physician, Immigration and Customs Enforcement agent, etc.).

The fact of the matter is that legislation does not seem to mention how verification of eligibility will work. In light of the limited ability of the government currently to prevent undocumented workers from finding gainful employment, this becomes an interesting question. It is especially interesting given that the system to detect and eliminate this type of illegal activity is long standing and ever improving in its efforts to thwart employment of undocumented immigrants. The question remains as to whether a newly formed healthcare system would be able to detect and eliminate such fraud.

Reducing Costs

Certainly covering the 6.6 million uninsured illegal immigrants in the United States (Camarota, 2009) under healthcare reform will contribute to the already skyrocketing costs associated with the reform. One potential cost-saving avenue is to deny services to undocumented immigrants. In fact, a fairly comprehensive analysis (see Camarota, 2009), based upon the Congressional Budget Office cost estimates and the current healthcare legislation, suggests a wide degree of variability (although significant) in fiscal savings (estimated costs range from $4.3 billion to $30.8 billion annually) for service denial.

Camarota (2009) discusses a critical flaw in any cost-saving measure that seeks to save costs through service denial considering that (as mentioned before) the legislation does not specify or fund any mechanism of verification and enforcement. Additionally, Camarota discusses the wide array of unknown variables that could impact the true cost and savings for undocumented immigrants (e.g., costs covered by employers, potential increases in wages through a corresponding amnesty, the number who will actually seek services or enroll, etc.).

Nonetheless, one would be hard-pressed to argue that covering undocumented immigrants under healthcare reform would not cost money. The following sections provide a concrete example of the cost increases specific to behavioral healthcare. Because we are describing an integrative healthcare system, we must consider the implications for untreated Axis I disorders, such as schizophrenia, mood disorders, and anxiety disorders. We know that the prognosis for these disorders is best with early intervention. If we look at just schizophrenia, which has a relatively small prevalence rate (1.5%; McGrath et al., 2004), the most conservative estimate would suggest that, for this population alone, an additional 99,000 individuals would require behavioral healthcare services that would most likely be paid for by taxpayers.

Considerations for Undocumented Immigrants if They Are Included in the Reform

While it is unclear if undocumented immigrants will be covered under the healthcare reform, the following is a discussion of considerations that are mostly relevant if undocumented immigrants do receive health insurance through the reform.

Undocumented immigrants are less likely to utilize services and healthcare coverage than their legal counterparts (Hubbell et al., 1991). Specifically, in states like California (where some of our largest populations of undocumented immigrants reside), utilization by undocumented immigrants has been primarily shown to be dependent upon whether or not the individual has healthcare coverage (Chavez et al., 1985; Chavez, Cornelius, & Jones, 1986; Hubbell et al., 1991).

This is particularly problematic because undocumented individuals are less likely to receive preventive services, such as mammograms and Pap smears for detecting cancer, as well as follow-up care after procedures when they do utilize services, like doctor visits after a caesarean delivery (Chavez et al., 1986). While childbirth is one circumstance where utilization of the healthcare system seems to be more common, children of undocumented immigrants are still at a higher risk for healthcare issues in general, due to the status of their parents (Berk, Schur, Chavez, & Frankel, 2000), and they are still subject to the same culture stigmas and barriers discussed in the previous section.

In fact, we previously discussed the stigma and reluctance to seek preventive care, some of which includes the prenatal care already discussed, but we must also acknowledge the potential for the children of these undocumented immigrants (who are citizens) to petition for their parents to become naturalized. Given the age at which this is possible, our nation could potentially see an onslaught of new citizens with the health problems (e.g., diabetes, COPD, hypertension, etc.) of older Americans who have not had preventive care. They then have the potential to become the high healthcare utilizers.

A big challenge for the integrative system is that most services for undocumented immigrants are not sought in traditional outpatient settings, but rather are much more likely to occur in medical settings, particularly emergency rooms (Chavez et al., 1986), thus suggesting a need to incorporate a behavioral healthcare specialist for acute care facilities. While the issue of providing insurance coverage for undocumented immigrants may be politically unattainable, the research clearly demonstrates areas where integrative care can maximize benefits while decreasing costs—at substantial health benefits for the undocumented individuals as well as their U.S.-born children. The first step for integrative care would be to provide targeted psychoeducation focused on the benefits of preventive care and screening, as well as easily accessible follow-up care (perhaps via telehealth or Internet-based means) when services *are* utilized. Additionally, it appears that the provision of this education would be maximally beneficial at emergency or urgent care sites, as well as in community-based clinics.

Recommendations

The issue of whether or not to cover undocumented immigrants under the healthcare reform is a terrible quandary and a simple solution is not attainable. At this point, the number of unknown variables is large (e.g., exact costs of healthcare reform, who will pay what portions—employers, employees, tax money—how eligibility will be determined, etc.), making it difficult to provide specific recommendations aimed at answering this very complicated question.

Integrated Care and Women

Considering that the healthcare system currently emphasizes preventive care for women (e.g., clinics for free mammograms and Pap smears), the implementation of integrative care in such settings would allow for higher accessibility to behavioral healthcare. Additionally, behavioral healthcare specialists placed in such settings could receive specialized training for identifying disorders that plague women at higher rates than men and disorders that only impact women (e.g., postpartum depression).

INTEGRATED HEALTHCARE IN PRACTICE

The literature reviewed in this chapter has provided a framework for discussing the specific issues faced by ethnic minorities and women as they pertain to mental and behavioral healthcare. Recommendations for addressing these issues from an integrated care perspective have been offered. The following vignette illustrates how the use of integrated care can practically reduce many of the issues described in this chapter.

Jorge is a 35-year-old Mexican male who believes his symptoms are related to a medical condition. He often ruminates over the prospect that he has chronic heart problems, emphysema, asthma, etc. He is plagued by incidents in which his palms begin to sweat, his heart beats rapidly, his blood pressure increases, and he feels as though he cannot breathe. He has been rushed to the emergency room on multiple occasions and leaves there each time with a large bill and feelings of hopeless because, each time he sees the doctor, he is told that nothing is wrong. His stress level increases because he is certain that there is something wrong with his heart that doctors have been unable to identify. He is afraid he will die.

In an integrated care system, the doctor would ask a behavioral healthcare specialist to assess Jorge's symptoms. After careful assessment, the behavioral healthcare specialist might come to the conclusion that Jorge is suffering from panic disorder and prescribe cognitive behavioral therapy (including relaxation training) via an Internet intervention. A follow-up meeting would be scheduled to reassess Jorge's symptoms a few weeks later.

Clearly, this vignette illustrates the efficiency and effectiveness of integrated care combined with evidenced-based treatments and the use of bibliotherapy and/or the delivery of treatments via the Internet.

CONCLUSIONS

Initially, we provided five recommendations associated with problems we identified within the current behavioral healthcare field (relevant to cultural minorities). They were as follows:

- That researchers begin conducting outcome studies to establish what treatments work with cultural minorities
- That as a field we become more proactive and solution focused
- That behavioral healthcare specialists recognize and make use of cultural factors that may act as facilitators in the treatment of cultural minorities
- That as a field we establish how exhaustive we need to be when considering the range of possible cultural group permutations
- That behavioral healthcare specialists use evidence-based treatments when working with cultural minorities

We then discussed how the largest barriers to the provision of services for women and ethnic minorities are access and the availability of coverage. The limitation of access is typically due to logistical limitations and provider skills, as well as a lack of culturally and linguistically appropriate instruments. The current legislation appears to address the issue of limited coverage through a mix of penalties (through tax penalties for those that fail to obtain coverage) as well as incentives (tax credits for small businesses). While not specifically mentioned in behavioral health in the legislation, access as discussed can be increased through a manner similar to that proposed for the traditional medical model. This is accomplished through a mix of more community-based centers as well as the utilization of available and developing technology (e.g., Web-based services).

The focus on technology and innovation may increase access and reduce the question of how to maximize resources. The common decision is often one of choosing between socio-economic class and cultural considerations. However, as newer technology is more easily modified and disseminated in conjunction with the increased utilization and availability of technology such as broadband Internet access, this decision becomes less critical as electronic services are more readily and cost effectively adapted. Additionally, technology, such as Web-based behavioral healthcare, can help overcome the stigma associated with seeking behavioral health services. However, a key component of the human factor is still relevant. An integrative setting that encompasses both behavioral health and primary care physicians can further reduce costs (e.g., consolidated training, reduced equipment setup costs) and increase access for these populations through the shared utilization of these technological resources.

This legislation and related budgetary considerations will need to incorporate knowledgeable staff who have the appropriate training and resources to differentiate culturally unique symptom presentation, in order to maximize resource utilization (through appropriate referrals that are currently best utilized in integrative healthcare settings) and to decrease waste, which may come from misdiagnosis or prescription of treatments unlikely to be utilized. Behavioral healthcare specialists should be aware of the culturally relevant issues related to the provision of these services (e.g., differential symptom presentation, linguistic issues, etc.).

The legislation fails to provide specific language with regard to undocumented immigrants. We have shown the potential for integrative care to increase overall health while holding and potentially reducing costs. Yet, the exclusion of this specific population from coverage may be the largest challenge to the comprehensive provision of services as proposed. It is unknown how employers will differentiate documented from undocumented workers in a manner that is distinct from current employment practices, thus suggesting that the same means utilized to obtain employment would also allow these individuals to receive coverage via their employers.

The current legislation has a high potential to address the common issues in the health system faced by women and ethnic minorities. For an integrative healthcare system, coverage would appear no longer to be an obstacle, thus freeing these healthcare systems to focus on improving access and technology utilization within a model of healthcare that has already demonstrated improved efficacy. In conjunction with empirically based training on cultural considerations for providers, we should see an improvement within the integrative healthcare system in the utilization of and outcomes for women and ethnic minorities that addresses many of the domains and goals set forth in the present legislation.

REFERENCES

Akutsu, P., Snowden, L., & Organista, K. (1996). Referral patterns in ethnic-specific and mainstream programs for ethnic minorities and Whites. *Journal of Counseling Psychology, 43*(1), 56–64.

Alvidrez, J., & Azocar, F. (1999b). Distressed women's clinic patients: Preferences for mental health treatments and perceived obstacles. *General Hospital Psychiatry, 21*(5), 340–347.

Barrett, B., Shadick, K., Schilling, R., Spencer, L., del Rosario, S., Moua, K., & Vang M. (1998). Hmong/medicine interactions: Improving cross-cultural health care. *Family Medicine, 30*(3), 179–184.

Berk, M. L., Schur, C. L., Chavez, L. R., & Frankel, M. (2000). Health care use among undocumented Latino immigrants. *Health Affairs, 19,* 51–64.

Betancourt, H., & Lopez, S. R. (1993). The study of culture, ethnicity, and race in American psychology. *American Psychologist, 48,* 629–637.

BigFoot, D. S., & Schmidt, S. R. (2010). Honoring children, mending the circle: Cultural adaptation of trauma-focused cognitive-behavioral therapy for American Indian and Alaska Native children. *Journal of Clinical Psychology, 66*(8), 847–856.

Bolen, J., Rhodes, L., Powell-Griner, E., Bland, S., & Holtzman, D. (2000). State-specific prevalence of selected behaviors, by race and ethnicity—Behavioral risk factors surveillance system, 1997. *Mortality and Morbidity Weekly Report Surveillance Survey, 49*(SSO2), 1–60.

Bower, P., & Gilbody, S. (2005). Stepped care in psychological therapies: Access, effectiveness and efficiency narrative literature review. *British Journal of Psychiatry, 186,* 11–17.

Camarota, S. (2009). Illegal immigrants and HR 3200: Estimate of potential costs to taxpayers. Retrieved from http://www.cis.org/illegalsAndHealthCareHR3200

Cardemil, E. V. (2010). Cultural adaptations to empirically supported treatments: A research agenda. *Scientific Review of Mental Health Practice.*

Chavez, L. R., Cornelius, W. A., & Jones, O. W. (1985). Mexican immigrants and the utilization of U.S. health services: The case of San Diego. *Social Science & Medicine, 21,* 93–102.

Chavez, L. R., Cornelius, W. A., & Jones, O. W. (1986). Utilization of health services by Mexican immigrant women in San Diego. *Women & Health, 11,* 3–20.

Conner, K. O., Koeske, G., & Brown, C. (2009). Racial differences in attitudes toward professional mental health treatment: The mediating effect of stigma. *Journal of Gerontological Social Work, 52*(7), 695–712.

Cummings, N. A., O'Donohue, W. T., & Cummings, J. L. (2009). The financial dimension of integrated behavioral/primary care. *Journal of Clinical Psychology in Medical Settings, 16*(1), 31–39.

DeBell, M., and Chapman, C. (2003). *Computer and Internet use by children and adolescents in the United States, 2001* (NCES 2004-014). Washington, DC: U.S. Department of Education, National Center for Education Statistics.

Eiraldi, R. B., Mazzuca, L. B., Clarke, A. T., & Power, T. J. (2006). Service utilization among ethnic minority children with ADHD: A model of help-seeking behavior. *Administration and Policy in Mental Health and Mental Health Services Research, 33,* 607–622.

El-Kebbi, I. M., Bacha, G. A., Ziemer, D. C., et al. (1996). Diabetes in urban African Americans: Use of discussion groups to identify barriers to dietary therapy among low-income individuals with non-insulin-dependent diabetes mellitus. *Diabetes Education, 22,* 488–492.

Falicov, C. (1996). Mexican families. In *Ethnicity and family therapy* (2nd ed.) (pp. 169–182). New York, NY: Guilford Press.

Flores, G., & Vega, L. R. (1998). Barriers to health care access for Latino children: A review. *Family Medicine, 30,* 196–205.

Foa, E., Hembree, E., & Rothbaum, B. O. (2007). *Prolonged exposure therapy for PTSD: Emotional processing of traumatic experiences: Therapist guide.* New York, NY: Oxford University Press.

Fox, S., & Fallows, D. (2003). Internet health resources, Pew Internet. Retrieved April 1, 2010, from http://news.ninemsn.com.au/health/story_13178.asp

Friman, P. C. (1986). A preventive context for enuresis. *Pediatric Clinics of North America, 33,* 871–886.

Garrett, C. R., Treichel, C. J., & Ohmans, P. (1998). Barriers to health care for immigrants and nonimmigrants: A comparative study. *Minnesota Medicine, 81,* 52–55.

Garrett, M. T., & Carroll, J. J. (2000). Mending the broken circle: Treatment of substance dependence among Native Americans. *Journal of Counseling & Development, 78*(4), 379–388.

Garrett, M. T., Garrett, J. T., & Brotherton, D. (2001). Inner circle/outer circle: A group technique based on Native American healing circles. *Journal for Specialists in Group Work, 26*(1), 17–30.

Garrett, M. W., & Osborne, W. L. (1995). The Native American sweat lodge as metaphor for group work. *Journal for Specialists in Group Work, 20*(1), 33–39.

Givens, J., Houston, T., Van Voorhees, B., Ford, D., & Cooper, L. (2007). Ethnicity and preferences for depression treatment. *General Hospital Psychiatry, 29*(3), 182–191.

Hamrick, K. (2005). Rural America at a glance. Economic information bulletin no. (EIB4). Retrieved April 1, 2010, from http://www.ers.usda.gov/publications/EIB4/EIB4.pdf

Harrell, J., & Carrasquillo, O. (2003). The Latino disparity in health coverage. Retrieved April 30, 2010, from http://jama.ama-assn.org/cgi/content/full/289/9/1167

Heilbron, C. L., & Guttman, M. A. J. (2000). Traditional healing methods with First Nation's women in group counseling. *Canadian Journal of Counseling, 34*(1), 3–13.

Hubbell, F. A., Waitzkin, H., Mishra, S. I., Dombrink, J., & Chavez, L. R. (1991). Access to medical care for documented and undocumented Latinos in a Southern California county. *Western Journal of Medicine, 154,* 414–417.

Jenkins, C. N., Le, T., McPhee, S. J., Stewart, S., & Ha, N. T. (1996). Health care access and preventive care among Vietnamese immigrants: Do traditional beliefs and practices pose barriers? *Social Science Medicine, 43*(7), 1049–1056.

Jones, E., Cason, C., & Bond, M. (2002). Access to preventive health care: Is method of payment a barrier for immigrant Hispanic women? *Women's Health Issues, 12,* 129–137.

Klein, B., & Richards, J. C. (2001). A brief Internet-based treatment for panic disorder. *Behavioral and Cognitive Psychotherapy, 29*(1), 113–117.

Koenig, H. G. (2010). Spirituality and mental health. *International Journal of Applied Psychoanalytic Studies, 7,* 116–122. doi: 10.1002/aps.239

Leaf, P. J., Bruce, M. L., & Tischler, G. L. (1986). The differential effect of attitudes on the use of mental health services. *Social Psychiatry, 21,* 187–192.

Lipton, R., Losey, L., Giachello, A., Mendez, J., & Girotti, M. (1998). Attitudes and issues in treating Latino patients with type 2 diabetes: Views of health-care providers. *Diabetes Education, 24,* 67–71.

McGrath, J., Saha, S., Welham, J., El Saadi, O., MacCauley, C., & Chant, D. (2004). A systematic review of the incidence of schizophrenia: The distribution of rates and the influence of sex, urbanicity, migrant status and methodology. *BMC Medicine, 2*(13), doi:10.1186/1741-7015-2-13

Moody, J. (1995). Art therapy: Bridging barriers with Native American clients. *Art Therapy, 12*(4), 220–226.

Morgan, M. (1996). Prenatal care of African American women in selected USA urban and rural cultural contexts. *Journal of Transcultural Nursing, 7,* 3–9.

Mossberger, K., Tolbert, C., & Gilbert M. (2006). Race, place, and information technology. *Urban Affairs Review, 41*(5), 583–620.

Mouton-Odum, S., Keuthen, N., Wagener, P., Stanley, M., & DeBakey, M. (2006). StopPulling.com: An interactive, self-help program for trichotillomania. *Cognitive and Behavioral Practice, 13*(3), 215–226.

NAS. (2009). Internet usage in the United States. Retrieved April 28, 2010, from http://www.nasrecruitment.com/docs/white_papers/Internet_Usage_United_States.pdf

O'Donohue, W., & Benuto, L. (2010). The many problems with cultural sensitivity. *Scientific Review of Mental Health Practice.*

O'Donohue, W. T. (1995). Cultural sensitivity: A critical examination. In R. H. Wright & N. A. Cummings (Eds.), *Destructive trends in mental health* (pp. 29–44). New York, NY: Routledge.

Passel, J., & Cohn, D. (2009). A portrait of unauthorized immigrants in the United States. A report by the Pew Hispanic Center. http://pewhispanic.org/files/reports/107.pdf

Quinn, K. (2000). Working without benefits: The health insurance crisis confronting Hispanic Americans. Retrieved May 20, 2010, from http://www.commonwealthfund.org/~/media/Files/Publications/Fund%20Report/2000/Mar/Working%20Without%20Benefits%20%20The%20Health%20Insurance%20Crisis%20Confronting%20Hispanic%20Americans/quinn_wobenefits_370%20pdf.pdf

Rhinehart, L. M., & Engelhorn, P. (1984). The full rainbow: Symbol of individuation. *Arts in Psychotherapy, 11*(1), 37–42.

Sackett, D. L., Straus, S. E., Richardson, W. S., Rosenberg, W., & Haynes, R. B. (2000). *Evidence-based medicine: How to practice and teach EBM* (2nd ed.). Edinburgh, Scotland: Churchill Livingstone.

Scheppers, E., van Dongen, E., Dekker, J., Geertzen, J., & Dekker, J. (2006). Potential barriers to the use of health services among ethnic minorities: A review. *Family Practice, 23*(3), 325–348.

Sciamanna, C. N., Nicholson, R. A., Lofland, J. H., Manocchia, M., Mui, S., & Hartman, C. W. (2006). Effects of a Web site designed to improve the management of migraines. *Headache: The Journal of Head and Face Pain, 46*(1), 92–100.

Shore, J., Savin, D., Novins, D., & Manson, S. (2006). Cultural aspects of telepsychiatry. *Journal of Telemedicine and Telecare, 12*(3), 116–121.

Smith, M., Kreutzer, R., Goldman, L., Casey-Paal, A., & Kizer, K. (1996). How economic demand influences access to medical care for rural Hispanic children. *Medical Care, 34,* 1135–1148.

Snowden, L. R. (1998). Racial differences in informal help seeking for mental health problems. *Journal of Community Psychology, 26*(5), 429–438.

Strecher, V., Shiffman, S., & West, R. (2005). Randomized controlled trial of a Web-based computer-tailored smoking cessation program as a supplement to nicotine patch therapy. *Addiction, 100*(5), 682–688.

Tafoya, T. (1989). Circles and cedar: Native Americans and family therapy. *Journal of Psychotherapy & the Family, 6*(1–2), 71–98.

Trupin, E., Forsyth-Stephens, A., & Low, B. (1991). Service needs of severely disturbed children. *American Journal of Public Health, 7,* 975–980.

U.S. Census. (2002). Health insurance coverage in the United States: 2002, consumer invoice. Retrieved April 30, 2010 from http://www.census.gov/prod/2003pubs/p60-223.pdf

U.S. Congress. (2010). House. The Patient Protection and Affordable Care Act. H.R. 3950. 111th Cong. 2nd sess. (January 5, 2010). http://frwebgate.access.gpo.gov/cgi-bin/getdoc.cgi?dbname=111_cong_bills&docid=f:h3590enr.txt.pdf (accessed June 22, 2010).

U.S. Department of Health and Human Services, United States Public Health Service Office of the Surgeon General. (2001). *Mental health: Culture, race, and ethnicity: A supplement to mental health: A report of the Surgeon General.* Rockville, MD: U.S. Public Health Service.

Yellowlees, P., Marks, S., Hilty, D., & Shore, J. (2008). Using e-health to enable culturally appropriate mental healthcare in rural areas. *Telemedicine and e-Health, 14*(5), 486–492.

Seventeen

Wellness and Prevention
Key Elements in the Next Generation of Behavioral Health Service Delivery Systems

MONICA E. OSS

INTRODUCTION

An integral part of the next generation of treatments for mental illnesses, addictions, and cognitive disabilities will be the incorporation of wellness and prevention tools (Oss, n.d. [b]). A recent report by the National Research Council and the Institute of Medicine, "Preventing Mental, Emotional, and Behavioral Disorders Among Young People: Progress and Possibilities," suggested that lack of prevention costs the U.S. healthcare system an estimated $247 billion. The report highlights a number of prevention initiatives, such as the Strengthening Families Program for Parents and Youth 10-14 (SFP 10-14) and the Adolescent Transitions Program (ATP), which report an estimated savings of anywhere from $386 to $650 for every dollar spent on prevention (O'Connell, Boat, & Warner, 2009).

Only a decade ago, it was typical to attend meetings in which any discussion of wellness and health promotion was relatively short and that concluded with the overall concurrence that there was little to be done with prevention in particular. What a difference a decade makes. A variety of industry factors are now converging to shape innovations in wellness and prevention and pushing their increasing availability in the service delivery system. Four particular factors are having the greatest impact on this expansion:

- Behavioral health parity
- Healthcare reform
- New scientific discoveries
- New information technology

The first two factors—parity and healthcare reform—will fundamentally change access to services for all consumers, and this change has spurred a greater interest in moving new scientific discoveries to commercially viable treatment (and prevention) methodologies. New opportunities in the prevention and wellness arena are being found by the field of neuroscience. Our changing understanding of the brain—and of the brain–body connection—is reshaping perceptions about the possibilities of preventive medicine among industry thought leaders. For example, one of the most important recent discoveries is the ability of the body to generate new brain cells; previously, scientific understanding was that the number of brain cells was static. This creates new possibilities for early intervention and return to wellness. Finally, new information technology is making the delivery of prevention services more affordable and more consumer centric. In this chapter, I want to explore each of these four factors and examine how they are shaping the role of prevention in the field of behavioral health.

BEHAVIORAL HEALTH PARITY REMOVES THE STIGMA OF MENTAL ILLNESS AND FOSTERS INTEGRATION

The passage of the Wellstone–Domenici Mental Health Parity and Addiction Equity Act of 2008 has set the stage for a new era in behavioral health service delivery, and the prospect of parity in behavioral health benefits has changed stakeholder perceptions in two important ways. The fundamental premise of the behavioral health parity laws passed by Congress and enacted by the Medicare program is that beneficiaries cannot pay more for behavioral health services than for other health services offered within the same health plan (i.e., if a copayment for a physician visit for a physical health condition is

$25, the copayment for a physician visit for a behavioral disorder must be the same).

First, because the treatment of mental illnesses and addictions will be covered at the same financial level as other healthcare conditions, the stigma among financial institutions in funding treatments and services in this sector has been removed. Second and equally important, parity will foster the growing integration of service delivery—from prevention to diagnosis to long-term disability supports.

HEALTHCARE REFORM AND ITS PREVENTION PROVISIONS CHANGE THE SERVICE DELIVERY LANDSCAPE

Soon after the passage of the parity legislation, the Patient Protection and Affordable Care Act (PPACA) made its way through Congress and was signed by President Obama in March 2010. Healthcare reform legislation accepted the provisions of the Wellstone–Domenici Mental Health Parity and Addiction Equity Act and extended them to all health plans envisioned in the legislation. The combination of these two landmark pieces of legislation will go a long way toward ensuring that Americans have not only basic physical health services, but also basic behavioral health treatment services. This change has also increased the availability of investment capital in new science-based behavioral health treatment solutions and fostered a new era of service integration.

The Strategic Implications of Healthcare Reform

After analyzing the many facets of the healthcare reform legislation and the multitude of other changes facing the field over the next 3 years, it seems that there are four key strategic implications for behavioral health provider organizations:

- The majority of behavioral health dollars will flow through health plans.
- The changes in finance and technology will increase the proportion of behavioral health services provided via "primary care."
- Health-plan-based financing will draw clearer lines of distinction between "health" services and "social" services.

- Comparative effectiveness initiatives will increase the private pay market in behavioral health.

In addition to these four industry-specific factors, two other aspects of the legislation will likely have direct effects on the issue of prevention of behavioral disorders and their integration in overall healthcare. The first is the extensive coverage of general preventive services within the legislation. The other is the provisions of the legislation that promote the integration of service management and delivery for individuals with chronic health conditions.

The Majority of Behavioral Health Dollars Will Flow Through Health Plans

The combination of parity and a greatly reduced uninsured population will translate into a shift wherein most behavioral health treatment will be funded by health plans (private, Medicaid, Medicare, etc.). This, in turn, will cause federal grants and state program dollars that make up traditional "safety net" funding for behavioral health to diminish. The management implications of this shift are many, including the following key considerations:

- Successful provider organizations will need an "expert" process in working with third-party payers: automated systems for health plan management such as eligibility determinations, care authorizations, and billing.
- Financing of delayed cash flow will be a growing issue because federal/state "safety net" funding has been typically prepaid while health plans generally pay within 30–60 days after service billing.
- A key focus of marketing efforts will need to be the optimization of fee-for-service reimbursement in health plans.

Changes in Finance and Technology Will Increase Proportion of Behavioral Health Services Provided via "Primary Care"

Parity provides equal coverage of behavioral health services, and the healthcare reform legislation encourages integration of primary care with all specialty care. The synchronistic combination of these factors—along with new service delivery technologies and new clinical interventions based on brain science—will encourage an increase in the delivery of behavioral health services in primary care settings. These will not be the services required for consumers with disabilities and complex conditions, but rather the "standard" behavioral health services needed by the other 80% of the population.

Primary care settings should not be confused with primary care physicians (PCPs). While PCPs will certainly be providing more behavioral health services in their office settings, the largest expansion of behavioral health services will be in retail clinics, online in consumers' homes, and in health clinics via e-health technologies.

What will remain for behavioral health services outside primary care settings? Generally, only clinical services for consumers with chronic and complex behavioral health conditions will be left. It is likely that services for these consumers will be channeled into highly specialized organizations with the ability to provide a wide array of services to this specific population using some type of risk-based financing. A number of models can provide coordinated and specialized management of care for individuals with disabling behavioral disorders: disease management models, specialty medical home models, and assertive community treatment models. When these models are combined with a pooled financing approach that gives flexibility in service array, consumers have the opportunity for a personalized approach to their care that is also more cost effective.

For executives of behavioral health provider organizations, this is a call for new strategy—and a decision on whether an integrated service model or a disease management model will be the direction for their organizations.

Health-Plan-Based Financing Will Draw Clearer Lines of Distinction Between "Health" and "Social" Services

One clear effect of the increased financing of health benefits through health plans (and the very likely increase in the use of managed care financing models) is that there will be a clear definition of what constitutes "healthcare" services. We will see more medical necessity criteria used for standard behavioral healthcare for the majority of consumers.

Services that are considered "social supports" (those not meeting medical necessity criteria such as peer supports and vocational training) will likely only be available for consumers with chronic and complex behavioral health conditions—and likely only under risk-based financing. For most behavioral health provider organizations, this likely future situation demands a scenario-based analysis of their current consumer base and service array. How many consumers will meet the chronic/complex case definition? What services will clearly meet the "medical necessity" test? Of the services, how would their utilization change in an environment with risk-based financing models such as case rates, episodic payments, or population-based payments?

Comparative Effectiveness Initiatives Will Increase the Behavioral Health Private Pay Market

The last of the implications of healthcare reform for our field is the likelihood that the use of comparative effectiveness analysis will increase the promotion of behavioral health funding from private pay. Comparative effectiveness analysis, which is essentially a meta-analysis of evidence-based practices specific to disease state, "recommends" clinical protocols based on outcome and cost. Two groups of services will likely be in the private pay domain. The first includes more expensive treatment approaches that do not have good cost-offset data and are not likely to be "recommended" competitive effectiveness analysis. The second group is new treatment technologies that are not included in the competitive effectiveness evaluation process. As a result, the private pay market will change dramatically: It will likely include many traditional therapies preferred by consumers as well as emerging technologies. To address this increase in private pay, many provider organizations will need enhanced intake billing and market functions.

The magnitude of the market impact of these four factors is unknown right now. While the legislation has passed, the regulations are still being crafted at this very moment—the devil is in the proverbial details. Ultimately, determining how beneficial this legislation is for behavioral health consumers and the implications for behavioral health professions and provider organizations will be a function of these regulations.

Expanded Coverage of Prevention in an Era After Healthcare Reform

Healthcare reform legislation is decidedly pro-prevention. There are seven key provisions of health prevention that have been included in the legislation; most of them have been recognized by both healthcare leaders and legislators as an important step forward in shifting healthcare strategies toward more proactive care. These initiatives include:

- Coverage of a wide array of preventive services
- Development of a national health promotion plan
- Enhanced health promotion research
- Technical assistance to enhance evaluation of workplace health promotion programs
- Regular periodic surveys on workplace health program prevalence and components
- Grants to pay a portion of the cost of comprehensive workplace health promotion programs for small employers
- Ability of employers to offer employees a premium discount of up to 30% (increased from the current 20%) for positive lifestyle practices or engagement in health promotion programs (The secretary of HHS will also initiate research studies to determine the cost effectiveness of increasing this premium discount to 50%.)

With regard to the coverage of prevention services, the Departments of Health and Human Services (HHS), Labor, and Treasury issued new Patient Protection and Affordable Care Act (PPACA) regulations on July 14, 2010. These required that private health plans cover evidence-based preventive services and immunization with no cost sharing. Services that must be covered with no cost sharing fall in four categories:

- Evidence-based preventive services
- Routine immunizations
- Preventive services for children
- Preventive services for women

Evidence-Based Preventive (EBP) Services

Health plans are required to provide evidence-based preventive services that have received a rating of "grade A" or "grade B," as determined by the U.S. Preventive Services Task Force (USPSTF), an independent panel of experts. The USPSTF bases its ratings on scientific evidence documenting the benefits of the EBP. The current covered benefits include preventive services such as:

- Certain screenings for cancer
- Vitamin deficiencies during pregnancy
- Diabetes
- High cholesterol

- High blood pressure
- Depression
- Counseling for tobacco cessation

Routine Immunizations

Health plans will cover a set of standard vaccines recommended by the Advisory Committee on Immunization Practices (ACIP) for routine use, ranging from childhood immunizations to periodic tetanus shots for adults.

Preventive Services for Children

Health plans will cover preventive care for children up to age 21 as described in guidelines from the Health Resources and Services Administration (HRSA) and the American Academy of Pediatrics, including:

- Regular pediatrician visits
- Vision and hearing screening
- Developmental assessments
- Immunizations and screening
- Counseling to address obesity

Preventive Services for Women

Health plans will cover preventive care and screening provided to women according to guidelines supported by HRSA that are not otherwise addressed by the USPSTF recommendations. HHS is developing further guidance on this requirement, which it expects to issue by August 1, 2011.

Focus on Integrated Management of Chronic Health Conditions

The final area of influence that healthcare reform will have on the field is the focus on integrated management of services for consumers with all types of chronic conditions. The move toward the integration of service delivery is not new—over half of prescriptions for psychotropic medications are written by prescribers who are not behavioral health specialists, and three quarters of federally qualified healthcare centers (FQHCs) offer behavioral health services (Lo Sasso & Byck, 2010). In 1996, mental health treatment and counseling was offered by 47% of FQHCs, 15% offered 24-hour crisis intervention and counseling, and 40% offered addiction treatment and counseling. In

2006, 76% provided mental health treatment and counseling, 20% provided 24-hour crisis intervention, and 51% provided addiction treatment (Lo Sasso & Byck, 2010).

There are numerous market factors supporting integrated delivery models for behavioral health services. Payers want integration because they believe it will result in more effective disease state management at a lower cost, and consumers are favorably disposed to integrated models because of convenience. New information technologies are proving to be disruptive innovations in the healthcare field, enabling services previously delivered by specialists to be delivered just as effectively in primary care settings (Oss, n.d. [c]). Many provisions of the healthcare reform bill build on this evolving trend in service delivery and provide additional incentives for integration. These provisions include the following:

- The *Medicaid state balancing incentive payments program* increases the portion of Medicaid beneficiaries who receive long-term care outside institutional settings. For states that qualify, increased federal share for expenditures for long-term-care services and supports is provided to Medicaid beneficiaries outside institutional settings (Section 10202 of the PPACA).
- The *Medicaid community first choice option* allows state Medicaid programs to offer community-based attendant services and supports to beneficiaries who otherwise would require the level of care offered in a hospital, nursing home, or intermediate care facility for the developmentally disabled (Section 2401, begins on October 1, 2011).
- The *Medicaid medical home model* allows states to enroll Medicaid beneficiaries with chronic conditions, including severe and persistent mental illness (SPMI), into medical homes as part of pilot projects. It authorizes grants of $25 million to help states plan and implement these projects (Section 2703, starts January 1, 2011).
- The *Medicare medical homes* establishes a program to create and fund the development of community health teams to support the creation of medical homes through increased access to comprehensive, community-based, and coordinated care (Section 3502, starts January 1, 2012).

NEW SCIENTIFIC DISCOVERIES EXTEND THE FRONTIERS FOR PREVENTION

While parity and healthcare reform legislation set the table for innovation in prevention, it is the new scientific discoveries about the brain and behavioral health that provide the raw material behind the innovation. These discoveries need refinement in order to be useful; the scientific information needs to be utilized to achieve a cost-effective outcome on a large scale. Those discoveries with the greatest implications for prevention and wellness include:

- Longer brain development process (NIMH, 2008)
- The possibility of generation of new brain cells (Bjornebekk, Mathé, & Brené, 2005; Bryner, 2007)
- Diagnostic blood tests and brain scans to identify disease and progress in recovery

Some of the recent work by Thomas Insel, MD, director of the National Institute of Mental Health, addresses the evolution of scientific understanding and of healthcare practice (Insel & Wang, n.d.). Dr. Insel stresses the importance of the revolution of understanding about the relationship between the mind and the body (and our ability to draw links between them) to the scientific and healthcare communities. He believes that "new discoveries" are shaping practice—while being quick to point out that we are "only 10%" on the way to understanding complex brain functioning.

Dr. Insel's work illustrates how even the most basic assumptions in behavioral health have changed, due to neuroscience, over the past three decades. These new understandings have served to end three great myths in the field:

- *Myth 1: Brain development is complete at birth.* It is now known that brain development is not complete until approximately age 25. From that point forth, we lose brain cells at the rate of 50,000 or so per day, but the human body continues to generate new brain cells throughout our lifetime.
- *Myth 2: The brain is an organ with static functioning.* It is now known that the brain is "plastic" and capable of change. In fact, new research indicates that the cells and size of the hippocampus actually grow when adults engage in new learning.

- *Myth 3: Specific human functions happen in specific regions of the brain.* We now know that brain functioning is not limited to a single location. For example, "vision" happens in many coordinated locations of the brain, as does language. Old models of the brain (remember junior high health class...)—where a specific spot in the brain controlled a certain function—just are not accurate.

Dr. Insel believes that this new knowledge has already affected the treatment of behavioral and neurological disorders (Oss, n.d. [a])—that we are moving from the study of treatment of these diseases using psychological principles alone to combining knowledge of psychology and behavior with neuroscience. However, our current treatments are still quite primitive. We know that medication is necessary, but not sufficient alone. We are certainly headed toward linking neuroscience to prevention by harnessing the brain's ability to continue to create new cells. Dr. Insel suggested three likely future effects of neuroscience on treatment:

- Treatments will develop based on our understanding of the difference in behavioral/neurological diseases in terms of the death of cells versus the faulty circuitry of cells. A whole group of conditions is related to the death of cells (Parkinson's disease, ALS, Alzheimer's), while others (schizophrenia, bipolar disorder) are a function of faulty communication/circuitry between cells. This understanding will drive new treatment approaches.
- Developments in neuroscience will eventually allow mental health professionals to move "upstream" in preventing mental illness, much like the treatment of heart disease. New scanning technologies will allow us to detect changes in brain cells earlier and to intervene to prevent (or delay) symptomatology. Although there is currently no predictive testing (via scanning, genomics, or biological testing) available for mental illnesses, addictions, or Alzheimer's disease, such testing is in the research pipeline and may be a reality sooner than anyone would have thought possible.
- The future of mental health treatment is to direct the development of new brain cells. New research shows us that the most serious mental illnesses start (though

they may not be diagnosed) before human brains are fully developed. The ability to detect and prevent brain development from going off course would be a form of preventive medicine that has not yet been experienced in the behavioral healthcare field.

What does this mean for organizations paying for or providing treatment services for behavioral disorders? Dr. Insel's work has two important management implications. First, clinical directors need to embrace emerging scientific findings and adopt a program development framework with the assumption that neuroscience will enhance—rather than conflict with—current psychological and social approaches. Second, in the near future, brain scanning technology is going to be central to state-of-the-art programming for the prevention, diagnosis, and treatment of behavioral disorders. To keep up with new developments and treatments, most programs in the field will need to develop collaborations with professionals who have brain scanning expertise.

NEW INFORMATION TECHNOLOGY MAKES PREVENTION FEASIBLE

With new science pointing to new opportunities for prevention and a regulatory and reimbursement framework that supports prevention, the one remaining issue is closing the science-to-service gap with a scalable cost-effective means for bringing new prevention services to market. The evolution of the Internet into Web 2.0 and a parallel increase in remote healthcare service delivery tools is making access to behavioral health services in general—and preventive and wellness services in particular—both scalable and affordable.

A number of studies (McGinty, Saeed, Simmons, & Yildirim, 2006) have identified e-health as a solution to the problem of access to behavioral health services (see, for example, O'Donohue & Draper, in press). One particular study examined the issue of access in the remote landscape of Australia, and Web-based mental health services were recommended as a way for Australia to boost access to prevention and early intervention services (Christensen & Hickie, 2010) and to correct a fundamental lack of access to mental health services. The Australia assessment concluded that Web-based services would reduce barriers to care, delivery costs, and demands on the clinical workforce.

Early intervention services for youth are most neglected by the current arrangements in Australia, and the study noted that young people with difficulties are increasingly seeking informal and formal help online.

Over the past decade, the tools for Web-enabled access to health services have increased. A wide range of technologies is available, such as text-based communication, video/audio Web communication that is both synchronous and asynchronous, consumer self-help services based on expert systems logic, applications for smart phones (California HealthCare Foundation, n.d.), remote monitoring tools, and smart home models. The ability of the Internet to provide the platform for these tools is enhanced by the evolution of Web 2.0—the term given to describe a second generation of the World Wide Web focused on the ability of people to collaborate and share information online. Web 2.0 basically refers to the transition from static HTML Web pages to a more dynamic Internet platform based on serving Web applications to users (Webopedia, n.d.).

Examples of these tech-enabled prevention programs are described in the following sections. And while these wellness and prevention programs are in early stages of development, they represent the future of reinventing prevention of, early diagnosis of, management of, and recovery from behavioral disorders.

Perfect Depression Care Initiative

The Perfect Depression Care Initiative of the Behavioral Health Services (BHS) Division of the Henry Ford Health System (HFHS) reported in early 2010 that its patient suicide rate had dropped to zero since 2008 (*Journal of the American Medical Association,* 2010). Before starting the initiative, BHS reported a suicide rate of 89 per 100,000 patients; by 2004, the rate had dropped by 75% to 22 per 100,000 patients. To date, the average national suicide rate is estimated at about 230 per 100,000 in patient populations.

These are the findings of a report, titled "Depression Care Effort Brings Dramatic Drop in Large HMO Population's Suicide Rate," by Tracy Hampton, PhD. The Perfect Depression Care Initiative currently utilized includes the following aspects:

- A clear vision of how each patient's care will change is developed by staff members. While working with the patients, staff members make sure that the care

patients receive meets their needs. Staff members design and test strategies for improvements, and they share results, analyses, and lessons learned with other staff members to improve patient care.
- Patients have access to a depression care Web site created and maintained by the program.
- Patients can communicate with behavioral health professionals via e-mail.
- The outpatient sites offer at least one drop-in outpatient group appointment every week that is led by a psychiatrist and social worker.
- BHS staff must go through annual staff training where they must score a 100% on a follow-up test or receive additional education after completing a suicide risk and prevention course.
- Physician extenders, which can include nurses, social workers, or physician assistants, were hired for patient outreach to support patients and call them periodically to check on how they were doing.
- Intranet sites for staff include depression guidelines, the patient registry, and electronic tools to improve quality and efficiency of care.

BHS has been operating a large integrated mental health and substance abuse system that has two inpatient hospitals and 10 clinics. The Perfect Depression Care Initiative was designed by HFHS in 2001. With the support of HFHS, BHS selected the goal of redesigning delivery of care for depression. The division wanted to improve depression care by six different ways that were mentioned in a report by the Institute of Medicine (IOM): safety, effectiveness, patient centeredness, timeliness, efficiency, and equity.

The IOM's report called for changes in the U.S. healthcare delivery system and suggested a strategy for building a stronger health system, along with praising advances in medical science in the United States. BHS's chief executive officer and HFHS's vice president, C. Edward Coffey, MD, personally led the Perfect Depression Care Initiative. He said that the approach could be applied to a range of general medical issues, including violence prevention, infection control, and medication safety. Principles of the Perfect Depression Care Initiative are already being applied to the care of patients at BHS with other psychiatric disorders, such as anxiety and psychotic disorders.

HealthMedia Digital Coaching Programs

HealthMedia, Inc., part of the Johnson & Johnson Family of Companies and the wellness and prevention business, introduced two new "digital coaching" programs to reduce cardiovascular disease risk in 2010 (*OPEN MINDS On-Line News*, 2010). The programs—HealthMedia® ACHIEVE™ and HealthMedia® CONTROL™—provide comprehensive and scalable digital health coaching that focuses on behavior change and motivation to help users improve their self-management of high cholesterol and/or high blood pressure and reach recommended cholesterol and blood pressure ranges. The programs simulate live health coaching sessions and promote medication adherence, more effective working relationships with healthcare providers, better weight control, stress management, improved nutrition, and increased physical activity.

A digital coaching program starts with an online consultation. The digital coach collects information about the individual, motivation for change, and perceived barriers. A personalized plan addresses the person's history, goals, emotional triggers, barriers, willpower, and current stage of change. Each participant receives personalized communications that are tailored to connect with his or her unique characteristics and lifestyle to create an emotional connection that builds motivation and improves outcomes.

HealthMedia offers its digital coaching programs to a wide range of employers and health plans. The programs can be bundled with 15 other HealthMedia digital health coaching programs. The per-person cost to employers and health plans varies depending on the number of people covered, the number of programs selected, and the length of time the company will offer the programs. Aggregate, "de-identified" outcomes reporting helps employers and health plans measure behavior change and productivity improvement.

UnitedHealth Invests in Telehealth

UnitedHealth Group is getting into telehealth in a big way. In early 2010, OptumHealth, (a division of UnitedHealth) announced its launch of "NowClinic," an e-health service connecting consumers to providers via video chat. NowClinic will be available to anyone for a flat registration fee; licensed physicians and clinicians are encouraged to register for NowClinic credentialing to deliver services to states in which they are licensed to practice. The initiative will begin in Texas and has plans for national expansion.

In addition, UnitedHealth announced a partnership with Cisco Systems Inc. to build the first national telehealth network, called "Connected Care," which will be used in a New Mexico Project HOPE program to expand healthcare access. Connected Care combines audio and video technology and health resources to expand physicians' reach into rural, urban, and other underserved areas. The Project HOPE program is funded by a $4.5 million, 3-year grant from UnitedHealth Group, which will also provide technology and technical support. Project HOPE will apply its knowledge of and experience in implementing healthcare training programs that address chronic diseases. The Project HOPE program will start in the first quarter of 2010 in New Mexico's rural southwestern Hidalgo and Doña Ana counties. A Connected Care mobile clinic will help residents obtain health screenings and treatment.

Services will expand over the 3 years to the central Albuquerque region, as well as to the southeast and northern regions. The program will have a focus on identifying and addressing diabetes and other chronic diseases, and will also provide treatment for common conditions, follow-up exams, wellness programs for employees and patients, and acute care. A "train-the-trainer" component will advance local health worker capacity, further helping to improve care quality for the long term.

Connected Care is built on an open network that integrates multiple vendors' technologies with electronic health records and other information technology platforms. Cisco's HealthPresence is one of the principal technologies enabling Connected Care; it uses video, audio, and medical information to create an experience similar to an in-person visit with a physician. The program will enable real-time connectivity and consultations among doctors, nurses, and health system professionals across the country, creating a more connected system of healthcare.

Intel Health Guide Launched in United States

On November 10, 2008, Intel Corporation announced the launch of the Intel Health Guide in the United States. The health guide is able to connect patients and their healthcare teams via 3G wireless and phone lines, in addition to the standard cable/DSL broadband connection already available. The Intel Health Guide is a personal health system that combines the Intel Health Guide PHS6000 in-home device with an online interface, the Intel Health Care Management Suite. It allows healthcare providers to customize care, gather timely information about the status of their patients, and collect and prioritize patient data.

After completing a small-scale pilot in the United Kingdom to demonstrate the health guide's clinical benefits, NHS Lothian is now rolling out 400 Intel Health Guide units across Edinburgh and the Lothian regions in a large-scale telehealth program. Another small-scale pilot was completed by the Academic Medical Center, Amsterdam, and the Institute for Prevention and Telemedicine in the Netherlands.

TRICARE Launches Web-Based Demo Project

On August 1, 2009, TRICARE launched its Web-based behavioral health demonstration project in its three U.S. regions. The project will provide Web-based behavioral health and related services and the use of video teleconferencing to deliver real-time mental health services to active duty service members and their families and to National Guard and Reserve members and their families enrolled in TRICARE Reserve Select. The demonstration project is designed to test the feasibility of using audio and visual technologies, including Web-based services, on a permanent basis.

TRICARE currently provides an array of text and multimedia-based educational materials targeting predeployment, deployment, and postdeployment adjustment concerns. The demonstration project will expand ways to access behavioral healthcare to include Web-based tools, audiovisual telecommunications, e-mail, instant messaging, and live chat. The demonstration project is funded by the fiscal year 2009 Department of Defense (DoD) appropriations. In the appropriation, DoD was directed to establish and use a Web-based clinical mental health services program as a way to deliver clinical mental health services to service members and their families in rural areas.

Google Health Teams Up With MDLiveCare

On October 7, 2009, Google Health announced a partnership with MDLiveCare as its first telehealth service provider. Google Health users accessing telehealth services through MDLiveCare will be able to share their Google Health personal health record (PHR) with the physician prior to the teleconsultation appointment. Following the appointment, MDLiveCare will automatically add the physician's clinical notes to the PHR. MDLiveCare provides HIPAA-compliant medical and behavioral health consultations through live, secure video feed; e-mail; or telephone.

Providers in a variety of medical specialties have been credentialed by MDLiveCare. Physician visits can take place by phone or via members' Internet connection and Webcam. Membership offers unlimited phone and e-mail advice. An adult wellness test that provides 23 blood tests to assess all major body systems is available with each plan. The plan also provides storage for the members' electronic medical records at the MDLiveVault, and members receive a card to enable emergency responder access to the record.

Ann-E Smartphone Application for Addiction

There are currently over 50,000 iPhone applications with various types of healthcare functionality. One example of this is the early November 2009 launch of a new Apple iPhone application, "Ann-e," created for people in addiction recovery who are following a 12-step program. This "app" helps them safely and anonymously connect with a support network of peers. Users can register their affiliation with a 12-step program and create an anonymous user name. The application supports text and live voice calls via anonymous conference lines. It also facilitates face-to-face meetings with selected trusted peers by disclosing proximity and location. Users who want to be available to help others can list themselves as "on call" and will be notified when other users need help.

The application's developer, "Annie," said recovery is strengthened in two ways: first by enabling people in 12-step programs to reach out for support and, second, by enabling them to serve as support for others, creating a safety net when cravings hit. Ann-e is available for the iPhone, iPhone 3G, iPhone 3GS, iPod touch, and the iPod touchG. The application is password protected, so casual viewing of owner contents or contact information is impossible.

Online Care Anywhere Launched by Minnesota Blue Cross and Blue Shield

On December 1, 2009, Blue Cross and Blue Shield (Blue Cross) of Minnesota and Fairview Health Services launched a pilot of Online Care Anywhere, a new telehealth care model that enables Blue Cross employees and their covered dependents to access medical care online or by telephone from physicians affiliated with Fairview Health Services. To facilitate workplace use of online care, Blue Cross created three secured "online care rooms" at two Minnesota campuses. Each room is equipped with a computer, a Webcam, and biometric devices to record weight, body mass index, and blood pressure, as well as other basic diagnostic tools. Employees can also access Online Care Anywhere from home with or without a Webcam. The secure system captures a complete, comprehensive record of each conversation that takes place between a consumer and physician. At the end of the conversation, consumers are encouraged to forward the record to their primary care physicians to ensure continuity of care.

As we move forward into the next generation of treatments for mental illnesses, addictions, and cognitive disabilities, preventive services will continue to increase in their importance. The expansion is being driven by industry factors that will shape innovations in wellness and prevention and increase their availability in the service delivery system. Behavioral health parity will remove the stigma of mental illness and foster the integration of behavioral and physical health; healthcare reform will impact the service delivery landscape in a variety of ways that are conducive to preventative services. New scientific discoveries will continue to expand the frontiers for prevention, and new information technology developments will make the delivery of preventive services more feasible. The convergence of these factors will ensure a large, permanent role for wellness and prevention in the field of behavioral healthcare.

REFERENCES

Bjornebekk, A., Mathé, A. A., & Brené, S. (2005). The antidepressant effect of running is associated with increased hippocampal cell proliferation. *International Journal of Neuropsychopharmacology, 8*(3), 357–368.

Bryner, J. (2007). Exercise grows new brain cells. Accessed at http://www.livescience.com/health/070628_exercise_brain.html

California HealthCare Foundation. (n.d.). How smartphones are changing health care for consumers and providers. Retrieved July 26, 2010, from the *OPEN MINDS* Industry Resources Library at http://www.openminds.com/circle-home/indres/040110smartphones.pdf

Care effort brings dramatic drop in large HMO population's suicide rate. (May 19, 2010). *Journal of the American Medical Association*. Retrieved June 7, 2010, from http://jama.ama-assn.org

Christensen, H., & Hickie, I. (2010). E-mental health: A new era in delivery of mental health services. *Medical Journal of Australia, 192*(11 Suppl), S2–3.

HealthMedia introduces two new digital coaching programs. (January 4, 2010). *OPEN MINDS* On-Line News. Retrieved July 26, 2010 from http://www.openminds.com/circle-home/eprint/omol/2010/010410strat2.htm

Insel, T. R., & Wang, P. S. (n.d.). Rethinking mental illness. Retrieved July 26, 2010, from the *OPEN MINDS* Industry Resources Library at http://www.openminds.com/circle-home/indres/050610rethinkingmentalillness.htm

Lo Sasso, A. T., & Byck, G. R. (2010). Funding growth drives community health center services. *Health Affairs, 29*(2), 289–296. Retrieved July 26, 2010, from http://content.healthaffairs.org/cgi/content/abstract/29/2/289?maxtoshow=&hits=10&RESULTFORMAT=&fulltext=funding+growth+drive+community+health+center+services&andorexactfulltext=and&searchid=1&FIRSTINDEX=0&resourcetype=HWCIT

McGinty, K. L., Saeed, S. A., Simmons, S. C., & Yildirim, Y. (2006). Telepsychiatry and e-mental health services: Potential for improving access to mental health care. *Psychiatric Quarterly, 77*(4), 335–342. Retrieved July 26, 2010, from https://springerlink3.metapress.com/content/70522w022nv57472/resource-secured/?target=fulltext.pdf&sid=iiwznc45a4vrm1bfiilhjeqt&sh=www.springerlink.com

NIMH (National Institute of Mental Health). (n.d.). Teenage brain: A work in progress. NIMH fact sheet, NIH publication no. 01-4929, 2008 at http://www.nimh.nih.gov/health/publications/teenage-brain-a-work-in-progress-fact-sheet/index.shtml

O'Connell, M. E., Boat, T., & Warner, K. E. (Eds.). (2009). Preventing mental, emotional, and behavioral disorders among young people: Progress and possibilities. Retrieved July 26, 2010, from the *OPEN MINDS* Industry Resources Library at http://www.openminds.com/circlehome/eprint/indres/020909natlacadprevention.pdf

O'Donohue, W., & Draper, C. (In press). *Evidence based e-health*. New York, NY: Springer.

Oss, M. E. (n.d. [a]). Be prepared for the revolution of mind & body understanding. Retrieved July 26, 2010 from the *OPEN MINDS* Industry Resources Library at http://www.openminds.com/circlehome/circle/content_chautauqua.htm

Oss, M. E. (n.d. [b]). Can we have parity for both behavioral health & coverage of prevention services in the health care reform mix? *OPEN MINDS* Circle. Retrieved July 26, 2010 from the *OPEN MINDS* Industry Resources Library at http://www.openminds.com/circlehome/circle/commentary_carlbellhcreform.htm

Oss, M. E. (n.d. [c]). Future trends in behavioral health care—Integration of behavioral health/primary health care, new technologies, health care reform, & more. Retrieved July 26, 2010, from the *OPEN MINDS* Industry Resources Library at http://www.openminds.com/circlehome/eprint/indres/051309ossmodels.htm

Webopedia. (n.d.). Retrieved July 26, 2010, from http://www.webopedia.com/TERM/W/Web_2_point_0.html

Eighteen

Reforms in Veteran and Military Behavioral Health*

R. BLAKE CHAFFEE

INTRODUCTION

The conflicts in Iraq and Afghanistan have catapulted behavioral health issues into prominence for their beneficial or deleterious contributions to fitness for duty and the performance of active-duty service members. These fitness-for-duty and performance concerns led armed forces leadership to focus on how service members and their families manage stress (i.e., their capacity for adaptive coping or "resiliency") and to ensure their access to information and resources when they need additional help. This focus has been the stimulus for innovation in the TRICARE Behavioral Health Program. The purpose of this chapter is to discuss those innovations. Some background on the military health system (MHS) and behavioral health issues in the military are presented to provide context for the rationale and development of these innovations.

THE MILITARY HEALTH SYSTEM

The TRICARE managed care support contractors (MCSCs) supplement the services available through the military treatment facilities (MTFs) and the Veterans Administration, together referred to as the "direct care system." Collectively, the MTFs, the VA, and the MCSC networks comprise the MHS. The

---

* Disclaimer: The views and opinions expressed in this chapter are those of the author and do not represent the position of the Department of Defense, the TRICARE Management Activity, or TriWest Healthcare Alliance.

MCSCs develop and administer networks of civilian healthcare facilities and providers that make healthcare services available to service members and their families nationwide. The MCSC networks provide additional capacity to the direct care system for services that the direct care system is unable to provide.

The current TRICARE Program was created by the National Defense Authorization Act of 1994. It replaced the previous Civilian Health and Medical Program of the Uniformed Services (CHAMPUS) created by Congress in 1966. TRICARE provides healthcare benefits to the dependents of active-duty service members, retirees and their dependents, surviving family members, and certain other categories of eligibles designated by the assistant secretary of defense for health affairs. TRICARE benefits extend to members of the seven uniformed services: Army, Navy, Air Force, Marine Corps, Coast Guard, National Oceanic and Atmospheric Administration, and the United States Public Health Service. Approximately 9.6 million service members and their families are eligible for TRICARE (TRICARE Management Activity Web site, 2010).

The role of the MCSCs has changed in several significant respects as a result of the current conflicts in Afghanistan and Iraq. First, MCSC network providers now serve more national guard and reserve (reserve component) members who have been activated for service in Operation Enduring Freedom (OEF) and Operation Iraqi Freedom (OIF). When a reserve component member is activated, he or she receives healthcare services through the direct care system and his or her family members become eligible for TRICARE. When he or she is deactivated and returns to civilian life, he or she and his or her family are TRICARE eligible for 6 months to facilitate transition back to civilian health plan coverage. About 1.9 million U.S. troops have been deployed to Operation Enduring Freedom (OEF), which began in Afghanistan on October 7, 2001, and Operation Iraqi Freedom (OIF), which began in Iraq on March 19, 2003 (Institute of Medicine, 2010). Reserve Component members represent approximately 45% of the total deployed forces (Powers, 2008).

Second, the MCSCs are an option for continued care for wounded service members who are medically discharged. As of April 15, 2010, wounded service members who were not returned to duty totaled 13,936 in OIF and 3,159 in OEF (Defenselink Casualty Report, 2010).

DEPLOYMENT, POSTTRAUMATIC STRESS, AND RESILIENCY

Research has shown that approximately 11–17% of service members report symptoms consistent with mental disorders postdeployment, including posttraumatic stress disorder (PTSD), anxiety, and depression (Hoge et al., 2004). Family members and significant others have been less well studied, but some preliminary evidence indicates that parental deployment may present challenges to the emotional well-being of their children and those challenges increase when the nondeployed parent has emotional difficulty (Chandra et al., 2009).

The fact that approximately 70% of deployed service members do not report clinically significant symptoms of mental disorder following deployment (Office of the Surgeon General U.S. Army Medical Command, 2008b) has led to the hypothesis that they may differ physiologically and psychologically in their responses to the prolonged stress of deployment. These differences have led to the assumption that exposure to stress may not be inherently pathological. In fact, some service members appear to "rise to the occasion" repeatedly and cope exceedingly well with stress. This has been referred to as "postadversity growth," "posttraumatic growth," or "resiliency" (Wikipedia, 2010)

Understanding both posttraumatic stress and resiliency is not a matter of studying either one in isolation, but rather of studying both within the context in which they occur. Both active-duty service members and their families are involved in the military lifestyle and culture, which can influence their beliefs, values, and behaviors, including their adaptation to stress and help-seeking behavior.

STIGMA, ACCESS TO BEHAVIORAL HEALTHCARE, AND FITNESS FOR DUTY

Although stigma associated with behavioral health (BH) consultation and treatment is not unique to the military population, it can be a significant barrier to access to appropriate behavioral healthcare for active-duty service members (ADSMs) and may negatively impact fitness for duty, operational readiness, and retention. Recent studies of returning service members expand what is known about their reports of symptoms of mental disorder, their attitudes toward BH consultation, the impact of their attitudes on access to appropriate BH care, and their actual utilization of BH services.

The initial study of soldiers and marines returning from deployment to Iraq and Afghanistan indicates that while stigma is of greatest concern for those who screened positive for a mental disorder, even those who did not meet the screening criteria for mental disorder frequently expressed concern (Hoge et al., 2004). Hoge et al. (2004) studied large samples of soldiers and marines prior to their deployment ($N = 2,530$) and 3–4 months following their return ($N = 3,671$). The percentage of subjects who met the criteria for major depression, generalized anxiety, and PTSD was significantly higher after duty in Iraq (15.6–17.1%) than after duty in Afghanistan (11.2%) or before deployment to Iraq (9.3%). The perceived barriers to seeking mental health services included the following:

	Screening ($N = 731$)	Screening ($N = 5,422$)
It would be too embarrassing	41%	18%
It would harm my career	50%	24%
Members of my unit would have less confidence in me	59%	31%
My unit leadership might treat me differently	63%	33%
My leaders would blame me for the problem	51%	20%
I would be seen as weak	65%	31%
Mental healthcare does not work	25%	9%

These results indicate that those soldiers and marines who screened positive for mental disorder (PTSD, generalized anxiety disorder, and depression) were twice as likely to express concern about being stigmatized and about other barriers to access to care. Only small percentages of the samples making up this group (23–40%) actually sought mental healthcare; in other words, those most in need of care are not likely to seek it.

In another study of all army soldiers and marines who completed the postdeployment health assessment on returning from OEF in Afghanistan ($N = 16,318$), OIF ($N = 222,620$), and other locations ($N = 64,967$), Hoge et al. (2006) found that 35% of OIF veterans accessed mental health services in their first year after deployment. Two thirds of service members who accessed mental healthcare did so within 2 months of returning home. This study used healthcare utilization data from the defense medical surveillance system (DMSS), which included all permanent U.S. military medical facilities, as well as care at other healthcare facilities reimbursed by the military. These data would not include veterans who seek mental health services outside the direct care system—for example, Military OneSource community-based services. Military OneSource is a program funded by a separate DoD contract that provides a broad range of services similar to those offered by commercial employee assistance programs (EAPs).

Elsewhere, Hoge, Auchterlonie, and Milliken (2006) studied the relationship between psychiatric hospitalization, involuntary separation, and disability. They found that the rate of service separation 6 months after first hospitalization was 45% among personnel whose primary hospital discharge diagnosis was a mental disorder, 27% among those with a secondary mental disorder discharge diagnosis, and 11% among those hospitalized for all other medical conditions.

Overall, the rate of medical disability separation from the service for mental disorders was twice that of those hospitalized for other conditions (8% vs. 4%). This is often quite expensive for the military, given costs of training and replacement, as well as disruptive for the service member, who might have been planning a military career. Hoge et al. (2005) suggest that possible contributing factors include higher levels of disability or disease chronicity for mental disorders than for other illness categories, the career-stigmatizing effects of mental disorders, and associations between mental disorders and behavioral problems that may not be conducive to military service.

Other studies of returning service members contribute the following findings:

- National guard (6.6%) and active-duty army (6.2%) service members reported three or more symptoms on the PTSD screen of the Post-Deployment Health Assessment (PDHA) at similar rates but diverged on the Post-Deployment Health Reassessment (PDHRA) with national guard (14.3%) higher than army (9.1%) members (Milliken, Auchterlonie, & Hoge, 2007).
- Of soldiers who reported a high rate of PTSD symptoms on the PDHA, 49.4% of national guard and army reserve soldiers and 59.2% of active soldiers reported symptomatic improvement by the time of the PDHRA approximately 6 months later. However, more than

twice as many new cases were identified among soldiers who did not have a high PTSD score initially on the PDHA (Milliken et al., 2007).
- The percentage of soldiers and marines who report symptoms of mental disorders and PTSD increases as the number of deployments increases (MHAT V, 2008). The percentage of service members reporting symptoms of mental disorder increased from approximately 10% among those on their first deployment to over 25% among those with three or more deployments.
- Of returning service members, 69.3% report no emotional distress or traumatic brain injury (TBI) (Rand Center for Military Policy Research, 2008).
- Confidence in leadership is a mitigating factor in emotional distress reported (i.e., units with high combat exposure and high confidence in their leadership reported fewer symptoms than units with high combat exposure and low confidence in their leadership and units with low combat exposure and low confidence in their leadership) (Office of the Surgeon General U.S. Army Medical Command, 2008a).
- PTSD patients are six times more likely to attempt suicide than the general population: 19% of patients with PTSD attempt suicide (Kessler, Borges, & Walters, 1999).

While the studies differ considerably, these findings provide a basis for understanding the concept of behavioral health need as well as stigma in the military community. Before proceeding further, it is useful to note that stigma surrounding behavioral health consultation is by no means unique to the military. Kessler (2000) reported that 23% of civilian men and 17% of civilian women reported stigma as a barrier to seeking behavioral health services.

Koffman (2002) discusses the management of combat stress reactions in the expeditionary forces. Focusing on forward-deployed operating forces and medical resources, he states:

> Commanders who can effectively limit the wide range of potentially avoidable serious stress reactions in their units maintain a decisive fighting edge. Managing operational stress is a significant force multiplier. The severe stress encountered by the Iraqi forces during Operation Desert Storm contributed to their quick defeat and widespread combat stress reactions were noted in scores of surrendering Iraqi soldiers. Conversely,

familiarity with superior equipment, realistic training, unit integrity, esprit de corps, and a decisive, unopposed victory led to a paucity of U.S. combat stress casualties. The nature of combat is a strong predictor of combat stress. The psychiatric morbidity found in Russians following guerilla-style urban combat in Chechnya was as high as 75% of the total force.

As Koffman (2002) notes, however, if managing operational stress is a force multiplier, the military may have more at stake in countering stigma than the civilian sector does.

In reality, mild to moderate mental disorders are managed by both military members and civilians as a matter of course in everyday life, treated or untreated, with varying degrees of disruption and success. Membership in a military unit, however, entails a level of scrutiny, continual functional demands, and stress rarely involved in civilian employment. Koffman (2002) notes the importance of unit integrity and esprit de corps as factors contributing to the relatively low rate of combat stress casualties in Operation Desert Storm. Hoge et al. (2004) report concerns about losing the confidence of unit members and being treated differently by unit leadership as elements of the stigma surrounding behavioral health consultation.

Both of these concerns indicate the importance of unit cohesion to the individual service member. Being seen as a stable, reliable, trustworthy member of the unit may be as essential to the success of the individual as it is to that of the unit. As Hoge et al. (2005) note, mental disorders are often associated with behavioral problems that are not conducive to military service. Symptoms of mental disorder such as fatigue, memory problems/forgetfulness, indecision, irritability, and impulsiveness can certainly undermine a service member's reputation as a stable, reliable, trustworthy unit member and can be mistaken as "bad attitude" by unit members and leadership.

The studies of soldiers and marines returning from OIF and OEF previously discussed cast into bold relief the importance of managing combat stress and PTSD to operational readiness and retention. Although we have no research on the actual attitudes of ADSMs toward mental illness, the concerns expressed by the soldiers and marines studied by Hoge et al. (2004) indicate that being identified as in need of behavioral health services is clearly something to be avoided. More research is necessary to understand fully how this perception develops and the specific factors that sustain it within the military lifestyle and culture. Career concern and loss of unit and leadership confidence appear to be at the core of behavioral health stigma (Hoge et al., 2004).

As with any human organization, attitudes toward mental illness among members of the military are certainly not monolithic and may differ from those expressed in official policy. The reticence of soldiers and marines to be identified as in need of behavioral health services may reflect an adaptive posture to the current military environment in which they function. Disclosing mental health symptoms or disorder may be perfectly acceptable and encouraged by their current unit and leadership, but that disclosure becomes part of their permanent record, which is available to future leadership whose attitudes may be different.

Coincidentally, military leadership is faced with the challenge of recruiting, selecting, and assigning military personnel to myriad administrative, industrial, and operational roles, many of which cannot be adequately undertaken by anyone whose performance might be impaired by physical or mental disorder. Lack of disclosure of any such condition, upon recruitment or subsequently, presents a potentially dangerous situation for the organization and the individual. In the ideal military, service members would willingly acknowledge their physical and mental disabilities, secure in the knowledge that their skills and abilities were sufficiently valuable to win them challenging and rewarding career opportunities. The ideal may not be achievable, but approximating it more closely may be realistic and beneficial to readiness and retention.

SUICIDE IN THE MILITARY

Numbers and rates of completed suicide in the army have increased substantially since the beginning of OEF and OIF. In 2009, the army reported the following numbers of completed suicides for the three preceding years (Jelinek, 2009):

Year	Number of Completed Suicides	Rate/100,000
2008	128	20.2
2007	115	18.8
2006	102	17.5

The 2008 army rate exceeded the age-adjusted rate of completed suicide for the general civilian population for the first time since the Vietnam War and was more than double the army rate for 2002, the first year of the Afghan conflict. The civilian age-adjusted rate for 2008 was approximately 19.5. The number of completed suicides among army personnel in 2008 was also the highest since record keeping began in 1980. The Marine Corps reported 41 possible or confirmed suicides in 2008—a rate of 16.8 per 100,000 (Jelinek, 2009). This number represented an increase from 33 in 2007 and 25 in 2006 (*Federal Health Institute Newsletter,* 2009).

The Centers for Disease Control and Prevention (CDC) launched the National Violent Death Reporting System (NVDRS) in 2003 as a nationwide data collection and reporting system for information on the circumstances of violent deaths, including suicide. According to the CDC, suicide was the 11th leading cause of death in the United States in 2004, with 32,000 suicide deaths reported. Among younger adults, suicide is the second leading cause of death among 25- to 34-year-olds and the third leading cause of death among 15- to 25-year-olds.

The use of firearms is the most common method of suicide among males, and poisoning is the most common method among females. This difference in choice of method may account for the fact that male suicide deaths outnumber females by 4 to 1: Firearms are generally considered a more lethal means of suicide than poisoning. There is no comparable reporting system or any official statistics for suicide attempts in the United States, but the ratio of attempted to completed suicide is generally estimated to be 25 to 1, with three suicide attempts among females for every attempt among males (American Association of Suicidology, 2006).

Among the general U.S. population, risk factors for suicide include the following:

- Prior suicide attempt
- Depression
- Alcohol and substance abuse
- History of trauma or abuse
- Family history of suicide
- Job or financial stress
- Stigma associated with seeking mental healthcare
- Barriers to access to healthcare
- Easy access to lethal means

Protective factors include the following:

- Strong family or community connections
- Accessible and effective clinical care
- Skills in problem solving
- Conflict resolution
- Nonviolent handling of disputes
- Cultural and religious beliefs that discourage suicide

Comparing these findings to the active-duty military population or the population of military veterans is difficult for two reasons. First, there is no national tracking system for suicide and suicide attempts among veterans or active-duty military personnel. Second, data for the general population typically include veterans and samples excluding veterans are lacking (Sundararaman, Panangala, & Lister, 2008).

In 2005, the CDC NVDRS identified the following circumstances associated with the suicides of 1,622 former and current military personnel:

- Depression (47.2%); receiving mental health treatment (26.7%)
- Alcohol problem (17.2%); problem with other substances (7.7%)
- Problem with an intimate partner (24.5%)
- Physical health problem (38.4%)
- Experienced acute crisis during the prior 2 weeks (28.0%)
- Left a suicide note (33.9%)
- Previous suicide attempt (13.3%)
- Disclosed intent to commit suicide with enough time for someone to have intervened (29.0%)

The risk factors associated with suicide deaths among the general population and circumstances associated with suicides among current and former military personnel show a number of similarities. The facts that veterans are included in the civilian data and that military personnel are drawn from the civilian population and continue to experience many of the same stressors that affect their civilian counterparts may explain this overlap. The one civilian risk factor missing from the CDC military personnel sample is "job or financial stress." This is really two separate sources of stress, and military personnel not only are not immune, but also may arguably be prone to experience stress from both of these sources.

Holloway (2008) reported that the top five stressors associated with suicides among active-duty personnel were

1. Failed intimate relationship
2. Job problems
3. Article 15 (legal problems)
4. Debt
5. Psychiatric condition

The occupational stress that members of the military may be exposed to differs significantly from that which most civilian workers experience (excluding some civilian contractors in OEF and OIF). Depending on their occupational specialty, military members may be likely to be involved in combat as part of their job. As mentioned previously, Hoge et al. (2004) found that the percentage of service members screening positive for PTSD increased with increased combat exposure, peaking at between six and nine firefights and leveling off after 10 or more. The frequent use of improvised explosive devices (IEDs) in OEF and OIF has also exposed service members to blast and penetrating head injuries. Sundararaman et al. (2008) note that both traumatic brain injury (TBI) and PTSD are independent risk factors for suicide, possibly adding to the risk factors of military personnel.

The U.S. Army and Marine Corps response to their increasing suicide rates has been comprehensive and swift. Secretary of Defense Robert Gates and Marine Corps General James Cartwright, vice chairman of the Joint Chiefs of Staff, cited repeated deployments and the length of deployments as possible factors contributing to the strain on military personnel (McMichael, 2009). The defense secretary committed to extended "dwell time" at home between deployments in a Pentagon press conference. The MHS response has also been unprecedented. The Defense Centers of Excellence (DCOE) and the VA have developed and implemented multiple new programs to increase access to mental health services for military personnel and their families.

PROMOTING PSYCHOLOGICAL HEALTH AND COMBATING STIGMA

While the solution to BH stigma and increased suicide in the military involves organizational and cultural change, which are already underway but will take time, certain measures can be initiated and may promote change on a more local and personal level. The military can capitalize on its tradition of "taking care of its own" and the strength and cohesiveness of the military community in supporting the adaptation of service members and their families to deployment and reintegration. These measures include the following:

- The focus should be on psychological health and the development of a skill set to promote "optimal performance." The management of psychological health as well as physical health is essential to optimal performance, and skills that contribute to psychological health and resilience can be taught. When psychological health is treated in the same manner as physical health and conditioning and service members are given self-management skills (e.g., stress management, anger management, communications skills), maintaining it may be viewed as a necessary part of the daily routine.
- Education about the continuum of psychological health and disorder to normalize the concept for both service members and their families should take place. Extreme examples of psychotic and insane behavior are prevalent in the media and current colloquial concepts of mental disorder, which promote the illusion that all mental disorder is mysterious and threatening. In reality, most "normal" people will experience emotional stress, bereavement, and mild to moderate anxiety and depression that may affect their ability to function. Understanding the continuum of psychological health and disorder can allow them to put these experiences into context and to seek professional help when necessary, and can allay unnecessary concern.
- Suicide prevention training should be available for service members and families. Suicide is the second leading cause of death among male veterans and the first leading cause of death among female veterans. Of the 115 completed suicides in the army in 2007, 50% had a recent failed relationship, and drugs or alcohol were involved in 30% of cases. In this scenario, suicide is frequently preventable, and peer support can be extremely important (Holloway, 2008).
- Leadership training on the early identification of mental disorders and strategies for intervention needs to

occur at all levels. Knowing when and how to intervene personally and interpersonally can increase the early identification of mental disorder and promote improved personal and organizational effectiveness.
- The role of direct care BH professionals should be diversified from the occupational medicine role they currently perform in conducting fitness-for-duty evaluations, special program screenings, administrative separations for unsuitability, and medical boards for psychiatric disability. Psychological health promotion, self-management skill building, and consultation with commands can be undertaken.
- BH professionals need to be integrated into primary care settings to facilitate the early identification of service members with combat stress and PTSD. Service members frequently present in the primary care setting with the sleep disturbance associated with PTSD, and many consider primary care a "stigma-free zone" where they can discuss BH concerns (Chaffee & O'Donohue, 2007).
- Evidence-based treatment programs for PTSD (e.g., cognitive/behavioral approaches using prolonged exposure therapy) should be developed with the endorsement and support of leadership. The Institute of Medicine report on the readjustment needs of veterans, service members, and their families found a relative paucity of data on OEF and OIF populations that are adequate to support the development of evidence-based policy (Institute of Medicine, 2010). Service members meeting criteria should be encouraged to participate without penalty. These outpatient programs promote the concept that such symptoms and disorders can be successfully managed and the member can remain fit for duty.
- Reintegration programs aimed at reducing the "negative transfer of training" (i.e., the generalization of responses that are adaptive in theater to the home front, where they may be maladaptive) need to be developed.
- The combat stress experience should be normalized via presentations by senior officers and senior enlisted personnel about their experiences and their recovery.
- A "risk management" approach to combat stress disorders (PTSD, generalized anxiety, depression) that views them as occupational hazards needs to be developed.

- Extension of the research on attitudes toward mental illness among service members and leadership is needed to target educational interventions appropriately.
- Research on the 69% of service members who return from deployment reports no symptoms of mental disorder or combat stress (Rand Report, 2008). We may have something to learn from these personnel about adaptation to combat and from battlefront to home front.
- Conduct research and development on the effects of "stress inoculation" programs (e.g., Battlemind), on performance, reintegration, and retention. "Battlemind," now referred to as "Resilience Training," was the U.S. Army training system for supporting soldiers and their families across the phases of the deployment cycle (Army developing master resiliency training, 2009).

In many respects, the concepts employed by combat stress management teams in forward-deployed settings have application to the organization as a whole. Peer-to-peer education and training in coping skills that permeate the organization sufficiently to become routine, supported by leadership and professionals who determine "best practices," are realistic and achievable.

TRICARE INNOVATIONS

Innovations in TRICARE and the TRICARE Behavioral Health Program have focused on increasing access to BH information and services.

Extending TRICARE Eligibility

Recognizing the expanded role of reserve component members in OEF and OIF, the TRICARE management activity (TMA) initiated a program to facilitate the transition back to civilian healthcare coverage after demobilization. Historically, reserve component members became eligible for TRICARE when they were activated, and they and their family members remained eligible for TRICARE as long as the service member remained on active duty. Reserve component members discharged from active duty would, theoretically, regain their civilian healthcare coverage upon their discharge and/or return to their civilian employment.

In reality, the experience of reserve component members discharged after serving in OEF and OIF in transitioning back to civilian healthcare coverage was often not that simple or smooth. Because most healthcare coverage in the United States is employer based, those national guard and reserve members whose employers did not hold their positions for them were left without employment and healthcare coverage. Even when employers held their positions, healthcare coverage did not automatically resume with employment for some service members due to delays in effective dates, changes in health status, etc.

In response, TMA initiated two programs. The first, called the Temporary Assistance to Military Personnel (TAMP) Program, extended TRICARE eligibility for the service members and his or her dependents for 6 months to facilitate the transition to civilian healthcare coverage. The second program, called TRICARE Reserve Select (TRS), offered service members the option of purchasing continued TRICARE coverage for themselves and their dependents beyond the 6 months provided by TAMP. The optional coverage period was tied to the length of time the service member had been activated.

Telemental Health Services

TMA has also implemented a demonstration program designed to increase access to behavioral health information and services for active-duty service members and their dependents. The demonstration program had two components: (1) telemental health network development, and (2) Web-based, nonmedical, solution-focused counseling.

Telemental Health Network Development

Telemental health services have always been a benefit under the TRICARE Program, but TMA's demonstration sought to increase the availability of and access to those covered services. TMA required the MCSCs to develop networks of "originating sites" where TRICARE beneficiaries could go to receive telemental health services from "distant providers" via Web-based videoconferencing. Previously, most telemental health services provided under TRICARE involved "point-to-point" video teleconferencing (VTC) from one facility to another via telephone lines. The availability and utilization of VTC technology in private practice offices of BH professionals was limited by the cost of the equipment and telephone lines. The advent of Web-based systems for VTC (e.g., Skype and Adobe Connect) offers a lower cost alternative for telemental health services and the prospect of expansion beyond the limits of established point-to-point VTC networks.

TMA requested that the MCSCs establish networks of "originating sites" and "distant providers" consistent with the Medicare definitions of those terms. Medicare defines these as the following (www.cms.hhs.gov/Telemedicine):

> Distant or Hub Site means the site at which the physician or other licensed practitioner delivering the service is located at the time the service is provided via a telecommunications system.
> Originating or Spoke site means the location of the patient at the time the service being furnished via a telecommunications system occurs. Telepresenters may be needed to facilitate the delivery of this service.

Originating sites are further defined as any of the following:

- The office of a physician or practitioner
- A hospital
- A critical access hospital
- A rural health clinic
- A federally qualified health center

The demonstration project required the MCSCs to develop originating sites in all areas in which the TRICARE Prime option was offered to beneficiaries. The purpose of the originating site is to provide a private, secure environment for the telemental health session with access to appropriate support services. Telepresenters are originating site staff who may be administrative, technical, or clinical staff, depending on their function. Generally, telepresenters are utilized to ensure that the VTC equipment is functional, the connection is established, and the patient is introduced to the provider. In some situations—particularly telemental health consultations—the telepresenter may be a clinically trained clinician or nurse who presents the case to the distant provider.

The originating sites the MCSCs established were broadly distributed across the areas where military bases are located and active-duty service members tend to reside; this considerably expanded the availability of telemental health services for ADSMs and their family members. National guard and reserve members and their families were less likely to be covered in all cases by these networks because they are less likely to be located near military bases and are more widely distributed geographically.

Establishing the MCSC networks of originating sites and distant providers was enabled primarily by the availability of Web-based VTC applications, which reduced the equipment costs for originating sites and providers to a personal computer and a Webcam. The MCSCs had to recruit providers who were already utilizing Web-based or point-to-point VTC or who were willing to adopt the technology and be trained in the administrative, technical, and clinical protocols for delivering effective, quality Web-based telemental health services.

The demonstration also required the MCSCs to coordinate scheduling between the beneficiary, the distant provider, and the originating site. The American Telemedicine Association (ATA) Core Standards for Telemedicine Operations (2007) and Core Standards for Videoconferencing-Based Telemental Health (2009) detail the current standards of practice and the current status of research on practice issues. They are essential to developing an adequate knowledge base for delivering telemental health services.

Under TRICARE, telemental health services are considered clinical services. Active-duty dependents can access telemental health services in the same manner as face-to-face consultation via the "initial eight" policy for outpatient psychotherapy, which does not require an outpatient treatment request from the provider or an authorization for the first eight psychotherapy sessions. The initial evaluation, typically billed as a psychodiagnostic interview (90801) does not require prior authorization for active-duty family members (ADFMs) or retirees and their dependents.

Outpatient mental health services for ADSMs, however, require authorization by the military treatment facility to which the service member is assigned. The authorization requirement and the fact that mental health consultations become part of the service member's medical record can represent barriers to access to service. Increased availability and access do not remove the concerns among many ADSMs for career and BH stigma discussed earlier. Whether telemental health services under the TMA demonstration will be utilized by ADSMs remains to be seen.

The requirement to have TRICARE-certified originating sites in each PSA may be an unnecessary requirement and may inadvertently limit use of telepsych services. Eligible beneficiaries may find the requirement to travel to an originating site to be a disincentive to using such services. Beneficiaries living outside a PSA may have to travel significant distances to access these services. If these beneficiaries must drive a significant distance, then it may be just as easy to see a clinician in person.

Requiring beneficiaries to access telemental health services from originating sites is consistent with the current standard of care for telemental health services (American Telemedicine Association, 2009). Concerns for patient safety have limited telemental health services to provider offices, clinics, hospital locations, and other originating sites where professional support is available to the beneficiary in the event that the beneficiary experiences a crisis during the session. Provider liability in such scenarios is also a concern, and the ATA clinical practice guidelines contain provisions for developing provider and originating site plans for psychiatric emergencies.

Telemental health services accessed from the patient's home computer are technically possible and highly convenient and practical, but the necessary clinical trials have yet to be conducted to determine whether or how such services may be delivered safely and effectively. For example, Egede et al. (2009) describe a randomized clinical trial currently underway of behavioral activation for the treatment of depression in elderly veterans in the VA system; the project compares services via telepsychology to traditional face-to-face intervention.

TRICARE Assistance Program (TRIAP) Services

In addition to the telemental health networks, the TMA demonstration required the MCSCs to offer Web-based, short-term, nonclinical, solution-focused counseling services available 24 hours a day, 7 days a week. The Department of Defense (DoD) has had a separate contract in place offering telephone-based and face-to-face nonclinical counseling for up to 12 visits for psychosocial problems similar to those served by commercial employee assistance programs (EAPs) (e.g., stress management, anger management, marital counseling). The services offered under that DoD contract through the Military OneSource (MOS) Program are much broader than those typically offered by commercial EAPs and include such issues as finding child care services and financial counseling. The demonstration program services were not intended to replace the services offered through MOS, but rather to extend access to such services, particularly those that may develop into clinical issues requiring clinical intervention.

Historically, the lack of availability of nonclinical, solution-focused counseling in the TRICARE Program has limited how these issues can be adequately addressed. For example, marital issues could only be addressed in conjoint psychotherapy sessions with one member of the couple as the identified patient having been diagnosed with a mental disorder (e.g., an adjustment disorder or a mood disorder). This limitation has meant that only a small proportion of the TRICARE population who fit these criteria could receive marital therapy services. The larger proportion of cases in which neither partner fit the diagnostic criteria for a mental disorder had to be referred to MOS for these services.

While there is a clinical logic to this arrangement, that logic is not always apparent to TRICARE beneficiaries and that is not how TRICARE beneficiaries or other laymen typically seek medical and mental health services. To the layman, a mental health provider—counselor, social worker, psychologist, or psychiatrist—is a mental health provider, not a TRICARE or a MOS provider. While some providers are members of both the TRICARE and MOS networks, not all are, and offering nonclinical services through the TRICARE Program avoids referrals between networks and better serves the beneficiaries.

Among ADSMs, nonclinical services through MOS have been particularly popular because they do not require prior authorization and are confidential and nonreportable (i.e., do not require notification of the ADSM's command or entries into the ADSM's medical record). ADSMs are therefore more likely to seek services through the MOS network than through TRICARE for such issues as stress, regardless of the severity of their problems. This means that ADSMs with clinically significant levels of stress may seek services through the MOS network in an effort to maintain confidentiality.

Due to the fee-for-service (FFS) payment arrangements for outpatient mental health services in both the TRICARE and MOS networks, providers have no incentive to refer patients who are clinically inappropriate for their services to the other program. The contingencies of the present system are arranged in a manner that may encourage patients with clinically significant complaints to continue to be treated in the MOS system and those with psychosocial issues to continue to be treated clinically in the TRICARE system. This is a persistent barrier to getting both ADSMs and ADFMs the services most appropriate to their needs.

The TRICARE Assistance Program (TRIAP) services required by the demonstration were unique in that the beneficiary could access the Web-based VTC services from the home. TRIAP services are nonmedical, short-term, solution-focused counseling for psychosocial problems similar to those provided via commercial EAPs. The kinds of problems addressed (e.g., marital problems, occupational problems, and stress management) are typical of the V codes in the DSM-IV-TR, which, by definition, are not due to a mental disorder but are the focus of consultation. The target population for these services is therefore "normal" adults for whom these issues represent problems in living.

Many EAPs currently deliver their services via telephone, so moving to Web-based video teleconferencing represents a relatively small and logical next step. Web-based VTC counseling services offer significant advantages over telephone-based services—primarily the availability of a live video image of the beneficiary with all of the information that provides in addition to the audio transmission of voices. This offers both the beneficiary and the counselor live, real-time information and feedback about their interaction. Adding the visual dimension provides all of the changes in appearance, body language, facial expression, and gestures to both participants as their interview progresses; none of these is available via voice communication alone.

Depending on the Web-based application selected, the participants may also be able to share documents and graphic arts or visual aids, further enriching the experience. Visual images and the information they provide may also facilitate the development of rapport and communication between the counselor and the beneficiary by eliminating some of the "guesswork" that attends voice communication and may lead to uncertainty or misunderstanding of the intention of the speaker in using certain words or phrases. Facial expressions added to the tone of voice and the words themselves often clearly convey the speaker's intent.

The advantages of home access to TRIAP services for service members and their families seeking information and counseling on stress management, anger management, marital problems, communication issues, parenting issues, anxiety, and sleep problems are immediately apparent. Such access is not only convenient, but also confidential and nonreportable—a fact that means that service members and their family members can consult licensed mental health professionals 24 hours a day, 7 days a week, 365 days a year about their concerns. The 24/7/365 availability of the service means that information and counseling can be available whenever a service member or one of his or her family members is ready to access it. This feature is particularly important to increasing access to BH services and to preventing nonclinical issues from escalating into more serious problems.

Integration of Behavioral Health Into Primary Care

There are numerous advantages to including specially trained behavioral health providers in primary care settings in MTFs. A significant percentage of TRICARE beneficiaries choose to receive services in MTFs. Of primary importance to a military population, integrated care may reduce stigma because the individual is getting behavioral health concerns met in a medical setting rather than in a mental health setting.

TriWest Healthcare Alliance collaborated with the Hawaii Multi-Service Medical Management Office at Tripler Army Medical Center and CareIntegra to implement an integrated care demonstration project. The purpose of the Hawaii Integrated Care Demonstration Project was to test the feasibility and effectiveness of employing an integrated care model within MTFs (Chaffee & O'Donohue, 2007). After identifying a feasible funding mechanism to support the initiative, the project successfully hired, trained, and placed five integrated care clinicians in four MTFs throughout Oahu. Following implementation in 2006, the project quickly demonstrated favorable outcomes, including

- Increased access to behavioral health services
- Increased physician efficiency and leveraged physician capacity
- Improved access to effective care
- High patient and provider satisfaction
- High referral completion and feedback to referring physicians

These findings and the reduction of stigma when behavioral health services are accessible in primary care are strong arguments for broader implementation of integrated care delivery models in military medical settings.

CONCLUSION

The innovations in the TRICARE Behavioral Health Program in the first decade of the twenty-first century have been system-wide initiatives to expand access to behavioral health services to support the challenges ADSMs and ADFMs face in coping with deployments to OEF and OIF. The conflicts in Iraq and Afghanistan catapulted behavioral health issues into prominence for their beneficial or deleterious contributions to fitness for duty and the performance of active-duty service members. These fitness-for-duty and performance concerns led armed forces leadership to focus on how service members and their families manage stress (i.e., their capacity for adaptive coping or "resiliency") and to ensure their access to information and resources when they need additional help. This train of thought and focus may be the most significant innovation of all.

REFERENCES

American Association of Suicidology. (2006). Suicide in the U.S.A. Based on current (2006) Statistics. Retrieved February 15, 2010, from http://www.suicidology.org/c/document_library/get_file?folderId=232&name=DLFE-159.pdf

American Telemedicine Association. (November 2007). *Core standards for telemedicine operations*. Washington, DC.

American Telemedicine Association. (October 2009). *Practice guidelines for videoconferencing-based telemental health*. Washington, DC.

Army developing master resiliency training. (August 5, 2009). Retrieved April 16, 2010, from http://www.army.mil/-news/2009/08/05/25494-army-developing-master-resiliency-training/

Centers for Medicare and Medicaid Services (CMS) Web site: http://www.cms.hhs.gov/Telemedicine

Chaffee, R. B., & O'Donohue, W. (2007). *The TriWest Hawaii integrated care pilot project: Executive summary and final report*. Unpublished manuscript.

Chandra, A., Lara-Sinisomo, S., Jaycox, L. H., Tanielian, T., Burns, R. M., Ruder, T., & Han, B. (2009). Children on the home front: The experience of children from military families. *Pediatrics, 125*(1), 13–22.

Defenselink Casualty Report 2010. Retrieved April 15, 2010, from http://www.defenselink.gov/news/casualty.pdf

Egede, L. E., Frueh, C. B., Richardson, L. K., Acierno, R., Mauldin, P. D., Knapp, R. G., & Lejuez, C. (2009, April 20). Rationale and design: Telepsychology service delivery for depressed elderly veterans. Retrieved February 15, 2010, from http://www.trialsjournal.com/content/10/1/22

Federal Health Institute Newsletter. (2009, January 30). Retrieved February 17, 2009, from http://www.fedhealthinst.org/newsletter.html

Hoge, C. W., Auchterlonie, J. L., & Milliken, C. S. (2006). Mental health problems, use of mental health services, and attrition from military service after returning from deployment to Iraq and Afghanistan. *Journal of the American Medical Association, 295*(9), 1023–1032.

Hoge, C. W., Castro, C. A., Messer, S. C., McGurk, D., Cotting, D. I., & Koffman, R. L. (2004). Combat duty in Iraq and Afghanistan, mental health problems, and barriers to care. *New England Journal of Medicine, 351,* 13–22.

Hoge, C. W., Toboni, H. E., Messer, S. C., Bell, N., Amoroso, P., & Orman, D. T. (2005). The occupational burden of mental disorders in the U.S. military: Psychiatric hospitalizations, involuntary separations, and disability. *American Journal of Psychiatry, 162*(3), 585–591.

Holloway, M. G. (2008, September). Assessment and treatment of suicide behavior. Presented at the TRICARE Provider Education Conference, San Diego, CA.

Institute of Medicine. (2010). Returning home from Iraq and Afghanistan: Preliminary assessment of readjustment needs of veterans, service members, and their families. Washington, DC: The National Academies Press.

Jelinek, P. (2009, January 30). Officials: Army suicides at 3-decade high. *Army Times.* Retrieved January 30, 2009, from http://www.armytimes.com/news/2009/01/1p_army_suicides_012909/

Kessler, R. C., Borges, G., & Walters, E. E. (1999). Prevalence of and risk factors for lifetime suicide attempts in the National Comorbidity Survey. *Archives of General Psychiatry, 56,* 617–626.

Koffman, R. L. (2002). *Management of combat stress reactions in the expeditionary operational forces: An assessment of deficiencies and capabilities.* Unpublished manuscript.

McMichael, W. H. (2009, February 11). DoD leaders seek clues to Army suicide spike. *Army Times.* Retrieved February 17, 2009, from http://www.armytimes.com/news/2009/02/military_armysuicides_021109w/

Office of the Surgeon General U.S. Army Medical Command. (2008a). Mental Health Advisory Team (MHAT) IV.

Office of the Surgeon General U.S. Army Medical Command. (2008b). Mental Health Advisory Team (MHAT) V.

Powers, R. (2008, September 7). The cost of war. Retrieved April 15, 2010, from About.com. (U.S. Military) http://usmilitary.about.com/od/terrorism/a/iraqdeath1000.htm?p=1

Rand Center for Military Policy Research. (2008). Invisible wounds: Mental health and cognitive care needs of America's returning veterans.

Sundararaman, R., Panangala, S. V., & Lister, S. A. (2008). CRS report for Congress: Suicide prevention among veterans. Washington, DC: Congressional Research Service, Domestic Social Policy Division, Order code RL34471.

TRICARE Management Activity (TMA) Web site. TRICARE and national health reform. Retrieved April 15, 2010, from the: http://www.tricare.mil

Wikipedia. http://en.wikipedia.org/wiki/Psychological_resilience

Nineteen

Biofeedback

JAMES LAWRENCE THOMAS

INTRODUCTION

Biofeedback is a method of treatment in which the patients are trained to control their own physiological variables in order to improve physical and psychological health. For example, a patient who is trained to control his or her temperature can help such diverse disorders as headaches, hypertension, anxiety, and tinnitus, as well as enhance general relaxation.

The use of biofeedback covers a wide span of medical disorders, as indicated later in the chapter. In this chapter, I will try to stay away from detailed explanations of physiological and medical terms; I will also stay away from the technical aspects of biofeedback. The equipment and software are usually complex, and there are several equipment systems, each one challenging to learn. A great deal of training is necessary to learn any given system, and the costs incurred for all of this are substantial. I see this chapter as an introduction to biofeedback and, if I succeed in getting across some major concepts with illustrations as to its utility, my goal will have been reached.

Because of this focus, I have also included a short list of important texts in the field, the major professional organizations, use of CPT (current procedural terminology) codes in billing insurance, major manufacturers of biofeedback equipment, and a table of biofeedback modalities and their use with medical and psychological disorders with ratings of their efficacy. These are provided so that if the reader is interested in pursuing this fascinating area of treating others, these resources will be at hand.

Some commonly used methods of biofeedback include temperature training, skin conductance (also known as galvanic skin response), respiration, heart rate variability, electromyography, and electroencephalography biofeedback. Each one will be briefly explained and then how they are used for different disorders will be discussed. If patients can learn to control their own physiology to the extent that their health improves, it follows that the use of medical care will be less than for similar patients not employing these methods.

Some common medical disorders can be successfully treated with biofeedback. Hypertension, migraine and tension headaches, chronic pain, attention deficit disorder, epilepsy, anxiety, children's stomach pain, and temporomandibular joint disorders (TMDs) are all rated as having "efficacious" levels of research to support their use in clinical work. This rating follows the Chambless and Hollon (1998) recommendations, updated for biofeedback by the two professional organizations Association for Applied Psychophysiology and Biofeedback (AAPB) and International Society for Neurofeedback and Research (ISNR) (Moss & Gunkelman, 2002). Biofeedback can save resources in healthcare and is underutilized, especially considering that an overall goal of biofeedback is giving patients control over their own physiology so that their health can be improved.

I would first like to explain some of the different modalities or methods of biofeedback so that as they are mentioned, there might be a rough idea as to what is going on in the treatment. In all cases, electronic instruments are used to measure the physiology of the patient, and this information is fed back in some sort of display, typically a computer display. Sometimes the display is only auditory, and at other times the display can be complex visual animations with sound. Some displays employ the ability to watch a movie, as in the hemoencephalography (HEG) system.

BIOFEEDBACK EQUIPMENT

The current equipment in the field of biofeedback is very sophisticated and, combined with modern and powerful computers, things can be done that were not available even 5 years ago. The major manufacturers are noted in the appendix at the end of this chapter; the most well known are Thought Technology, J & J Engineering, and Nexus. Biofeedback systems cost from $1,500 to $10,000 and can do all the modalities described in the following sections. One can also measure and provide biofeedback in several modalities at once, as well as customize the software to meet the needs of the situation and the patient. However, the software is very complex and takes substantial training and practice to learn.

COMMON MODALITIES USED IN BIOFEEDBACK

I have listed the major biofeedback modalities in the following sections. These are explained in isolation so that, as they are mentioned with regard to treatment of disorders, the reader might have a rough sense of the procedure.

Electromyography Biofeedback

EMG uses a surface electrode to measure muscle tension; by displaying this information, patients can see directly their muscle tension on a display and learn how to reduce the tension. In most systems, the resolution is one microvolt or better, which is one millionth of a volt. This very small amount of electricity indicates more muscle tension with more microvolts. By learning to relax one's own musculature, physical tension can be brought under control. This can be especially helpful for those suffering with tension headaches or any disorder in which muscle tension release would be helpful (e.g., arthritis).

Temperature Training

This training can be very useful for general relaxation, hypertension, headaches, and tinnitus. The sensor is sometimes called a "thermistor" and can measure temperature to a very fine degree. This is taped to the skin, usually on one of the fingers. A display shows how the temperature changes. A lower temperature usually indicates anxiety, while higher temperature correlates with being relaxed. The patient is trained to increase the temperature by imagining the hand getting warmer; by various autogenic phrases, such as "My hand is getting warm and heavy"; or by visualizing himself or herself on a pleasantly warm beach.

The patient is asked to practice such exercises at home, sometimes with a small handheld temperature device that can be purchased in an electronics store. The goal can be to get to 95° for 10 minutes in a row; a patient may have to practice every day, twice per day, for a number of weeks before achieving this on a regular basis. Temperature training has been used successfully with hypertension, Raynaud's disease, migraines, and anxiety. As with many biofeedback techniques, temperature training is often combined with other modalities.

Skin Conductance

Biofeedback measures the electricity emitted from the skin. This is accomplished by putting two sensors on the skin (often two fingers separated by one finger). This is also known as galvanic skin response (GSR) or electrodermal activity (EDA). This electrical activity is produced by sweat from the skin and is correlated with relaxation as this measure goes down and with anxiety as the measure goes up. If a practitioner mentions something stressful, for example, this very sensitive measure of emotion will register, providing a measure of stress or emotional reactivity. Learning to calm one's skin conductance in the context of some stressful suggestion can result in relaxation and desensitization.

Heart Rate Variability

In HRV training, the measure is the variability of the heart rate, which in healthy people varies as much as 10 beats from the lowest (often on the exhale) to the highest (often as one inhales). Experts in HRV training assert that, by learning to coordinate one's respiration with the heart rate variability, a physiological coherence is attained that can be very therapeutic (Lehrer, 2007). (A previous conceptualization was termed respiratory sinus arrhythmia, or RSA.) A simple sensor is attached to a finger or an ear lobe; this measures the pulse and a display shows the heart rate. For young people, a display of an animation is sometimes used. By employing relaxed breathing and coordinating this with the HRV, a calmness can result and produce an autonomic balance of the parasympathetic and sympathetic nervous systems. In many disorders, including cardiac conditions, hypertension, anxiety, and any disorder that involves chronic maladjustment of the autonomic nervous system, this kind of training can be helpful.

Respiration

The patient is trained to control his or her breathing. This can be very helpful for pulmonary diseases and is often utilized with heart rate variability training (noted previously). This will not be discussed in detail; more information can be found in the text *Biofeedback* by Schwartz and Andrasik (2003).

EEG Biofeedback

This is also known as neurofeedback or neurotherapy. It is when patients are trained to control their own brain waves, or what is called the EEG (electroencephalograph). The patient often obtains a quantitative EEG in order to identify where the brain waves need to be trained or changed. The electrode is then placed in one or more areas, and the patient is displayed a feedback so that the dysfunctional frequencies are trained down and the "good" waves are trained up. The display can be the brain waves themselves (good for some patients) or a display generated by the computer. The patient is asked to keep the animation going (for example) and, by operant conditioning, the patient trains his or her brain waves to be more normal.

Neurofeedback is considerably more complex than most other biofeedback modalities and is the newest modality in the field of biofeedback. Nonetheless, there is a fair amount of research regarding its effectiveness (see Monastra, 2005; Thompson & Thompson, 2003; Yucha & Montgomery, 2008). Neurofeedback has been shown to be effective for attention deficit disorder, chronic pain, traumatic brain injury, and other brain disorders (Yucha & Montgomery, 2008). Frank Duffy, a well-known neurologist, stated in a special issue of the journal *Clinical Electroencephalography* devoted to neurofeedback, "If any medication had demonstrated such a wide spectrum of efficacy, it would be universally accepted and widely used" (2000, p. v).

Hemoencephalography

HEG biofeedback trains the patient to control the cerebral blood flow in the frontal lobes. An infrared camera sensor is placed on the forehead and reads the cerebral blood flow (actually, a close correlate of the blood flow), and the patient learns to control the blood flow by watching the display. In the case of the passive infrared (pIR) HEG, the display is a movie—any DVD that the patient wishes to see. If the frontal lobe blood flow remains high, the patient can continue to watch the movie. When the temperature drops (believed to be in the anterior cingulate gyrus), then the movie stops; by focusing on a bar graph display, the patient can increase the cortical activity such that the movie starts again.

Other methods of biofeedback include capnometer, which measures the CO_2 from the breath, and pelvic floor EMG rehabilitation, an effective treatment for pelvic floor training for female urinary incontinence and vulvodynia (Glazer, 2000; Glazer & Laine, 2006). This latter method of biofeedback has proven so successful that Medicare pays for this treatment.

Sessions of biofeedback are usually once per week for several weeks and can even extend to a few months. The patient is expected to practice the exercises given in the sessions. Neurofeedback, however, can extend for 40–100 sessions or more for some difficult cases of brain dysfunction, and the number of sessions is usually two to three per week.

Details of these instruments and their electronics can be found in biofeedback textbooks (e.g., Schwartz & Andrasik, 2003; Thompson & Thompson, 2003). As might be expected, a great deal of technical knowledge goes into these methods of treatment. References for the use of biofeedback with many disorders can be found in these textbooks as well as in Yucha and Montgomery's *Evidence-Based Practice in Biofeedback and Neurofeedback* (2008).

There are some general aspects of biofeedback treatment that are important to keep in mind. The first is that a goal of biofeedback is to train the patients to practice the exercises on their own, to develop their ability to regulate their own physiology in the service of improving their health. This aspect alone can result in reduced medical costs and medication. Because a person learns skills that can be applied for a lifetime, the long-term effects of self-regulation therapies can result in a continuing reduction in medical costs.

Another aspect of biofeedback treatment is that the practitioner often uses several modalities to help the patient. Thus, temperature training, relaxation, and heart rate variability training might all be used to help the sufferer of migraines in addition to using HEG biofeedback (see later discussion). This kind of multimodality is also found in much of biofeedback research. Often, experimental groups consist of one group with a few components of treatment and another group with the added treatment being investigated (in addition to a wait list control group and/or medication).

This highlights the fact that biofeedback is an important component of behavioral medicine considered in the broadest sense. Indeed, many studies in biofeedback place it under the overall rubric of behavioral treatments or behavioral medicine. The special contribution of biofeedback is that it feeds back to patients important information about their own physiology so that they have the option to control their symptoms. This is done in a way that is precise beyond our usual capabilities. For example, a patient is able to control muscle to the extent of 1/10 of a microvolt—one ten-millionth of a volt. Currently, almost all biofeedback equipment has this degree of resolution. Controlling this level of muscle tension has also been one aspect of why Olympic athletes attribute some of their success to training with biofeedback instruments.

A final aspect of biofeedback is worth mentioning. In dealing with patients learning to control their physiological behavior, being psychologically minded is not necessary. Indeed, one is able to control one's own physiology without having any psychological insights. For some patients, this could be a very attractive aspect. It could be especially important in treating those with limited language abilities with respect to the therapist or uncomfortable with the usual psychological treatment situation, such as those with combat- and trauma-related disorders.

MEDICAL DISORDERS HELPED BY BIOFEEDBACK

The brief descriptions of medical disorders and their treatments that follow are selected from a larger list of disorders known to be amenable to biofeedback and related behavioral interventions. As research and the technological capabilities improve over the coming decades, we can expect more treatments that involve people learning to control their own physiology. This will reduce the utilization of healthcare services and reduce the medical costs overall. Much of the research noted in the following sections has a tentative quality to it. Strict randomized placebo controlled studies are rare; however, because there is so much promise, we can expect more rigorous studies to appear in these areas. Finally, in a chapter like this one, only the briefest review of the literature concerning these areas can be done; more extensive resources can be consulted, such as the annotated bibliography of biofeedback texts found in the appendix at the end of the chapter.

Hypertension

This disorder is one of the most common and vexing medical disorders in the Western world. Untreated hypertension (HT) is a contributing factor in premature death from stroke, kidney disease, and heart attack; elevated blood pressure affects some 50 million people in this country (Burt et al., 1995). Increased blood pressure (BP) risk factors include increasing age, diabetes, obesity, lifestyle factors such as alcohol use, lack of exercise, high-sodium diet, and chronic psychological stress (McGrady & Linden, 2003). There are significant gender and ethnic differences as well: Men have higher BP than women, and African Americans have higher BP than Caucasians.

The explanation of the physiology of BP can be found in the book *Biofeedback* (Schwartz & Andrasik, 2003, p. 383 ff); it is too complex to review here. Briefly, baroreceptors (BR), located in the heart and its arterial walls, are sensitive to stretching, which is a major factor in elevated BP. These send messages to the medulla of the brain (which itself is a feedback loop). This is an important system because the BR can influence the hypertension within 5–10 seconds (see Schwartz & Andrasik, 2003, p. 383). What this means in terms of biofeedback is that training the person's behavior and including the brain in such training can positively influence HT.

The Joint National Committee (JNC, 1997) meets every few years to classify the levels of HT as follows (for systolic BP):

Less than 130 is normal.
From 130 to 139 is high normal.
Over 140 is hypertension (HT), with the following categorizations: 140–159 = Stage 1; 160–179 = Stage 2; 180–209 = Stage 3; ≥210 = Stage 4.

Over a decade ago, the 130 level would have been considered normal, but all too often the level of >130 has warranted attention because of the prospect of future disease (JNC, 1997).

Although biofeedback has been known to be effective in lowering BP for several decades, it seems to play a minor role in the medical treatment of cardiovascular disorders. Several meta-analytic studies have been done showing the effectiveness of biofeedback and other behavioral treatments. The review by Yucha and her colleagues (2001) revealed that both biofeedback and other active behavioral interventions resulted in lower systolic blood pressure (SBP) and/or diastolic blood pressure (DBP), with all treatments equally effective compared to no-treatment controls. The average reduction was modest but meaningful (6.7 mmHg for SBP and 4.8 mmHg for DBP; Yucha et al., 2001). Another meta-analysis by Nakao, Yano, Nomura, and Kuboki (2003) supported this conclusion; they reviewed 22 randomized controlled studies in which they found that biofeedback reduced DBP by 7.3 mmHg and DBP by 5.8 mmHg. Again, these results were equal to those of other behavioral treatments.

Lifestyle modification is commonly included in most biofeedback treatment; a good example of this is the treatment of HT. The JNC (1997) recommends the following for such patients:

Lose weight if overweight.
Limit alcohol to once per day (8 oz wine, 24 oz beer, or 2 oz liquor).
Exercise aerobically on a regular basis.
Reduce sodium intake to less than 100 mmol per day (<6 g of salt).
Do not smoke.
Reduce dietary saturated fat and cholesterol intake.
Maintain adequate dietary potassium, calcium, and magnesium intake.

Explaining the rationale for each component of a lifestyle change can be helpful in gaining cooperation of the patient. For example, it could be explained that increased sodium causes retention of water and thereby increases BP because of the increased fluid in the body. Aggressive treatment of high BP decreases the incidence of morbidity and mortality from cardiovascular events (McGrady & Linden, 2003). The preceding lifestyle recommendations are often considered an integral part of the office practice of biofeedback, and the ones noted for hypertension could apply to many disorders.

Biofeedback is considered one component of many possible biobehavioral interventions. Early studies reported the effectiveness in biofeedback alone or combined with other relaxation treatments in lowering BP in those with hypertension (Benson, Shapiro, Tulsky, & Schwartz, 1971; McGrady, Yonker, Tan, Fine, & Woerner, 1981; Patel, 1973; Weaver & McGrady, 1995). What predicts whether a patient will be successful with biofeedback treatment for hypertension? Higher neurogenic tone (Cottier, Shapiro, & Julius, 1984) and higher anxiety, forehead muscle tension, and cortisol levels have been reported (McGrady, Utz, Woerner, Bernal, & Higgins, 1986).

An important issue in hypertension treatment research is how high the BP is when treatment is started. For example, subjects who enter an hypertension study with very high BP can be expected to show a more dramatic drop in blood pressure with treatment, thereby distorting the percentage of success in the study. Still, biofeedback has been found to be helpful at all levels of hypertension (Linden & Chambers, 1994; Linden & Moseley, 2006).

Migraines and Tension Headaches

Biofeedback treatment for migraines and other kinds of headaches has been known to be helpful for several decades. In a

2002 review, Penzien, Rains, and Andrasik noted that even by 1980 there were enough studies to conduct a meta-analysis (Blanchard, Andrasik, Ahles, Teders, & O'Keefe, 1980). This revealed that over the 16 studies, behavioral treatment of migraines showed promise. By 1999, Goslin and colleagues had identified 355 articles describing behavioral and physical treatment for migraines, and the 70 controlled studies of behavioral treatments for migraines meeting strict criteria for inclusion in this meta-analysis resulted in reductions in migraines of 32–49%. The treatments included EMG training, relaxation therapy, combined EMG and relaxation, and cognitive-behavioral therapy. All were more effective than wait list controls.

Neurofeedback has also been used to treat migraine headaches. Although it is quite new, this research is promising (Siniatchkin et al., 2000).

In a new kind of biofeedback treatment called hemoencephalography (HEG), the patient learns to train the frontal lobe cerebral blood flow. As described earlier, an infrared camera reads the temperature of the blood flow of the frontal lobe beneath the skull. If the patient keeps the temperature above the threshold level, the movie continues to play. If the temperature drops in the frontal lobe, then the movie stops. By focusing on a bar graph, the patient can bring up the temperature and the movie continues. This biofeedback system was originally designed for migraine headache treatment and has shown promising results. Carmen (2004) took 100 migraine patients who had been through many previous treatments, including many trying several medications, with little success. Positive results were usually seen in six HEG sessions, and over 90% of the patients reported significantly positive results, according to their own report. Although much more research needs to be done with this method, such dramatic results are promising.

Chronic Pain

The term "chronic pain" covers a vast area, from very specific sites of pain to more global pain experienced by the patient all over the body. More than one third of the population experiences chronic pain in their lives at some noticeable level (Bonica, 1992). Biofeedback has been found to help at both levels of chronic pain; some techniques are understood to influence the whole physiology and some methods are more focused on the parameters of the particular disorder.

Flor and Birbaumer (1993) reported that in treating back pain and temporomandibular joint pain, both with biofeedback and relaxation therapy, biofeedback had the greatest positive effect on several aspects of pain and the effects lasted at a 24-month follow-up. Stinson (2003) reviewed 18 randomized, controlled studies in a meta-analysis (from Eccleston et al., 2002), and patients in the treatment groups had a greater than 50% reduction in pain compared to the controls.

In a study by Qi and Ng (2007), two treatment groups were created for patellofemoral pain patients. One used exercise only and one had exercise plus biofeedback. After the 8-week home program, the biofeedback group had significantly reduced pain.

In a study involving pain patients wearing an ambulatory monitor for 4 weeks (Voerman, Vollenbroek-Hutten, & Hermens, 2006), measures of muscle activation and relaxation were recorded, and feedback was provided when relaxation was less than it should be. Pain in the neck, shoulders, and upper back, as well as activation patterns in typing, rest, and stress tasks, was measured. The intensity of the pain reduced after the training.

Lebovits (2007) summarized a comprehensive review by the National Institutes of Health Technology of several behavioral approaches. The overall conclusion was that specific relaxation methods (including relaxation training, biofeedback, hypnosis, meditation, and guided imagery) had the highest rating for effectiveness.

As noted before, it is hard to tease out the exact contribution of biofeedback in many of these studies because there are often combined treatment modalities in many of the experimental conditions.

There are significant limitations in much of the medical treatment of chronic pain, according to Singh (2005), who states that "the therapeutic response of pharmacology in chronic pain at the present time remains unsatisfactory at best and refractory at the worst. Multidisciplinary pain management has not only brought new hope, but has also increased the therapeutic response in general." The references cited in this chapter and in this section in particular should give an indication that behavioral methods should be included in the medical treatment of chronic pain.

Epilepsy

Neurofeedback was discovered as a treatment for epilepsy in the late 1960s by Barry Sterman, a UCLA physiological psychologist. He was asked to determine why fighter pilots sometimes went into seizures while flying their planes, and he discovered that a chemical in the jet fuel (hydrazine) triggered the seizures. In working on this project, he tried to induce seizures into some cats he had in his lab; some cats went into seizures but others did not. He learned that the cats that did not go into seizures (when they should have) were ones that had been trained previously to increase certain brain waves in previous experiments. Sterman concluded that the place and frequency at which he had trained the cats (12–15 Hz at C4) seemed to be protective of seizures. His continued work eventually led to working with people, helping many to eliminate seizures in their life. The scientific details, theory, and references of this work can be found in other sources (Sterman & Egner, 2006; Sterman, 2000; Thompson & Thompson, 2003). Neurofeedback continues to be a viable method of treatment for epilepsy (Monastra, 2003; Yucha & Montgomery, 2008).

Temporomandibular Disorder

Temporomandibular joint disorders (TMJDs), commonly called TMDs or TMJs, are a collection of poorly understood conditions characterized by pain in the jaw and surrounding tissues accompanied by limitations in jaw movements. Injury and conditions that routinely affect other joints in the body, such as arthritis, also affect the temporomandibular joint. Approximately 35 million people in the United States suffer from TMD. While both men and women experience TMD, the majority of those seeking treatment are women in their childbearing years.

Used alone, biofeedback can improve pain, pain-related disability, and mandibular functioning (Gardea, Gatchel, & Mishra, 2001). A meta-analysis of 13 studies of EMG biofeedback treatment showed biofeedback was superior to no treatment or psychological placebo control for patient pain reports, clinical exam findings, and/or ratings of global improvement (Crider & Glaros, 1999).

In a recent review of the literature, Crider, Glaros, and Gevirtz (2005) reported on 14 controlled and uncontrolled outcome evaluations of biofeedback-based treatments for TMD published since 1978. The authors concluded that surface electromyographic (SEMG) training of the masticatory muscles combined with adjunctive cognitive-behavioral therapy (CBT) techniques is an efficacious treatment for TMD. Myers (2007) reported on a systematic review of TMD treatments and, based on a collection of previously reviewed studies and yet to be reviewed studies, concluded that biofeedback has been shown to be consistently superior to placebo or no-treatment controls. The texts *Biofeedback* (Schwartz & Andrasik, 2003) and *Mind–Body Medicine for Primary Care* (Moss, McGrady, Davies, & Wickramasekera, 2003) can give a more detailed review and explanation of treating these disorders.

Traumatic Brain Injury

Traumatic brain injury (TBI) can result in problems of cognition, behavior, emotional sensitivity, and attention. Patients can frequently become much more impulsive, appear to have poor judgment, have memory and word-finding problems, and often not be very aware of their problems. Planning and organizing can also be significant deficits (Varney & Roberts, 1999). There are some two million brain injuries every year in the United States, and while most people appear to recover completely, a substantial minority—up to 50%—can have enduring symptoms 6 months or more after the injury (Jacobson, 1995).

The vast majority of brain injuries are mild cases. By definition, mild TBI means a loss of consciousness of less than 20 minutes, with a posttraumatic amnesia (PTA) of less than 24 hours. Posttraumatic amnesia is defined as the period of time from the accident until there is reliable and consistent memory. Brain injuries with longer durations of these variables are considered to be moderate or severe.

Neurofeedback is the biofeedback modality most commonly used to treat traumatic brain injury. It is almost always the case that mild TBI is the level seen by the private practitioner; severe cases of brain injury are usually not treated with neurofeedback, although there are exceptions (Larsen, 2009).

Thatcher (1999, 2000) advocates obtaining a quantitative electroencephalograph (QEEG) in order to determine which of the 2,500 variables to focus on with respect to the neurofeedback. When the problematic sites are determined, these variables become the focus of targeted treatment. The QEEG then can be a means of scientifically noting progress in the TBI patient.

One interesting form of neurofeedback is called the low energy neurofeedback system, or LENS, which tracks the dominant brain wave frequency of the site where the electrode is placed and delivers a tiny electromagnetic pulse to the brain at a prescribed difference from that dominant frequency (Larsen,

2006, 2009; Schoenberger, Shiflett, Esty, Ochs, & Matheis, 2001). This method results in the brain responding to the tiny stimulus, and the brain physiology appears to move toward a healthier homeostasis, sometimes with dramatic results (Larsen, 2006).

Attention Deficit Disorder

Neurofeedback is the primary modality for treating attention deficit disorder (ADD) with regard to biofeedback. A large number of studies can be found in review articles by Monastra (2005) and in Yucha and Montgomery (2008). The early term of EEG biofeedback has been updated to be called neurofeedback in most publications. A variety of protocols have been used over the last three decades, so it is hard to summarize them in a brief review. The overall trend is to train the patient to lower the slow waves (especially theta) and increase the fast waves (beta) in the frontal regions of the brain (i.e., the frontal lobes).

Joel Lubar and his colleagues did the earliest studies (Lubar & Shouse, 1976, 1977) and showed that, in training down the slow activity and training up the beta or faster brain activity, behaviors improved in the ADD children. Lubar followed 52 patients over 10 years, and the gains were maintained over time. In another study (Linden, Habib, & Radojevic, 1996), the children with attention deficit disorder who received neurofeedback showed better control over their attentiveness and a full scale IQ gain of 10 points, while the control groups showed no gains. In a large study by Kaiser and Othmer (2000), significant improvements were found on the TOVA continuous performance test, as well as gains of 10 points in verbal and performance IQs.

A randomized, placebo, control group study done by Levesque, Beauregard, and Mensour (2006) showed that, with neurofeedback training, the experimental group of ADD children improved on neuropsychological measures as well as pre- and post-fMRI measures of the anterior cingulate cortex, indicating that functional neuroanatomical changes occur with neurofeedback training.

Neurofeedback as a treatment model has expanded into Asian countries. In a study by Zhang, Zhang, and Jin (2006), ADD children were randomly assigned to a medication group (methylphenidate) or EEG biofeedback. They were rated pre- and posttreatment, and at 1-, 3-, and 6-month intervals. The EEG group showed substantially improved scores on the Conners parent rating scale and at 6-month follow-up. In a study by Zhong-Gui, Hai-Qing, and Shu-Hua (2006), those children who did EEG biofeedback training showed significant improvements on the TOVA continuous performance test after 40 sessions.

Many more studies of improved functioning in ADD can be found in other references (Lubar, 2003; Monastra, 2003; Carmody, Radvanski, Wadhwani, Sabo, and Vergara, 2001; Thompson & Thompson, 1998; Rossiter & LaVaque, 1995; Rossiter, 2004; Yucha & Montgomery, 2008); and it has been shown that the positive results remain long after treatment has been completed (Lubar, 2003; Monastra, 2003; Yucha & Montgomery, 2008). Yucha and Montgomery (2008) concluded that the use of neurofeedback is strongly supported in the treatment of ADD, despite the fact that treatment protocols vary widely. In addition, several studies have shown that the treatment effects last over time.

Anxiety

Anxiety is one of the most frequently observed categories of emotional disorders in the American population and often seriously interferes with the quality of everyday life. All of the anxiety disorders are defined by the dual characteristics of physiologic hyperarousal and excessive emotional fear. A variety of modalities have been used in treating anxiety, including GSR, temperature training, EMG, and neurofeedback (Yucha & Montgomery, 2008).

Biofeedback is one of the most useful adjuncts in treating the physiologic hyperarousal, both episodic and chronic, seen in anxiety disorders. Biofeedback has demonstrated value for hyperarousal reduction training in generalized anxiety disorder (GAD) and exposure desensitization in panic disorder (PD) and PTSD (Goodwin & Montgomery, 2006; Rice, Blanchard, & Purcell, 1993; Sarkar, Rathee, & Neera, 1999; Vanathy, Sharma, & Kumar, 1998). In the Rice et al. study (1993), the group who used the alpha increase neurofeedback condition experienced reduced heart rate reactivity to stressors, an unexpected benefit.

In a two-treatment group comparison study ($n = 50$) of anxiety in individuals with chronic pain, Corrado, Gottlieb, and Abdelhamid (2003) reported a significant improvement in anxiety and somatic complaints in the group who received biofeedback of finger temperature training and muscle tension reduction when compared to a pain education group. From a group of 312 high school students in Shanghai, Dong and Bao (2005) recruited 70 students who met criteria for high levels of anxiety and assigned 35 students to a group who were treated with biofeedback and 35 to a group of no-treatment controls. They reported a significant improvement in anxiety, somatization, and depression in the treatment group when compared to the controls. Cory Hammond (2003) used QEEG-guided neurofeedback protocols to help patients with OCD, which resulted in significant improvements.

Several biofeedback modalities are effective for anxiety reduction. Most are found to compare favorably with other behavioral techniques, including relaxation training and cognitive restructuring, and occasionally found to be superior to medication alone. As noted before, the most common biofeedback modality used for anxiety is temperature training; however, evidence indicates that heart rate variability training is also effective (Berger & Gevirtz, 2001; Clark & Hirschman, 1999). For more details using biofeedback for anxiety disorders, see Donald Moss's chapter on anxiety in *Handbook of Mind–Body Medicine for Primary Care* (Moss, 2003).

Functional Abdominal Pain in Children

Functional abdominal pain (FAP) is one of a group of functional gastroenterological disorders (FGDs), which include irritable bowel syndrome (IBS) and functional dyspepsia (FD). FAP has been identified as recurrent episodes of abdominal pain severe enough to interfere with a patient's usual activities but not caused by an identifiable organic disease and unrelated to bowel function (Sanders, Shepherd, Cleghorn, & Woolford, 1994). Minimal criteria for patient inclusion in studies of FAP consist of at least three bouts of pain severe enough to affect activities during a period of not less than 3 months, with episodes occurring in the year preceding the examination (Clouse et al., 2006). FAP affects approximately 10–15% of the pediatric population (Apley & Naish, 1958; Kristjansdottir, 1996; Oster, 1972; Parcel, Nader, & Meyer, 1977). FAP causes disruption of daily activities and missed school days, overutilization of healthcare (Hyams, Burke, Davis, Rzepski, & Andrulonis, 1996), unnecessary surgeries, learning difficulties (DiPalma & DiPalma, 1997), and anxiety (Jansdottir, 1997). There is good evidence to support using behavioral interventions, such as biofeedback, in reducing or eliminating FAP.

Treatment, including temperature and breathing training biofeedback (along with adding fiber to the diet), has been shown to be more effective than adding fiber alone (Humphreys

& Gevirtz, 2000). Investigators have found that after completing six sessions of HRV biofeedback, a sample of children with FAP was able to reduce symptoms significantly in relation to increasing their autonomic nervous system balance significantly (Sowder, Gevirtz, Shapiro, & Ebert, 2010).

Other disorders that can be helped by biofeedback include vulvidynia, stroke, tinnitus, urinary incontinence, insomnia, coronary heart disease, and arthritis. Yucha and Montgomery (2008) and Schwartz and Andrasik (2003) can be consulted regarding these and other disorders for their treatment.

CONCLUDING REMARKS

Given the preceding applications of biofeedback in the treatment of medical and psychological disorders, it is amazing that this expertise is not available in every healthcare office. Although the research is far from definitive with most disorders, there is certainly evidence that such therapeutic work can be beneficial. We owe it to our patients to offer these treatment methods, which may help their health through self-regulation of their own physiology. The result would be improved health and lower medical care costs.

APPENDIX: RESOURCES

Major Manufacturers of Biofeedback Equipment

Thought Technology: www.thoughtechology.com, (800) 361-3651

J & J Engineering: www.jjengineering.com, (888) 550-8300

Nexus www.stens-biofeedback.com, (800) 257-8367

Biofeedback Organizations

The Biofeedback Certification Institute of America (303/420-2902, BCIA@resourcenter.com) organization certifies practitioners on biofeedback (board certified in biofeedback, or BCB) and neurofeedback (BCN). It also publishes some training materials and books.

The Association for Applied Psychophysiology and Biofeedback (AAPB), 10200 W 44th Ave, #304, Wheat Ridge, CO, 80033 (303/422-8436, www.aapb.org. aapb@resourcenter.com), is the principal professional organization for biofeedback.

Important Recommended Texts in Biofeedback With Behavioral Healthcare

Lehrer, P., Woolfolk, R., & Simes, W. (2007). *Principles and practice of stress management.* New York, NY: Guilford. Although this text focuses on stress management, biofeedback is a featured modality of treatment throughout. In addition to biofeedback, methods described include Eastern approaches such as yoga and Qi Gong, music therapy, sports psychophysiology and peak performance, mindfulness, and autogenic training.

Moss, D., McGrady, A., Davies, T., & Wickramasekera, I. (Eds.). (2003). *Handbook of mind–body medicine for primary care.* Thousand Oaks, CA: Sage. This deals with many behavioral and medical disorders, with an emphasis on biofeedback, but also included are acupuncture, hypnotherapy, spirituality and healing, and dealing with associated personnel such as nurses and physician assistants.

Schwartz, M., & Andrasik, F. (2003). *Biofeedback: A practitioner's guide.* New York, NY: Guilford. This is the main text in the field and contains detailed explanations of the equipment, physiology of the disorders most commonly treated, and an extensive review of the literature, as well as ethical and office practices for professionals. It is currently under revision with the fourth edition coming out probably in late 2010 or in 2011.

Thompson, M., & Thompson, L. (2003). *The neurofeedback book.* Wheat Ridge, CO: AAPB. This book is the most thorough text on neurofeedback to date, written by experienced neurofeedback practitioners, a psychologist and psychiatrist, with a detailed background in neuroanatomy and neurophysiology.

Yucha, C., & Montgomery, D. (2008). *Evidence-based practice in biofeedback and neurofeedback.* Wheat Ridge, CO: AAPB. In this short book, disorders are reviewed in which biofeedback and other behavioral interventions are reviewed and rated according to the Chambless and Hollon (1998) level of efficacy. Ratings by these authors do not necessarily agree with others rating the utility of biofeedback (e.g., Schwartz & Andrasik, 2003, p. 107).

CPT Codes Used for Biofeedback

Overall code for biofeedback: 90901. This is for all modalities.

Health psychology interventions (including psychophysiological interventions): 96152. This could also be used for biofeedback, as well as other behavioral interventions. However, 96152 is meant for diagnoses that *do not* have a psychiatric diagnosis. This CPT code was designed for psychologists working with medical disorders.

Feedback Modalities, Treatments, With Level of Efficacy

In Table 19.1, the feedback modality is briefly explained and the associated disorders are noted, with their level of efficacy supported by empirical research as rated by Yucha and Montgomery (2008).

Table 19.1 Feedback Modalities and Disorders Treated

Feedback Modalities	Disorders Treated
Temperature training: The goal is to teach the learner to warm his or her peripheral extremities. In order to raise skin temperature, one must relax skeletal muscles as well as the muscles within the walls of the blood vessels. A thermal sensor, called a thermistor, is taped to the skin, usually on the palmar surface of one of the fingers. The temperature of the skin changes the resistance of the thermistor, thereby altering the electrical signal in proportion to the temperature.	Anxiety,[4] hypertension,[4] chronic pain,[4] Raynaud's disease,[4] arthritis,[3] headache,[3] diabetes mellitus,[3] alcoholism/substance abuse,[3] irritable bowel syndrome,[2] repetitive strain injury[2]
Heart rate variability (HRV): HRV refers to the rise and fall of heart rate synchronized with each breath (faster on the inhale, slower on the exhale). The magnitude of this systematic variability seems to reflect a healthy alternation between two autonomic influences on the heartbeat: sympathetic and parasympathetic. The biofeedback setup involves monitoring heart rate alone or heart rate plus respiration. Heart rate may be detected from plethysmographic sensors on the finger or earlobe or via EKG monitors.	Asthma,[2] chronic obstructive pulmonary disease (COPD),[2] coronary artery disease,[2] depressive disorders,[2] fibromyalgia/chronic fatigue syndrome[2]
Electromyography (EMG): The goal is to provide the learner with enhanced information about his or her muscle tension in a particular area in the hope that this will facilitate learning control of the muscle. Relaxation of excess and inappropriate tension is the usual goal.	Anxiety,[4] chronic pain,[4] hypertension,[4] temporomandibular disorder (TMD),[4] constipation (adults),[4] headache,[3] arthritis,[3] urinary incontinence (females,[5] males,[3] children[2]), fecal incontinence (adults),[3] vulvar vestibulitis (vulvodynia),[3] asthma,[2] Bell's palsy,[2] cerebral palsy,[2] coronary artery disease,[2] stroke (cardiovascular accident),[2] fibromyalgia/chronic fatigue syndrome,[2] hand dystonia,[2] repetitive strain injury,[2] respiratory failure (mechanical ventilation),[2] tinnitus,[2] spinal cord injury,[1] syncope (neurocardiogenic)[1]
Skin conductance training: This provides feedback information about sweat gland activity on the hand, which is closely correlated with sympathetic nervous system activity. Sensors are attached to fingers or two sites on the palm.	Anxiety,[4] epilepsy,[4] hypertension,[4] motion sickness,[4] irritable bowel syndrome,[2] eating disorders[1]

Table 19.1 (*Continued*)   Feedback Modalities and Disorders Treated

Feedback Modalities	Disorders Treated
Neurofeedback: Surface sensors are placed on selected areas of the head and ears. Brain wave changes in the desired direction are rewarded with feedback.	Anxiety,[4] ADHD,[4] epilepsy,[4] traumatic brain injury (TBI),[3] alcoholism/substance abuse,[3] autism,[2] chronic pain,[4] depressive disorders,[2] fibromyalgia/chronic fatigue syndrome,[2] posttraumatic stress disorder (PTSD),[2] tinnitus[2]
Hemoencephalography (HEG): In this method, the patient is trained to increase the frontal cerebral blood flow, which is the area of the brain that manages the brain itself. Although research has yet to be published, this method has been helpful for migraines, attention deficit disorder, and endogenous depression.	Migraines,[2] ADHD, and depression are possible applications

Note: Superscripts indicate the level of efficacy. Level 1: not empirically supported; level 2: possibly efficacious; level 3: probably efficacious; level 4: efficacious; level 5: efficacious and specific. These are rated by Yucha, C., and Montgomery, D. (2008). *Evidence-based practice in biofeedback and neurofeedback.* Wheat Ridge, CO: AAPB.

REFERENCES

Apley, J., & Naish, N. (1958). Recurrent abdominal pains: A field survey of 1,000 school children. *Archives of Disease in Childhood, 33*(168), 165–170.

Benzon, H., Shapiro, D., Tursky, B., & Schwartz, G. (1971). Decreased systolic blood pressure through operant conditioning techniques in patients with essential hypertension. *Science, 173*, 740–741.

Berger, B., & Gevirtz, R. (20001). The treatment of panic disorder: A comparison between breathing retraining and cognitive behavior therapy. *Applied Psychophysiology and Biofeedback, 26*(3), 227–228.

Blanchard, E., Andrasik, F., Ahles, T., Teders, S., & O'Keefe, D. (1980). Migraine and tension-type headache: A meta-analytic review. *Behavior Therapy, 11*, 613–631.

Bonica, J. (1992). Preface. In G. Aronoff (Ed.), *Evaluation and treatment of chronic pain* (2nd ed.) (p. xx). Baltimore, MD: Williams & Williams.

Burt, V., Cutler, J., Higgins, M., Horan, M., Labarthe, D., Whelton, P., et al. (1995). Trends in the prevalence, awareness, treatment, and control of hypertension in the adult US population. *Hypertension, 26*, 60–69.

Carmen, J. (2004). Passive infrared hemoencephalography: Four years and 100 migraines. *Journal of Neurotherapy, 8*(3), 23–51.

Carmody, D., Radvanski, D., Wadhwani, S., Sabo, M., & Vergara, L. (2001). EEG biofeedback training and attention deficit/hyperactivity disorder in an elementary school setting. *Journal of Neurotherapy, 4*(3), 5–27.

Chambless, D., & Hollon, S. (1998). Defining empirically supported therapies. *Journal of Consulting & Clinical Psychology, 66,* 7–18.

Clark, M., & Hirschman, R. (1999). Effects of paced breathing on anxiety reduction in a clinical population. *Biofeedback and Self-Regulation, 15*(3), 273–284.

Clouse, R., Mayer, E., Aziz, Q., Drossman, D., Dumitrascu, D., Monnikes, H., et al. (2006). Functional abdominal pain syndrome. *Gastroenterology, 130*(5), 1492–1497.

Corrado, P., Gottlieb, H., & Abdelhamid, M. (2003). The effect of biofeedback and relaxation training on anxiety and somatic complaints in chronic pain patients. *American Journal of Pain Management, 13*(4), 133–139.

Cottier, C., Shapiro, K., & Julius, S. (1984). Treatment of mild hypertension and emerging treatment considerations. *Archives of Internal Medicine, 144,* 1954–1958.

Crider, A., & Glaros, A. (1999). A meta-analysis of EMG biofeedback treatment of temporomandibular disorders. *Journal of Orofacial Pain, 13*(1), 29–37.

Crider, A., Glaros, A., & Gevirtz, R. (2005). Efficacy of biofeedback-based treatments for temporomandibular disorders. *Applied Psychophysiology and Biofeedback, 30*(4), 333–345.

DiPalma, A., & DiPalma, J. (1997). Recurrent abdominal pain and lactose maldigestion in school-aged children. *Gastroenterology Nursing, 20*(5), 180–183.

Dong, W., & Bao, F. (2005). Effects of biofeedback therapy on the intervention of examination-caused anxiety. *Chinese Journal of Rehabilitation, 9*(32), 17–19.

Duffy, F. (2000). The state of EEG biofeedback therapy (EEG operant conditioning) in 2000: An editor's opinion. *Clinical Electroencephalography, 31*(1), v–vii.

Eccleston, C., Morley, S., Williams, A., et al., (2002). Systematic review of randomized controlled trials of psychological therapy for chronic pain I children and adolescents, with a subset meta-analysis of pain relief. *Pain, 99,* 157–165.

Egner, T., & Sterman, M. B. (2006). Neurofeedback treatment of epilepsy: From basic rationale to practical application. *Expert Review of Neurotherapeutics, 6*(2), 247–257.

Flor, H., & Birbaumer, N. (1993). Comparison of the efficacy of electromyographic biofeedback, cognitive-behavior therapy and conservative medical interventions in the treatment of chronic musculoskeletal pain. *Journal of Consulting and Clinical Psychology, 61*(4), 653–658.

Gardea, M., Gatchel, R., & Mishra, K. (2001). Long-term efficacy of biobehavioral treatment of temporomandibular disorders. *Journal of Behavioral Medicine, 24*(4), 34–59.

Glazer, H. (2000). Dysethetic vulvodynia: Long-term follow-up after treatment with surface electromyography-assisted pelvic floor rehabilitation. *Journal of Reproductive Medicine, 45,* 798–802.

Glazer, H., & Laine, C. (2006). Pelvic floor muscle biofeedback in the treatment of urinary incontinence: A literature review. *Applied Psychophysiology and Biofeedback, 31*(3), 187–201.

Goodwin, E., & Montgomery, D. (2006). A cognitive-behavioral, biofeedback-assisted relaxation treatment for panic disorder with agoraphobia. *Clinical Case Studies, 5*(2), 112–125.

Goslin, R., Gray, R., McCrory, D., Eberlin, K., Tulsky, J., & Hasselblad, V. (1999). *Behavioral and physical treatments for migraine headache* (technical review 2.2). Prepared for the Agency for Health Care Policy and Research under contract no. 290-94-2025 (NTIS accession no. 127946).

Hammond, C. (2003). QEEG-guided neurofeedback in the treatment of obsessive-compulsive disorder. *Journal of Neurotherapy, 7*(2), 25–52.

Humphreys, P. A., & Gevirtz, R. N. (2000). Treatment of recurrent abdominal pain: Components analysis of four treatment protocols. *Journal of Pediatric Gastroenterology and Nutrition, 31*(1), 47–51.

Hyams, J. S., Burke, G., Davis, P. M., Rzepski, B., & Andrulonis, P. A. (1996). Abdominal pain and irritable bowel syndrome in adolescents: A community-based study. *Journal of Pediatrics, 129*(2), 220–226.

Jacobson, R. (1995). The postconcussional syndrome: Physiogenesis, psychogenesis, and malingering: An integrative model. *Journal of Psychosomatic Research, 39,* 675–693.

Jansdottir, G. (1997). The relationship between pains and various discomforts in school children. *Childhood: Global Journal of Child Research, 4,* 491–504.

JNC (Joint National Committee on Detection, Evaluation and Treatment of High Blood Pressure). (1997). The sixth report of the Joint National Committee on Detection, Evaluation and Treatment of High Blood Pressure: JNC VI. *Archives of Internal Medicine, 157,* 2413–2446.

Kaiser, D., & Othmer, S. (2000). Effect of neurofeedback variables of attention in a large multicenter trial. *Journal of Neurotherapy, 4*(3), 5–15.

Kristjansdottir, G. (1996). Sociodemographic differences in the prevalence of self-reported stomach pain in school children. *European Journal of Pediatrics, 155*(11), 981–983.

Larsen, S. (Ed.). (2006). *The healing power of neurofeedback.* Rochester, VT: Healing Arts Press.

Larsen, S. (2009). The special applicability of the low energy neurofeedback system form of neurofeedback to traumatic brain injury: I. The theory. *Biofeedback, 37*(3), 104–107.

Lebovits, A. (2007). Cognitive-behavioral approaches to chronic pain. *Primary Psychiatry, 14*(9), 48–54.

Lehrer, P. (2007). Biofeedback training to increase heart rate variability. In P. Lehrer, R. Woolfolk, & W. Simes (Eds.), *Principles and practice of stress management* (pp. 227–248). New York, NY: Guilford.

Levesque, J., Beauregard, M., & Mensour, B. (2006). Effect of neurofeedback training on the neural substrates of selective attention in children with attention-deficit/hyperactivity disorder: A functional magnetic resonance imaging study. *Neuroscience Letters, 394,* 216–221.

Linden, M., Habib, T., & Radojevic, V. (1996). A controlled study of the effects of EEG biofeedback on cognition and behavior of children with attention deficit disorder and learning disabilities. *Biofeedback and Self-Regulation, 21*(1), 35–49.

Linden, W., & Chambers, L. (1994). Clinical effectiveness of non-drug therapies for hypertension: A meta-analysis. *Annals of Behavioral Medicine, 16,* 35–45.

Linden, W., & Moseley, J. (2006). The efficacy of behavioral treatments for hypertension. *Applied Psychophysiology and Biofeedback, 31*(1), 51–63.

Lubar, J. (2003). Neurofeedback for attention deficit disorders. In M. Schwartz & F. Andrasik (Eds.), *Biofeedback: A practitioner's guide* (3rd ed.) (pp. 409–437). New York, NY: Guilford.

Lubar, J., & Shouse, M. (1976). EEG and behavioral changes in hyperkinetic child concurrent with training of the sensorimotor rhythm (SMR): A preliminary report. *Biofeedback and Self-Regulation, 3,* 293–306.

Lubar, J., & Shouse, M. (1977). Use of biofeedback in the treatment of seizure disorders and hyperactivity. In B. B. Lacey & A. E. Kazdin (Eds.), *Advances in clinical child psychology* (p. 1). New York, NY: Plenum.

McGrady, A., & Linden, W. (2003). Biobehavioral treatment of essential hypertension. In M. Schwartz & F. Andrasik (Eds.), *Biofeedback* (pp. 382–407). New York, NY: Guilford.

McGrady, A., Utz, S., Woerner, M., Bernal, G., & Higgins, J. (1986). Predictors of success in hypertensives treated with biofeedback-assisted relaxation. *Biofeedback and Self-Regulation, 11*(23), 95–103.

McGrady, A., Yonker, R., Tan, S., Fine, T., & Woerner, M. (1981). The effect of biofeedback-assisted relaxation training on blood pressure and selected biochemical parameters in patients with essential hypertension. *Biofeedback and Self-Regulation, 6*(3), 343–353.

Monastra, V. (2003). Clinical applications of EEG biofeedback. In M. Schwartz & F. Andrasik (Eds.), *Biofeedback: A practitioner's guide* (3rd ed.) (pp. 438–463). New York, NY: Guilford.

Monastra, V. (2005). Electroencephalographic biofeedback (neurotherapy) as a treatment for attention deficit hyperactivity disorder: Rationale and empirical foundations. *Child and Adolescent Psychiatric Clinics of North America, 14*(1), 55–82.

Moss, D. (2003). Anxiety. In D. Moss, A. McGrady, T. Davies, & I. Wickramasekera (Eds.), *Handbook of mind–body medicine for primary care* (pp. 359–375). Thousand Oaks, CA: Sage.

Moss, D., & Gunkelman, J. (2002). Task force report on methodology and empirically supported treatments: Introduction and summary. *Applied Psychophysiology and Biofeedback, 27*(4), 261–262.

Myers, C. (2007). Complementary and alternative medicine for persistent facial pain. *Dental Clinics of North America, 51*(1), 263–274.

Nakao, M., Yano, E., Nomura, S., & Kuboki, T. (2003). Blood pressure-lowering effects of biofeedback treatment in hypertension: A meta-analysis of randomized controlled trials. *Hypertension Research, 26*(1), 37–46.

Oster, J. (1972). Recurrent abdominal pain, headache and limb pains in children and adolescents. *Pediatrics, 50*(3), 429–436.

Parcel, G. S., Nader, P. R., & Meyer, M. P. (1977). Adolescent health concerns, problems, and patterns of utilization in a triethnic urban population. *Pediatrics, 60*(2), 157–164.

Patel, C. (1973). Yoga and biofeedback in the management of hypertension. *Lancet, ii,* 1053–1055.

Penzien, D., Rains, J., & Andrasik, F. (2002). Behavioral management of recurrent headache: Three decades of experience and empiricism. *Applied Psychophysiology and Biofeedback, 27*(2), 163–181.

Qi, Z., & Ng, G. (2007). EMG analysis of vastus medialis obliquus/ vastus lateralis activities in subjects with patellofemoral pain syndrome before and after a home exercise program. *Journal of Physical Therapy Science, 19*(2), 131–137.

Rice, K., Blanchard, E., & Purcell, M. (1993). Biofeedback treatments of generalized anxiety disorder: Preliminary results. *Biofeedback & Self-Regulation, 18*(2), 93–105.

Rossiter, T. (2004). The effectiveness of EEG biofeedback and stimulant drugs in treating ADHD. Part II: Replication. *Applied Psychophysiology and Biofeedback, 29*(4), 233–243.

Rossiter, T., & LaVaque, T. (1995). A comparison of EEG biofeedback to psychostimulants in treating attention deficit/ hyperactivity disorders. *Journal of Neurotherapy, 1*(1), 54–63.

Sanders, M., Shepherd, R., Cleghorn, G., & Woolford, H. (1994). The treatment of recurrent abdominal pain in children: A controlled comparison of cognitive-behavioral family intervention and standard pediatric care. *Journal of Consulting and Clinical Psychology, 62*(2), 306–314.

Sarkar, P., Rathee, S., & Neera, N. (1999). Comparative efficacy of pharmacotherapy and biofeedback among cases of generalized anxiety disorder. *Journal of Projective Psychology & Mental Health, 6*(1), 69–77.

Schoenberger, N., Shiflett, S., Esty, M., Ochs, L., & Matheis, R. J. (2001). Flexyx neurotherapy system in the treatment of traumatic brain injury: An initial evaluation. *Journal of Head Trauma Rehabilitation, 16,* 260–274.

Schwartz, M., & Andrasik, F. (Eds.). (2003). *Biofeedback: A practitioner's guide* (3rd ed.). New York, NY: Guilford.

Singh, A. (2005). Multidisciplinary management of chronic pain. *International Medical Journal, 12*(2), 111–116.

Siniatchkin, M., Hicrundar, A., Kropp, P., Khunert, R., Gerber, W., & Staphani, U. (2000). Self-regulation of slow cortical potentials in children with migraine: An exploratory study. *Applied Psychophysiology and Biofeedback, 25,* 13–32.

Sowder, E., Gevirtz, R., Shapiro, W., & Ebert, C. (2010). Restoration of vagal tone: A possible mechanism for functional abdominal pain. *Applied Psychophysiology and Biofeedback, 35*(3), 199–206.

Sterman, M. B. (2000). Basic concepts and clinical findings in the treatment of seizure disorders with EEG operant conditioning. *Clinical Electroencephalography, 31*(1), 45–55.

Sterman, M. B., & Egner, T. (2006). Foundation and practice of neurofeedback therapy for epilepsy. From basic rationale to practical application. *Applied Psychophysiology and Biofeedback, 31*(1), 21–35.

Stinson, J. (2003). Review: Psychological interventions reduce the severity and frequency of chronic pain in children and adolescents. *Evidence-Based Nursing, 6*(2), 45.

Thatcher, R. (1999). EEG database guided neurotherapy. In J. R. Evans & A. Arbarbanel (Eds.), *Introduction to quantitative EEG and neurofeedback.* San Diego, CA: Academic Press.

Thatcher, R. (2000). EEG operant conditioning (biofeedback) and traumatic brain injury. *Clinical Electroencephalography, 31,* 38–44.

Thompson, L., & Thompson, M. (1998). Neurofeedback combined with training in metacognitive strategies: Effectiveness in students with ADD. *Applied Psychophysiology and Biofeedback, 23*(4), 243–263.

Thompson, M., & Thompson, L. (2003). *The neurofeedback book.* Wheat Ridge, CO: AAPB.

Vanathy, S., Sharma, P., & Kumar, K. (1998). The efficacy of alpha and theta neurofeedback training in treatment of generalized anxiety disorder. *Indian Journal of Clinical Psychology, 25*(2), 136–143.

Varney, N., & Roberts, R. (Eds.). (1999). *The evaluation and treatment of mild traumatic brain injury.* Mahwah, NJ: Lawrence Erlbaum Associates.

Voerman, G., Vollenbroek-Hutten, M., & Hermens, H. (2006). Changes in pain, disability, and activation patterns in chronic whiplash patients after ambulant myofeedback training. *The Clinical Journal of Pain, 22*(7), 656–663.

Weaver, M., & McGrady, A. (1995). A provisional model to predict blood pressure response to biofeedback-assisted relaxation. *Biofeedback and Self-Regulation, 20*(3), 229–240.

Yucha, C., Clark, L., Smith, M., Uris, P., Lafleur, B., & Duval, S. (2001). The effect of biofeedback in hypertension. *Applied Nursing Research, 14*(10), 29–35.

Yucha, C., & Montgomery, D. (2008). *Evidence-based practice in biofeedback and neurofeedback.* Wheat Ridge, CO: AAPB.

Zhang, F., Zhang, J., & Jin, X. (2006). Effect of electroencephalogram biofeedback on behavioral problems of children with attention deficit hyperactivity disorder. *Chinese Journal of Clinical Rehabilitation, 10*(10), 74–76.

Zhong-Gui, X., Hai-Qing, X., & Shu-Hua, S. (2006). The controlled study of effectiveness of EEG biofeedback training on children with attention deficit disorder. *Chinese Journal of Clinical Psychology, 14*(2), 207–208.

Index

A

AAPB, *see* Association for Applied Psychophysiology and Biofeedback (AAPB)
AARP, *see* American Association for Retired Persons (AARP)
ABBHP, *see* American Board of Behavioral Healthcare Practice (ABBHP)
Abdominal pain, children, 456–457
Accessibility of research, 189, 191–192
Access issues
  e-health and telehealth, 93–95
  healthcare crisis, 205
  integrated care, 382, 385–386
  language barriers, 381
  reforms, children/family treatment, 351–353
  rural communities, 381
  stigma, 382
  veteran/military behavioral health reforms, 419–424
  women's preventative care, 385–386
Accidents, motor vehicle, 89
Accountability, 261, 286
Accreditation guidelines, 188–189, 193
ACHIEVE (HealthMedia), 409
ACIP, *see* Advisory Committee on Immunization Practices (ACIP)
ACNP, *see* American College of Neuropsychopharmacology (ACNP)
Act, Deming's cycle, 214
Action lists, 216
Active duty service members (ADSM)
  attitudes toward mental illness, 423–424, 430
  nonclinical services, 435
  outpatient mental health services, 433
  posttraumatic stress disorder, 421, 422
  stigma as barrier, 419
  stressors associated with suicide, 427
  telemental health services, expansion, 432–433
  TriCare, 411
Activity, secondary aging, 307
AD, *see* Alzheimer's disease (AD)
ADD, *see* Attention deficit disorder (ADD)
Addiction, 412
ADHD, *see* Attention deficit hyperactivity disorder (ADHD)
Adjunctive services, 90–92
Adolescent Transitions Program (ATP), 395
Adoption, 50, 67–68
ADSM, *see* Active duty service members (ADSM)
"The Advanced Medical Home: A Patient-Centered, Physician-Guided Model of Health Care," 231
Adverse drug events reduction
  growing incidence, 329
  medication first-line treatment/misuse, 332–333
  older adults, 308
Advertising, 335–336

469

Advisory Committee on Immunization Practices (ACIP), 402
Age of Anxiety, 4–5
"Age of depression," 7
Age regression for sexual abuse, 209
Aging in place, service delivery, 314–315
Aging population
  aging in place, 314–315
  behavioral health, 304–309
  dementia, 303–304
  demographic shift, 299–300
  e-health, 313–314
  excess disability, 308–309
  fundamentals, 299
  future directions, 315
  healthcare spending, 300–302
  home-based services, 310
  integrated care, 310–312
  issues, health impact, 307–308
  life-history factors, 304–309
  Medicare, 300–302
  medications, first-line treatment/misuse, 340–341
  physical health, 302–303
  at risk population, 329
  service delivery, 309–315
  stepped care, 312–313
AHLTA, 68–69
AIDS/HIV, 354
AIG, see American International Group (AIG)
Aims, setting, 216
Alcohol, 375, 447
ALS (Amyotrophic lateral sclerosis) disease, 405
Alzheimer's disease (AD), 303–304, 405
American Academy of Family Physicians, 231
American Academy of Pediatrics, 230, 231, 338
American Association for Retired Persons (AARP), 287
American Biodyne, see also Biodyne
  historical developments, 36
  outpatient therapy, 25
  process vs. outcomes, 291–292
  quality assurance, 46
American Board of Behavioral Healthcare Practice (ABBHP), 291
American College of Neuro-psychopharmacology (ACNP), 137
American College of Physicians, 231
American Geriatric Society, 340
American Health Information Management Association, 76
American Indians, see Native American populations
American International Group (AIG), 280
American Journal of Psychotherapy, 38
American Medical Association (AMA), 301
American Osteopathic Association, 231
American Psychiatric Association (APA), 9, 76
American Psychological Association (APA)
  accreditation, 188–189, 260–261
  advocacy efforts, 344
  changes, 262–263
  costs, traditional therapy, 44
  credentials and credentialing, 260, 274
  curricula for training, 238
  education and training, 143, 172, 262–263
  evidence-based practice definition, 184–185, 195–196

Index 471

integrated care importance, 13
irrelevant course curriculum, 259
lack of blueprint, 14
lawsuit costs, 47
licensure, 262
Medicare access issues, 301
overarching problem, 204
process *vs.* outcomes, 290
psychiatry *vs.* psychology, 11
reforms, emerging, 262–263
research planning conference, 160
reticence on statistics, 1
salaries, 288
standards, 172
American Psychological Science (APS), 11
American Recovery and Reinvestment Act (ARRA), 60, 64
American Telemedicine Association (ATA), 433–434
American *vs.* Irish nuns, 28
Ammirati, Rachel, 203–222
Amyotrophic lateral sclerosis (ALS) disease, 405
Analyze, Deming's cycle, 214
Anchoring-and-adjustment heuristic, 175
Anecdotal descriptions, 61–62
Annapolis Coalition, 142, 238
Ann-E Smartphone application, 412
Anonymity, 86, 93
Antibusiness, antihealthcare agenda, 260
Antidepressant medications, *see also* Depression disorders
adolescent statistics, 131
"age of depression," 7
cautions, 139
first-line treatment/misuse, 334–335
religious beliefs, barrier *vs.* facilitation, 372

stepped care, 312–313
usage statistics, 99
Antipsychotic drugs, refilling, data, 67
Anxiety disorders
biofeedback treatment, 442, 455–456
computer-based treatment, 91
implications for untreated, 384
resiliency, 419
temperature training, 443
APA, *see* American Psychiatric Association (APA); American Psychological Association (APA)
Applications, mental health informatics
data complexity, 64–65
data range, 62–64
EHR in decision making, 65–68
exemplary programs, 68–69
APS, *see* American Psychological Science (APS); Association for Psychological Science (APS)
Arbitrary diagnostic thresholds, 154–157
Arizona State University, 258, 263
Aromatherapy, 210
ARRA, *see* American Recovery and Reinvestment Act (ARRA)
Arthritis, 303
Asperger's syndrome, 12
ASPPB, *see* Association of State and Provincial Psychology Boards (ASPPB)
Assessment separation, 162–163
Assisted living costs, 314
Association for Applied Psychophysiology and Biofeedback (AAPB), 442

Association for Behavioral and
    Cognitive Therapies,
    194, 357
Association for Psychological
    Science (APS), 262
Association of State and
    Provincial Psychology
    Boards (ASPPB), 262,
    274
ATA, see American
    Telemedicine
    Association (ATA)
ATP, see Adolescent Transitions
    Program (ATP)
Attention deficit disorder (ADD),
    see also Children
  biofeedback treatment, 442,
    454–455
  medicating children, 337,
    338, 339
Attention deficit hyperactivity
    disorder (ADHD), see
    also Children
  comparative effectiveness
    research, 348
  medicating children, 337,
    338, 339
Attitudes toward mental illness,
    423–424, 430
Australia, access issues, 406
Australian National Survey
    of Mental Health and
    Well-Being, 156
Autism spectrum disorders, 12,
    210
Automation, paper-based office,
    75
Availability heuristic, 175
Avoidance of care, 228
Axis I disorders, 384
Axis II disorders, 6

B

Baby Boomer generation, 106
Back pain, chronic, 100, 445,
    450
"Bad apples approach," 212, 213
Bad attitudes, 423

Barlow designations, 284
Barriers
  delivery of care, 83
  e-health and telehealth,
    92–93, 103–106, 377
  financing integrated care,
    248–249
  fundamentals, 369–371
  geographical remoteness, 90
  self-management programs,
    87
  technology, access to
    services, 376–380
Basing care on evidence,
    177–179
"Battlemind," 430
BDI, see Beck's Depression
    Inventory (BDI)
"Beating the Blues," 98, 99
Beck's Depression Inventory
    (BDI), 47, 52
Behavioral care providers
    (BCPs)
  cost savings, marketing tool,
    44–45
  funding integrated care, 50
  integration vs. collaboration,
    40
  laboratory model, integrated
    care, 51
  leveraging physicians' time,
    44
  physician group practices, 51
Behavioral healthcare crisis
  education and training,
    210–211
  empirically supported
    treatments, 208–210
  fundamentals, 207–208
  quality improvement agenda,
    207–211
  responses, 14
Behavioral health medical
    homes, see also Medical
    homes; Patient-centered
    medical/healthcare
    homes (PCMH/PCHH)
  barriers, 248–249
  blending healthcare, 227–229

Index   **473**

Cherokee Health Systems
  model, 243–247
 disincentives, 248–249
 future directions, 251–253
 integration, 239–242, 249–251
 intervention locus/mode,
   236–238
 paradigm shift, 236–238
 patient-centered healthcare
   home, 229–233
 payment systems, reforming,
   247–251
 primary care, behavioral
   nature, 233–236
Behavioral health practice, 348
Behavioral health programs,
  285–287
Benuto, Lorraine, 367–388
Berwick, Daniel, 14
Best available research
  evidence, 182–183
Biases, 174–176
"Biodyne Bootcamp," 46
Biodyne Institute, 39, see also
  American Biodyne
Biodyne model, 267, 272
Biofeedback, 444, 448, 453
Biofeedback treatment
 anxiety, 455–456
 attention deficit disorder,
   454–455
 chronic pain, 450–451
 CPT codes, 459
 electroencephalograph
   feedback, 444–445
 electromyography, 443
 epilepsy, 451–452
 equipment, 442–443, 457
 functional abdominal pain,
   children, 456–457
 fundamentals, 441–442, 457
 heart rate variability, 444
 hemoencephalography,
   445–447
 hypertension, 447–449
 medical disorders, treatment,
   447–457, 460–461
 migraines, 449–450
 modalities, 443–447, 459–461

 neurofeedback/neurotherapy,
   444–445
 organizations, 457
 recommended texts, 458
 resources, 457–459
 respiration, 444
 skin conductance, 444
 temperature training, 443
 temporomandibular disorder,
   452–453
 tension headaches, 449–450
 traumatic brain injury,
   453–454
 unvalidated treatments, 210
Biological psychiatry, 2
Biomedical revolution, 38
Bipolar disorder
 combined interventions, 134
 neuroscience impact, 405
 overdiagnosis, 338
 political correctness, 8
Blood pressure, *see*
  Hypertension
Blount, Alexander, 238
Blue Cross Blue Shield
 Cherokee Health System, 247
 historical developments, 35,
   36
 Online Care Anywhere,
   412–413
 pay for performance, 281
 quality assurance, 47
Blunders, 259–263
Body image dissatisfaction, 88
"Boulder model"/Boulder
  Conference, 172,
   185–186
Brain development, 404–405
Bray, James H., 289, 343–360
Breathing training biofeedback,
   456–457
Bridging the gap, science and
  practice, 188–192
British Association for
  Behavioral
  and Cognitive
  Psychotherapies, 105
British National Heath Service,
  217

"Broken leg" phenomenon, 176–177
"BT Steps," 98
Budget establishment, 75
Bulimia, 89, 192, *see also* Eating disorders
Bureau of Primary Health Care, 237
Business Wire, 282, 285
BuyerZone, 76

C

Caccavale, John L., 327–341
California HealthCare Foundation, 76
Cancer
  cultural sensitivity, 375
  evidence-based preventive services, 401
  Pap smears, 384, 385
Candy bar intervention, 22
Capnometer, 445
Car accidents, 89
Cardiovascular disorders, 240
Career opportunities, 274–275
CareIntegra, 437
Care management, 49
"Care," passive/one-directional process, 229
Cartwright, James (Marine Corps General), 427
Carve outs
  disincentives and barriers, 248–249
  elimination, mental health, 343
  private funding, 49
Casciani, Joseph, 327–341
Catholic school district case, 28
Catlin, Casey, 299–315
Cats experiment, 452
CDC, *see* Centers for Disease Control (CDC)
CDR, *see* Clinical data repository (CDR)
CD-ROM-based interventions, 98

Centers for Disease Control (CDC)
  antidepressant medication usage statistics, 99
  PEARLS intervention, 310
  suicide, 425
Centers for Medicare & Medicaid Services (CMS), 14, 59
CER, *see* Comparative effectiveness research (CER)
Cereal makers example, 336
Cerebral blood flow, 445, 450
Certification, 291, *see also* Credentials and credentialing
Chaffee, R. Blake, 417–438
Challenges, 142–143
CHAMPUS (Civilian Health and Medical Program of the Unformed Services), 44, 418
Characteristics of patients, evidence-based practice, 183–184
Cherokee Health Systems
  behavioral health medical homes, 243–247
  fully integrated, federally qualified, 132
  hallway handoff, 28
  integrated care provider, 235
  integration *vs.* collaboration, 40
Childbirth, 384
Children, *see also* Attention deficit disorder (ADD); Attention deficit hyperactivity disorder (ADHD)
  childcare, lack of, 95
  diabetes, 359
  early intervention, 407
  former foster care, 351
  insufficient specialists, 141
  medications, 337–339, 454–455

pediatric behavioral health disorders, 131–132
preventative services, 402
psychotropic drug use, 131
at risk population, 329
schizophrenia, 12
special needs, 230
stomach pain, biofeedback treatment, 442
undocumented immigrants, 384
Children/family treatment, reforms
access to care, 351–353
behavioral health practice, expanding, 348
CHIP/CHIPRA, 351–352
community prevention efforts, 353–354
comparative effectiveness research, 348
evidence-based practice, 348, 357–358
fundamentals, 343–344, 351
healthcare overview, 345–350
health disparities, 355
home visiting programs coverage, 354–355
insurance coverage, 354–355
integrated care, 349–350
patient-centered medical homes, 349–350
payment issues, 356
postpartum conditions, 353
pregnant women, 353
preventative services, 353–355
primary care, 346–348
school-based health centers, 352
technology integration, 350
training opportunities, 356–357
Children's Health Insurance Program/Reauthorization Act (CHIP/CHIPRA), 351–352, 356

China, quality transformation, 213
CHIP/CHIPRA, see Children's Health Insurance Program/Reauthorization Act (CHIP/CHIPRA)
Cholesterol, high, 401
Chronic back pain, 100, 445, 450
Chronic headaches, 88, see also Migraines; Tension headaches
Chronic health conditions, general, 354, 402–403
Chronic pain, 442, 450–451
Cigna care management organization, 47
Cisco Systems, Inc., 410
Clarification of definition, 195–196
Classifications, dimensional, 159–161, 162
Clergy, 305, 372–373, see also Psychoreligions; Religion
"Cleveland Clinic" model, 294
Clinical curriculum, 265–266, see also Education
Clinical data repository (CDR), 69
Clinical expertise
  vs. opinion/intuition, 183
  referring to as evidence, 185
  unchecked, 173–174
Clinically oriented computer systems, 73
Clinical needs, threshold establishment, 163
Clinical training, reforms, 261, see also Training
Clinical vs. statistical prediction, 176–177
CoA, see Committee on Accreditation (CoA)
Codes, see Current procedural terminology (CPT) codes; International Classification of Diseases (ICD)

Coffey, C. Edward, 408
Cognitive-behavioral therapy (CBT)
   DESTRESS program, 86–87
   drop-out rate, 92
   e-health treatment, 84, 91–92
   group permutations, 373
   insomnia, 91
   temporomandibular disorder, 452
Cognitive heuristics, 174–175
Collaboration
   IMPACT intervention, 310
   vs. integration, 40
   moving forward through, 344
   PROSPECT model, 311–312
Colocated models, 241–242, 349
Comanagement care model, 246
Combat stress reactions, management, 422–423, 429
Combined interventions, 133–136
Committee on Accreditation (CoA), 193
Communication, *see also* Diagnostic and Statistical Manual of Mental Disorders (DSM)
   breakdown, disparity of SES, 370
   facilitated, 174
   office, 75
Community health centers, 66, 355
Community mental health centers (CMHCs), 237
Community prevention efforts, 353–354
Comorbidity
   co-occurrence, 151–153, 235–236
   preventative care and services, 354
   research, 20
Comparative effectiveness initiatives, 400
Comparative effectiveness research (CER)
   data complexity, decision making, 64–65
   data range, decision making, 63–64
   healthcare overview, 348
Competence, 261, 271–273
Competition as driver, 49–50
Competitive effectiveness evaluation, 400
Computer-aided therapy, 88, *see also* E-health and telehealth
Computerized provider order entry systems, 67
"Conditions," 6–7
Confidentiality, e-health and telehealth, 106, *see also* Privacy
Connected Care, 410
Consensus Development Conference, 338
Constancy of purpose, 216
Consultation codes, payment, 53, *see also* Current procedural terminology (CPT) codes; International Classification of Diseases (ICD)
Consultation liaison models, 50
Consumer-centric approach, 216–218, *see also* Patient-centric approach
Consumer's Union, 134
Content of care, 65, 77
Context of care, 65, 77
Continuing education, 101–102, 194–195, *see also* Education; Training
CONTROL (HealthMedia), 409
Controls, treatment criteria, 178
Controversies, 262–263
Cookbooks (manuals), 284
"Cope," 98
Core Standards for Telemedicine Operations, 433

Index 477

Core Standards for Videoconferencing-Based Telemental Health, 433
Costs, *see also* Financial dimensions; Funding; Medical cost offset
  access issues, 381
  advertising, 335–336
  assisted living, 314
  barrier to healthcare, ethnic groups, 370
  chronic medical conditions, 236
  day care health centers, 314
  e-health and telehealth, 95–100
  fundamentals, 20
  healthcare crisis, 205
  immigration status, 383–384
  Internet-delivered therapy, 86
  lack of prevention, 395
  leveraging physicians time, 44
  medical, offset, 41–43
  nursing facilities, 314
  older Americans, 300
  professional education reforms, 267–268
  psychiatric hospitalization, 25
  reduction, 95–100, 383–384
  reform, 219, 221
  savings as marketing tool, 44–46
  technology, upfront, 95–97, 103–104, 109
  traditional therapy, 44
Coverage, denial of, 351
CPT codes, *see* Current procedural terminology (CPT) codes
Creativity, 33
"Credentialed Persons, Credentialed Knowledge," 173
Credentials and credentialing
  practicum program, 273–274
  process *vs.* outcomes, 290
  professional education reforms, 260–261
Credibility, intervention interfaces, 96
Crider Center, 132
Crisis intervention responsivity, 103
Critical incident stress debriefing, 173–174, 209
Cultural reforms, 218
Cultural sensitivity and issues
  attitudes, 382
  defining, 369
  evidence-based treatment, 368–369
  inclusion *vs.* exclusion, 373–374
  issues, 368–369
  technology, treatment delivery, 379–380
Cummings, Janet L., 33–54, 279–295
Cummings, Nicholas A., *xi*
  efficacy, effectiveness, and efficiency, 19–31
  failure to serve, 327–341
  financial dimension, 33–54
  historical developments, 1–16
  pay for performance and innovative reimbursement, 279–295
Current flawed approach, 212
Current healthcare system, 90–102
Current procedural terminology (CPT) codes, *see also* International Classification of Diseases (ICD)
  biofeedback treatment, 441, 459
  consultant codes, payment, 53
  financing structure, healthcare homes, 250
  lag behind delivery system, 249
  treating children, 358

Current status, pay for performance, 282–283
Curricula, 140–142, 238, 265–266, *see also* Education

D

Data
 complexity, 64–65
 formats, 73
 integration, 72–73
 range, decision making, 62–64
 storage, 106
 summary, medications, 331–341
Data Standards for Mental Health Decision Support, 60
Day care health center cost, 314
DBH, *see* Doctor of behavioral health (DBH) program
DCOE, *see* Defense Centers of Excellence (DCOE)
Decision making, data ranges, 62–64
Decoupling data, 73
Deep knowledge, 216
De facto mental health treatment system, 39–40, 233
Defense Centers of Excellence (DCOE), 427
Defense medical surveillance system (DMSS), 421
DeLeon, Patrick, 289
Delivery issues, 65, 83–84
Delusion, joining patient's inner world, 22–23
Dementia, 303–304
Deming's cycle, 213–214
Demographic shift, 63, 299–300
Dentistry, success, 216
Department of Family Medicine and Community Health, 238

Deployment, 419
"Depression Care Effort Brings Dramatic Drop in Large HMO Population's Suicide Rate," 407
Depression disorders, *see also* Antidepressant medications
 "age of depression," 7
 Biodyne model, 268
 complications from disease, 303
 computer-based therapy, 84, 88, 89, 91
 cultural sensitivity, 375
 declining with age, 305–306
 IMPACT intervention, 310, 312
 improving care, 408
 integrated care, 239–240
 military service, 94
 older adults, 305–306
 preventative care and services, 354
 resiliency, 419
 subthreshold, 155–156
Desensitization, 29
DESTRESS program, 86–87, 102
Determination of status, 373–374
Deviant peer involvement, 354
Diabetes
 biofeedback treatment, 447
 children, 359
 evidence-based preventive services, 401
 integrated care, 240
 statistics, 302–303
 telehealth, 410
Diagnoses
 arbitrariness, 9
 by ballot, 7
 by consensus, 8–10
 reports, historical, 4
Diagnosis-related groups (DRGs), 36

Index **479**

Diagnostic and Statistical Manual of Mental Disorders (DSM), *see also* Current procedural terminology (CPT) codes; International Classification of Diseases (ICD)
  Age of Anxiety, 4–5
  colocated providers, 242
  diagnostic system innovations, 149, 159–161
  fundamentals, 3–4, 330
  future changes and developments, 11–16
  personality disorders as mental illnesses, 6
  present state, 7–8
  "psychiatric bible," 3
  psychopathology, end of, 6–7
  target population, 436
Diagnostic co-occurrence, excessive, 151–154
Diagnostic systems
  arbitrary diagnostic thresholds, 154–157
  clinical needs, threshold establishment, 163
  Diagnostic and Statistical Manual of Disorders, 159–161
  dimensional classification, 159–161
  disorder *vs.* impairment, assessment separation, 162–163
  excessive diagnostic co-occurrence, 151–154
  fundamentals, 149–151
  ICD *vs.* DSM, 350
  intellectual disability, 157–159
  paradigm shift, implementation, 162
  recommendations, 162–163
  social needs, threshold establishment, 163
  threshold establishment, 163

Diagnostic thresholds, arbitrary *vs.* fixed, 154–157
Difficulties, financial dimension, 51–53
Digital coaching programs, 409
Dimensional classification, 159–161, 162
Dimensional proposals, 161
"Direct care system," 417
Disabilities as barrier, 95, 314
Disabling conditions, reducing, 194
"Disease mongering," 9
Disincentives, 248–249
Disorder *vs.* impairment, 162–163
Dissemination efforts
  as barrier, 105
  e-health potential, 84
  publication format, 191
  recommendations, 196–197
Dissociative identity disorder, 10
Distant providers, 432
DMSS, *see* Defense medical surveillance system (DMSS)
Doctoral psychologists, 3
Doctor of behavioral health (DBH) program
  career opportunities, 274–275
  clinical curriculum, 265–266
  competency assessment, 271–273
  credentials, 273–274
  culminating research project, 269
  efficiency and medical cost offset, 267–268
  fundamentals, 263–264
  macrocurriculum, 264–265
  medical literacy courses, 268
  overviews, 263–264, 269–270, 275
  practicum program, 269–275
  research courses, 269
  sites, 270–271
  supervision, 270
Domestic violence, 131

Draper, Crissa, 83–110
DRG, see Diagnosis-related groups (DRGs)
"Drum circle therapy," 375, 376
DSM, see Diagnostic and Statistical Manual of Mental Disorders (DSM)
Dynamic vs. static approach, 213
Dyspepsia, see Functional abdominal pain (FAP), children
Dysthymia, 8

E

Early sexual initiation, 354
Eating disorders, 88, 89, see also Bulimia
EBP, see Evidence-based practice (EBP)
EBT, see Evidence-based treatment (EBT)
ECA, see Epidemiologic catchment area (ECA)
Economic developments, 34–36
EDA, see Electrodermal activity (EDA)
Education, see also Continuing education; Training
  behavioral healthcare crisis, 210–211
  changes, 262–263
  continuing, 194–195
  continuum, psychological health/disorder, 428
  disseminating evidence-based care, 101–102
  preparing psychologists, 140–143
  public, 193–194
  recommendations, 192–193
  videoconferencing, 102
Education reforms
  antibusiness, antihealthcare agenda, 260
  blunders, 259–263
  career opportunities, 274–275
  clinical curriculum, 265–266
  clinical training, 261
  competence and competency assessment, 261, 271–273
  controversies, 262–263
  credentials and credentialing, 260–261, 273–274
  doctoral degree, 263–269
  efficiency, 267–268
  emerging reforms, 262–263
  fundamentals, 257–259, 275
  irrelevant course curriculum, 259–260
  licensure, 262
  macrocurriculum, 264–265
  medical cost offset, 267–268
  medical literacy courses, 268
  practicum program, 269–275
  research courses and research project, 269
  sites, 270–271
  supervision, 270
  "unblundering," 263–269
EEG, see Electroencephalograph (EEG) feedback
Effective Child Therapy Web site, 357, 358
Efficacy, effectiveness, and efficiency
  Biodyne model, 267
  cultural sensitivity, 375–376
  education reforms, 267–268
  evidence-based treatment, 284
  extending/denying treatment, 26
  failure to be, 206–207
  fundamentals, 19–20, 29–30
  hallway handoff, 27–28
  high utilizers, medical care, 24–25
  immediate group, 23–24
  inner world access, 22–23
  international impact, 28–29
  medical homes, 13
  outpatient therapy, hospital emergency room, 25–26

phobic patients, 29
research shortfalls, 109
therapeutic shopping spree, 29–30
training and competence, 261
unexpected places, 21–22
wait times, 382
E-health and telehealth
　access to care and services, 93–95, 376–377
　adjunctive services, 90–92
　barriers, 92–93, 103–106
　comparison, 100
　cost reduction, 95–100
　current healthcare system, 90–102
　delivery issues, 83–84
　dropout rates, 88
　ethnic minorities, 376–377
　evidence-based care, disseminating, 100–102
　fundamentals, 84–90, 107–110
　information technology, impact, 409–410
　integrating into practice, 350
　overview, 107–110
　reforms, ethnic minorities/women, 376–377
　reimbursement guidelines, 104
　service delivery, 313–314
　stepped care, 90–92
　treatment, barriers to seeking, 92–93
　using, 103–106
　Web site advantages, 89
　women, 376–377
eHealth Initiative, 70
Electrodermal activity (EDA), 444
Electroencephalograph (EEG) feedback, 444–445, 454–455
Electromyography (EMG) biofeedback, 443, 450, 455, 460
Electronic health records (EHR), *see also* Electronic medical record (EMR); Personal health records (PHRs)
　decision making, 65–68
　failure to use, 206
　future directions, 15
　implementation and integration, 75–76, 350
　limited movement toward, 13
　President Bush goal, 59
　start-up costs, 70
　vendors, 75
Electronic medical record (EMR), 66, 107, *see also* Electronic health records (EHR)
"Elephant in the room," 47–48
Eligibility, extending, 430–431
Eligibility determination, immigration status, 383
E-mails, insufficiency, 13
Emergency rooms, 355, 385
Emerging reforms, 262–263
EMG, *see* Electromyography (EMG) biofeedback
Empirical barriers, 103
Empirically supported treatments (EST), 208–211
Empirically validated psychotherapists, 294–295
Empirically validated therapists, 291
Employee assistance programs (EAPs), 421, 434, 436
Employer-paid healthcare, 35–36
EMR, *see* Electronic medical record (EMR)
Energy therapies, 210
Enuresis example, 372–373
Epidemiologic catchment area (ECA), 152–153, 154, 304
Epilepsy, 442, 451–452

EPPP, *see* Examination for professional practice in psychology (EPPP)
Equipment, biofeedback treatment, 442–443, 457
Errors and self-correction, 214–215
Espirit de corps, 423
EST, *see* Empirically supported treatments (EST)
Ethical concerns, 103
Ethnicity, 105–106, 355
Ethnic minorities/women, treatment reforms
  access issues, 376–386
  barriers, 369–371, 376–377
  cost of healthcare, 381
  cultural attitudes and sensitivity, 368–369, 374–376, 382
  determination of status, 373–374
  e-health access to services, 376–377
  evidence-based treatment, 368–369
  fundamentals, 367, 387–388
  health insurance coverage, lack, 381
  immigration status, 382–385
  integrated care, 382, 385–386
  Internet access, 377–379
  issues, 368–369
  language barriers, 381
  rural communities, 381
  stigma, 382
  technology, 376–380
  telehealth access to services, 376–377
  treatment delivery, 379–380
  two-faced cultural factors, 372–373
  women's preventative care, 385–386
Euro-Americans, 377
Everyday behavior, conversion to disease, 12
Evidence-based assessment, 50

Evidence-based care, 100–102, 177–179
Evidence-based groups, 50
Evidence-based interventions, 50
Evidence-based practice (EBP)
  APA definition, 184–185
  best available research evidence, 182–183
  clinical expertise, 183
  consensus components, 181–182
  five steps, 180–181
  fundamentals, 182
  healthcare overview, 348
  patient characteristics, 183–184
  reforms, children/family treatment, 357–358
Evidence-Based Practice in Biofeedback and Neurofeedback, 446
Evidence-based preventive services, 401–402
Evidence-based treatment (EBT)
  accessibility of research, 189, 191–192
  APA definition, 184–185
  basing care on evidence, 177–179
  best available research evidence, 182–183
  biases, 174–176
  bridging the gap, 188–192
  clarify definition, 195–196
  clinical expertise, 183
  clinical *vs.* statistical prediction, 176–177
  continuing education, 194–195
  cultural sensitivity, 368–369
  dissemination efforts, 196–197
  education, 192–193
  evidence-based practice, 182–185
  fundamentals, 171
  gap, science/practice, 185–192

heuristics, 174–176
historical developments, 171–172
insurance reimbursement, 194
McFall Manifesto, 177
patient characteristics, 183–184
pay for performance/innovative reimbursement, 283–284
practice/science integration, 171–172, 177–182
public education, 193–194
recommendations, 192–197
relevance of research, 189–191
science, importance, 172–177
science/practice integration, 171–172
scientific mentality, 179–182
training, 188–189, 192–193
unchecked clinical expertise, 173–174
understanding the gap, 188
Examination for professional practice in psychology (EPPP), 261, 262
Excess disability, dementia, 308–309
Excessive diagnostic co-occurrence, 151–154
Exclusion, groups, 373–374
Exemplary programs, 68–69
Exercise, lack of, 447
Expanded coverage, 400–402
Expensive treatment approaches, 400
Experimental design, treatment criteria, 178
Exponential growth, 77
Extending/denying treatment, 26

F

Failure to serve
adverse drug events reduction, 332–333
antidepressant medications, 334–335
children, medicating, 337–339
data summary, 331–341
evidence against primary care physicians, 331–332
fundamentals, 327, 341
harm, reducing, 336–337
healthcare cost reduction, 336–337
lack of prescription information, 335–336
long-term care, treatment of aged, 340–341
patient safety issues, 333
primary care issues, 333
psychiatry in crisis, 333
public healthcare policy issues, 333
statement of concern, 327–330
treatment by real doctors, 339
unlimited license to practice, 336–337
Fairview Health Services, 412–413
Family/children treatment, reforms, *see also* Children
access to care, 351–353
behavioral health practice, expanding, 348
CHIP/CHIPRA, 351–352
community prevention efforts, 353–354
comparative effectiveness research, 348
evidence-based practice, 348, 357–358
fundamentals, 343–344, 351
healthcare overview, 345–350
health disparities, 355
home visiting programs coverage, 354–355
insurance coverage, 354–355
integrated care, 349–350

patient-centered medical homes, 349–350
payment issues, 356
postpartum conditions, 353
pregnant women, 353
preventative services, 353–355
primary care, 346–348
school-based health centers, 352
technology integration, 350
training opportunities, 356–357
Family support, barrier *vs.* facilitation, 372
Fannie Mae, 280
FAP, *see* Functional abdominal pain (FAP), children
"Fear Fighter," 98
Federal Bureau of Prisons, 90
Federal Coordinating Council for Comparative Effectiveness Research, 70
Federal Food, Drug and Cosmetic Act, 98
Federally qualified health centers (FQHCs), 237, 243, 402
Federation of State Medical Boards (FSMB), 337
Fees, pay for performance, 287–288
Female urinary incontinence, 445
Fiber, 456–457
50-minute hour
　extending/denying treatment, 26
　fundamentals, 19–20, 29–30
　hallway handoff, 27–28
　high utilizers, medical care, 24–25
　immediate group, 23–24
　inner world access, 22–23
　international impact, 28–29
　medical homes, 13
　outpatient therapy, hospital emergency room, 25–26
　phobic patients, 29
　therapeutic shopping spree, 29–30
　unexpected places, 21–22
Financial dimensions, *see also* Costs; Funding; Medical cost offset
　barriers, 103–104
　biomedical revolution, 38
　cost savings as marketing tool, 44–46
　difficulties, 51–53
　fundamentals, 33–34, 53–54
　funding, integrated care, 49–51
　healthcare economic developments, 34–36
　inadequate implementation, 51–53
　integration, 40–44
　laboratory model, 51
　leveraging physician's time, 44
　medical cost offset, 41–43
　mental health silo funding, 38–40
　nonpsychiatric psychotherapy, 37
　outcomes, 52
　perverse incentives, 51–53
　physician group practices, 51
　private funding, 49
　public funding, 49
　quality assurance, 46–48
　service delivery, 398–400
　traditional therapy costs, 44
Financing integrated care
　barriers, 248–249
　disincentives, 248–249
　fundamentals, 247–248
　integration support, 249–251
Firearms, suicide, 425
Fire engine example, 175
First impressions, undoing, 175
First-line treatment/misuse, medications
　adverse drug events reduction, 332–333

Index

antidepressant medications, 334–335
children, medicating, 337–339
data summary, 331–341
evidence against primary care physicians, 331–332
fundamentals, 327, 341
harm, reducing, 336–337
healthcare cost reduction, 336–337
lack of prescription information, 335–336
long-term care, treatment of aged, 340–341
patient safety issues, 333
primary care issues, 333
psychiatry in crisis, 333
public healthcare policy issues, 333
statement of concern, 327–330
treatment by real doctors, 339
unlimited license to practice, 336–337
Fisher, Jane E., 299–315
Fitness for duty, 419–424
Flexner Report, 290
Follow-up care, videoconferencing, 90
Food and Drug Administration (FDA), 97–98, 338
Ford Motor Company, quality transformation, 213
Format of research, 191–192
Fort Bragg Champus Study, 44
Foster care children, former, 351
FQHC, *see* Federally qualified health centers (FQHCs)
Freddie Mac, 280
Freeman, Dennis, 227–253
Free-market healthcare continuation, 293–294
Freud, Sigmund, 6
Fromm-Reichmann, Frieda, 21–23
FSMB, *see* Federation of State Medical Boards (FSMB)

Functional abdominal pain (FAP), children, 456–457
Functionality, intervention interfaces, 96–97
Functionality, restoring, 50
Funding, *see also* Costs; Medical cost offset
integrated care, 49–51
lack, e-health and telehealth, 107
mental health silo, 38–40
private, 49
public, 49
Future changes and directions
classifications, 160
"Cleveland Clinic" model, 294
Diagnostic and Statistical Manual of Mental Disorders, 11–16
empirically validated psychotherapists, 294–295
free-market healthcare continuation, 293–294
lesser public ownership, healthcare delivery, 293
present system continuation, 292
trends, aging America, 315
universal healthcare, 293
"The Future of Family Medicine: A Collaborative Project of the Family Medicine Community," 230

G

GAD, *see* Generalized anxiety disorder (GAD)
Galvanic skin response (GSR), 444, 455, 460
GAO, *see* U.S. Government Accountability Office (GAO)

Gap, science and practice
  accessibility of research, 189, 191–192
  bridging, 188–192
  fundamentals, 185–187
  relevance of research, 189–191
  training, improving, 188–189
  understanding the gap, 188
Garrison-Diehn, Christina, 299–315
Gastrointestinal disorders, see Functional abdominal pain (FAP), children
Gates, Robert (Secretary of Defense), 427
Gehrig's (Lou) disease, see Amyotrophic lateral sclerosis (ALS) disease
Geisinger Health System, 283–284, 289
Gender, manipulation, 174–175
Generalized anxiety disorder (GAD), 455, see also Anxiety disorders
Geographical remoteness, 90, see also Barriers
Google Health, 411–412
Google Language Tools, 381
Graduate psychology education (GPE), 356–357
Grants and grant support
  graduate psychology education, 356–357
  Licensure Portability Grant Program, 108
  school-based health centers, 352
  technology transfer, 97
  telemedicine services, 108
Grassley, Senator Charles, 288
Great Depression, 34
Group disease programs, Biodyne model, 267–268
Group permutations, inclusion vs. exclusion, 373–374
GSR, see Galvanic skin response (GSR)
Guidelines, adherence, 74

H

Habits
Hallway handoff
  clinical curriculum, 265
  cost savings, marketing tool, 45, 46
  efficiency, 27–28
  laboratory model, integrated care, 51
  leveraging physicians' time, 44
  Medicaid billing, 53
  physician group practices, 51
Hampton, Tracy, 407
Hanson, Ardris, 59–77
Harm, reducing, 336–337
Hawaii Integrated Care Demonstration Project, 437
Hawaii Integrated Healthcare Project II, 40
Hawaii Medicaid Project, 39, 41–43, 267
Hawaii Multi-Service Medical Management Office, 437
HDR, see Health data repository (HDR)
Headaches, see Chronic headaches; Migraines; Tension headaches
Health and Human Services, see U.S. Department of Health and Human Services (HHS)
Health Care and Education Reconciliation Act, 343
Healthcare cost reduction, 336–337
Healthcare economic developments, 34–36
Health Care Financing Administration, 39
Healthcare home, see Medical homes; Patient-centered medical/healthcare homes (PCMH/PCHH)

Index 487

Healthcare Information and Management Systems Society (HIMSS), 61, 70, 73
Healthcare overview
  behavioral health practice, expanding, 348
  comparative effectiveness research, 348
  evidence-based practice, 348
  fundamentals, 345–346
  integrated care, 349–350
  patient-centered medical homes, 349–350
  primary care, 346–348
  technology integration, 350
Healthcare reform strategic implications, 397–400
Healthcare spending, 300–302
Healthcare system
  crisis, 204–207
  e-health and telehealth, 90–102
  pyramid, 345
Health data dictionary (HDD), 69
Health data repository (HDR), 69
Health disparities, 355
Health habits, poor, 228
Health information exchange, 72
Health Information Portability and Accountability Act (HIPAA), 60, 412
Health Information Technology for Economic and Clinical Health Act (HITECH Act)
  electronic medical records, 107
  historical developments, 60–61
  integrating technology into practice, 350
Health Information Technology (HIT), 59–60, 75
Health Information Technology Policy Committee, 70

Health insurance coverage, lack, 381
Health literacy, 228
Health maintenance organizations (HMO), 36
HealthMedia digital coaching programs, 409
Health on the Net Foundation, 313
Health performance questionnaire (HPQ), 273
Health-plan-based financing, 399–400
HealthPresence, 410
Health Resources and Services Administration (HRSA), 108, 354, 402
Health vs. social services, 399–400
Heart rate variability (HRV), 444, 460, 457444
HEG, see Hemoencephalography (HEG)
Hemoencephalography (HEG)
  biofeedback treatment, 445–447
  fundamentals, 461
  migraines and tension headaches, 450
  watching movies, 442
Henry Ford Health System (HFHS), 407–408
Herbal remedies, 210
Herd animals, 51
Heterogeneous vs. homogeneous data formats, 73
Heuristics, science importance, 174–176
HFHS, see Henry Ford Health System (HFHS)
High blood pressure, 401, see also Hypertension
High cholesterol, 401
High-sodium diet, 447
High utilizers, medical care, 24–25
Hildebrand, Joel, 33

HIMSS, see Healthcare Information and Management Systems Society (HIMSS)
HIPAA, see Health Information Portability and Accountability Act (HIPAA)
Hispanics, access to Internet, 377–378, see also Latino patients
Historical developments
  Age of Anxiety, 4–5
  diagnosis by consensus, 8–10
  Diagnostic and Statistical Manual of Mental Disorders, 3–8, 11–12
  evidence-based treatment, 171–172
  fundamentals, 1–3
  future changes and developments, 11–16
  managed behavioral health organizations, 283
  mental health informatics, 60–61
  pay for performance/innovative reimbursement, 280–281
  personality disorders as mental illnesses, 6
  political correctness vs. science, 8–10
  present state, 7–8
  psychology vs. psychiatry, 10–11
  psychopathology, end of, 6–7
  science/practice integration, 171–172
  TriCare Program, 435
HIT, see Health information technology (HIT)
HITECH, see Health Information Technology for Economic and Clinical Health Act (HITECH Act)
HIV/AIDS, 354

HMO, see Health maintenance organizations (HMO)
Home-based services, service delivery, 310
Homeopathy, 210
Home visiting programs coverage, 354–355
Homework, assigned, 26, 92
Homogeneous vs. heterogeneous data formats, 73
Homosexuality, normalizing, 9
Honda success, 216
Hospitals, HIT system, 70–71
HPQ, see Health performance questionnaire (HPQ)
HRSA, see Health Resources and Services Administration (HRSA)
HRV, see Heart rate variability (HRV)
Hub Site, 432
Hypertension
  biofeedback treatment, 442, 447–449
  evidence-based preventive services, 401
Hypnosis, 210
Hypnotherapy, 376
Hypotheses, judgments as, 180

I

ICD codes, see International Classification of Diseases (ICD)
Identify, Deming's cycle, 214
IED, see Improvised explosive devices (IED)
IHA, see Integrated Healthcare Association (IHA)
Illegal substance abuse, older adults, 306
Imago relationship therapy, 209
Immediate group, efficiency, 23–24
Immigration status
  considerations, 384–385
  cost reduction, 383–384
  eligibility determination, 383

Index   **489**

recommendations, 385
undocumented immigrants, 382, 384–385
Immunizations, routine, 402
IMPACT (improving mood-promoting access to collaborative treatment), 310, 312
Impairment *vs.* disorder, assessment separation, 162–163
Implementation, 51–53, 162
Implications, mental health informatics, 76–77
Improving Access to Psychological Therapies Program initiative, 196
Improving mood-promoting access to collaborative treatment (IMPACT), 310
Improvised explosive devices (IED), 427
Inadequate implementation, 51–53
Incident reporting, removing barriers, 218
Inclusion, groups, 373–374
Indian Health Care Improvement Act, 367, *see also* Native American populations
Inferential systems, 73
Information, undoing initial, 175
Information technology, impact addiction, 412
   Ann-E Smartphone application, 412
   digital coaching programs, 409
   fundamentals, 406–407
   Google Health, 411–412
   HealthMedia digital coaching programs, 409
   Intel Health Guide, 409–410
   MDLiveCare, 411–412
   Minnesota Blue Cross/Blue Shield, 412–413
   Online Care Anywhere, 412–413
   Perfect Depression Care Initiative, 407–408
   telehealth, 409–410
   TRICARE Web-based demo project, 411
   UnitedHealth, telehealth, 409–410
   Web-based demo project, 411
Informed culture, 218
Initial information, undoing, 175
Inner world access, 22–23
Innovation fatigue, 52
Innovative reimbursement and pay for performance (P4P)
   behavioral health programs, 285–287
   "Cleveland Clinic" model, 294
   current status, 282–283
   empirically validated psychotherapists, 294–295
   evidence-based treatment, 283–284
   fee scales, 287–288
   free-market healthcare continuation, 293–294
   fundamentals, 279–280, 295
   future developments, 292–295
   historical development, 280–281
   lesser public ownership, healthcare delivery, 293
   lessons learned, 284–285
   present system continuation, 292
   process *vs.* outcomes, 290–292
   salary models, 288–290
   universal healthcare, 293
Insel, Thomas, 404–406
Insomnia, 89, 134

INSR, *see* International Society for Neurofeedback and Research (ISNR)
Institute of Medicine (IOM)
  adverse drug event reduction, 332
  comparative effectiveness research, 348
  exposure therapy, 86
  improving depression care, 408
  lack of prevention, costs, 395
  readjustment needs, veterans, 429
  specialist shortage for aging adults, 340
Insurance coverage
  access issues, 381
  denial of, 351
  limits for, lifted, 352
  reforms, children/family treatment, 354–355
  telemedicine services, 108
Insurance reimbursement, 194, *see also* Reimbursement
Integrated care
  access issues, 385–386
  barriers, 248–249
  disincentives, 248–249
  fundamentals, 247–248
  healthcare overview, 349–350
  integration support, 249–251
  rating scales, 271–272
  service delivery, 310–312
Integrated Healthcare Association (IHA), 285
Integration
  basing care on evidence, 177–179
  care, reforms, 221
  financial issues, 40–44, 247–251
  fostering, wellness and prevention, 396–397
  fundamentals, 177, 180–182
  historical developments, 171–172
  primary care, 437
  scientific mentality, 179–182

Integrative care system implementation, 382
Intel Health Care Management Suite, 410
Intel Health Guide, 409–410
Intellectual disability, 157–159
Interapy, 101
International Classification of Diseases (ICD), 61, 154, 162, 330, *see also* Current procedural terminology (CPT) codes; *Diagnostic and Statistical Manual of Mental Disorders* (DSM)
International impact, 28–29
International Society for Neurofeedback and Research (ISNR), 442
Internet access, 106, 377–379, *see also* E-health and telehealth; Technology
Interventions, *see also specific interventions*
  CD-ROM-based, 98
  combined, prescribing psychologists, 133–136
  unvalidated, e-health and telehealth, 103
Intuition *vs.* clinical expertise, 183
IOM, *see* Institute of Medicine (IOM)
iPhone/iPod applications, 412
Irish *vs.* American nuns, 28
Irrelevant course curriculum, 259–260
Irritable bowel syndrome, *see* Functional abdominal pain (FAP), children
Issues, *see also specific issue or barrier*
  cultural sensitivity, 368–369
  health impact, behavioral health, 307–308
  mental health delivery, 83–84
IT systems, healthcare, 74

Index

J

Japan, quality transformation, 213
Jet fuel discovery, 452
JNC, see Joint National Committee (JNC)
Johnson & Johnson Family of Companies, 409
Joint National Committee (JNC), 448
"Joint Principles," 231
Jorge, vignette, 386
Journals, practitioner-oriented, 191
Judgments, 180, 193
Jungian sandtray therapy, 209
Just culture, 218

K

Kaiser, Henry J., 35–36
Kaiser Foundation, 335
Kaiser Permanente
 Biodyne model, integrated care, 267
 exemplary programs, 69
 funding integrated care, 49
 historical developments, 36
 immediate group, 22–23
 integration vs. collaboration, 40
 pay for performance, 280
 present free-market healthcare continuation, 283–284
 salaries, 289–290
Kaiser Permanente Health Plan, 44–45
Klonsky, E. David, 171–197
Knowledge gap, 65

L

Laboratory model, integrated care, 51
Lack of prescription information, 335–336
Language barriers, 371, 381
Latino patients, see also Undocumented immigrants
 access to Internet, 377–378
 depression treatment protocol, 268
 undocumented, 371
 vignette, 386
Leadership, 219, 428–429
Leany, Brian D., 367–388
Leaps of faith, 216
Learning culture, 218
Learning organizations, 213–216
"Lemon problem," 48
LENS, see Low energy neurofeedback system (LENS)
Lesser public ownership, healthcare delivery, 293
Less intensive treatments, 379
Lessons learned, 284–285
Leveraging physician's time, 44
Levin, Bruse Lubotsky, 59–77
Librium medication, 5, 7
Licensure
 fees, 98
 issues, 104
 professional education reforms, 262
 unlimited, 330, 336
Licensure Portability Grant Program, 108
Life-history factors, 304–309
LifeScape, 283, 284
Lifetime coverage, 352
Lilienfeld, Scott O., 203–222
Limited mobility, service delivery, 314
Literacy, low health, 228
L.L. Bean, 216
Long-term shortage, psychiatrists, 329
Lou Gehrig's disease, see Amyotrophic lateral sclerosis (ALS) disease
Love vs. rage, 21
Low energy neurofeedback system (LENS), 453

"Low hanging fruit," 13
Low health literacy, 228

M

Macrocurriculum, 264–265
Magellan care management organization, 47
Mammograms, 384, 385
Managed behavioral health organizations (MBHOs)
 evidence-based treatment, 283
 funding integrated care, 49
 historical developments, 36, 283
 pay for performance, 281
Managed care, 49
Managed care support contractors (MCSCs)
 fundamentals, 417–418
 telemental health network development, 431–433
 TriCare Assistance program services, 434
Mandated overtime, 290
"Manifesto for a Science of Clinical Psychology," 177
Manipulation of gender, 174–175
Manuals (cookbooks), 284
Marketing strategy, 336
Marriage and family therapy (MFT), 37
Masters-level psychotherapists, 3
May, Rollo, 5
Mayo Clinic, 283, 288
MBHO, *see* Managed behavioral health organizations (MBHOs)
McFall Manifesto, 177
MDLiveCare, 411–412
"Meaningful use," 72
The Meaning of Anxiety, 5
Medicaid, *see also* Medicare
 annual wellness visits, 354
 behavioral health treatment funding, 398

CHIP/CHIPRA, 352
 finance matters, 53
 foster children, 351
 hallway handoff, 28
 health disparities, 355
 integrated treatment, chronic health conditions, 403
 pay for performance, 282, 285
 payment issues, 356
 per-member-per-month rate, 250–251
 pregnant women, 353
 racheting down fees, 287–288
 reimbursement guidelines, 104
Medical cost offset, *see also* Costs; Funding
 efficiency measures, 272
 financial dimension, 41–43
 high utilizers of medical care, 24
 pay for performance, 281
 private pay domain, 400
 productivity measures, 272
 professional education reforms, 267–268
Medical disorders, 447–457, 460–461, *see also specific disorder*
Medical Expenditure Panel Survey, 131
Medical homes, *see also* Behavioral health medical homes; Patient-centered medical/healthcare homes (PCMH/PCHH)
 effectiveness *vs.* interest, 13
 integrated treatment, chronic health conditions, 403
 opportunities, 132
Medical literacy courses, 268
Medical News Today, 285
Medical records, 75, *see also* Electronic health records (EHR)
Medicare, *see also* Medicaid
 access to providers, 301
 annual wellness visits, 354

Index   493

behavioral health treatment
    funding, 398
biofeedback treatment, 445
cost, chronic medical
    condition, 236
"distant providers," 432
hallway handoff, 28
health disparities, 355
integrated treatment, chronic
    health conditions, 403
"originating sites," 432
payment issues, 356
racheting down fees,
    287–288
trends, aging America,
    300–302
Medicare Payment Advisory
    Commission (MEDPAC),
    301
Medicare Telehealth
    Enhancement Act
    (MTEA), 104, 108
Medications
    adverse drug events
        reduction, 332–333
    antidepressant medications,
        334–335
    attention deficit disorder, 454
    children, medicating,
        337–339
    combined interventions,
        133–136
    data summary, 331–341
    evidence against primary
        care physicians,
        331–332
    first-line treatment,
        unsupported, 329
    fundamentals, 327, 341
    harm, reducing, 336–337
    healthcare cost reduction,
        336–337
    lack of prescription
        information, 335–336
    long-term care, treatment of
        aged, 340–341
    patient safety issues, 333
    primary care issues, 333
    psychiatry in crisis, 333

    psychotherapy, combined
        intervention, 133–136
    public healthcare policy
        issues, 333
    secondary aging effects, 307
    statement of concern,
        327–330
    treatment by real doctors, 339
    unlimited license to practice,
        336–337
MEDPAC, see Medicare Payment
    Advisory Commission
    (MEDPAC)
Meehl, Paul, 173
Menninger, William (Will), 21,
    37
Menninger Clinic, 21
Mental health informatics
    applications, 62–69
    data complexity, 64–65
    data integration, 72–73
    data range, 62–64
    decision making, 62–68
    EHR, 65–68
    exemplary programs, 68–69
    fundamentals, 59
    historical developments,
        60–61
    implications, 76–77
    recommendations, 69–76
    return on investment, 39–72
    small group practices, 74–76
    solo practitioners, 74–76
    training/workforce
        development, 74
Mental health silo funding,
    38–40
Mental health statistics, 92,
    129–131
Mental Health Statistics
    Improvement Program
    (MHSIP), 60
Mental Parity and Addiction
    Equity Act, 343, 396,
    397
Mental retardation, 157, see also
    Intellectual disability
Meprobamate medication, 5
Merrill Lynch, 280

Meyer, Adolph, 6
MFT, see Marriage and family therapy (MFT)
Microcephaly, 159
Migraines, see also Chronic headaches; Tension headaches
  biofeedback treatment, 442, 449–450
  temperature training, 443
Military health system
  electronic health records, 15
  funding integrated care, 49
  prevalence, mental health problems, 94
  veteran/military behavioral health reforms, 417–418
Military OneSource (MOS), 421, 434–435
Military treatment facilities (MTFs), 417–418, 437
Milk example, 48
Milltown medication, 5, 7
Mind-Body Medicine for Primary Care, 453
Minnesota Blue Cross/Blue Shield, 412–413
Minorities, access issues, 205, see also Ethnic minorities/women, treatment reforms
Misuse/first-line treatment, medications
  adverse drug events reduction, 332–333
  antidepressant medications, 334–335
  children, medicating, 337–339
  data summary, 331–341
  evidence against primary care physicians, 331–332
  fundamentals, 327, 341
  harm, reducing, 336–337
  healthcare cost reduction, 336–337
  lack of prescription information, 335–336
  long-term care, treatment of aged, 340–341
  patient safety issues, 333
  primary care issues, 333
  psychiatry in crisis, 333
  public healthcare policy issues, 333
  statement of concern, 327–330
  treatment by real doctors, 339
  unlimited license to practice, 336–337
Mobile devices, 84
Modalities, biofeedback treatment, 443–447, 459–461
Moderators, therapy outcome, 190
Mood disorders, 384, see also *specific disorder*
MoodGym, 98
Morehouse School of Medicine, 236
Morris, Jerry, 327–341
MOS, see Military OneSource (MOS)
Mosaicism, 159
Motor vehicle accidents, 89
MTEA, see Medicare Telehealth Enhancement Act (MTEA)
MTF, see Military treatment facilities (MTFs)
Muda (waste), 15
Multiple personality disorder, 10
Multisystemic therapy, 354–355
Music therapy, 210
Myths, 404

N

National Alliance of Professional Psychology Providers (NAPPP), 11, 262, 273, see also Failure to Serve
National Center for Primary Care, 236

Index   495

National Child Traumatic Stress
    Network initiative, 196
National Committee for Quality
    Assurance (NCQA), 232,
    286, 290
National Comorbidity Survey
    (NCS), 152–153, 154, 156
National Comorbidity Survey
    Replication (NCS-R),
    233, 304–305
National Council for
    Community Behavioral
    Healthcare, 76, 238
National data infrastructure, 72
National Defense Authorization
    Act, 418
National Epidemiologic Survey
    on Alcohol and Related
    Conditions (NESARC),
    152
National Guard and Reserve
    members, 411, 421
National Information Standards
    Organization, 70
National Institute of Behavioral
    Health Quality
    (NIBHQ), 273
National Institute of Mental
    Health (NIMH)
  data complexity, decision
    making, 64
  epidemiologic catchment
    area, 152–153, 304
  historical developments, 60
  medical cost offset, 24
  research planning
    conference, 160
  research priorities, 110
  retrospective studies, 39
  scientific understanding and
    healthcare practice,
    404
  stipends/educational
    funding, 37
  training standards, 60
National Institutes of Health
    (NIH), 74, 338
National Institutes of Health
    Technology, 451

National Library of Medicine
    (NLM), 74
National Registry of Evidence-
    Based Programs and
    Practices, 358
National Research Council, 65,
    395
National Violent Death
    Reporting System
    (NVDRS), 425–426
Nationwide Health Information
    Network (NHIN), 70
Native American populations
  cultural sensitivity, 375
  depression treatment
    protocol, 268
  Indian Health Care
    Improvement Act, 367
  videoconferencing
    technology, 90, 100
Navy, *see* U.S. Navy
NCQA, *see* National Committee
    for Quality Assurance
    (NCQA)
NCS, *see* National Comorbidity
    Survey (NCS)
NCS-R, *see* National
    Comorbidity Survey
    Replication (NCS-R)
Negative transfer of training,
    429
Neo-Kraepelinian movement,
    155
"Nerves" diagnosis, 5
NESARC, *see* National
    Epidemiologic Survey
    on Alcohol and Related
    Conditions (NESARC)
Neurofeedback/neurotherapy,
    444–445, 460, *see also*
    Biofeedback treatment
Neurolinguistic programming,
    209
Neuropsychological assessment,
    90
Neuroscience effects,
    treatments, 405–406
New Hampshire Telemedicine
    Act, 108

Newly disabled, barriers for, 95
NHIN, see Nationwide Health Information Network (NHIN)
NIBHQ, see National Institute of Behavioral Health Quality (NIBHQ)
NIMH, see National Institute of Mental Health (NIMH)
NLM, see National Library of Medicine (NLM)
Nonpartisan Center for Public Integrity, 335
Nonphysician healthcare provider groups, 138
Nonpsychiatric psychotherapy, 37
Nonspecialty settings, successful treatment, 133
NOS, see "Not otherwise specified" (NOS)
"Not otherwise specified" (NOS), 155, 160
"NowClinic," 409
Nuns, Irish vs. American, 28
Nurse-drive disease management, 52–53
Nurse practitioners, substitution with, 138–139
Nursing facility costs, 314
NVDRS, see National Violent Death Reporting System (NVDRS)

O

Obesity
  aging population, 303
  biofeedback treatment, 447
  children, 348
  preventative care and services, 354
Objections, prescribing psychologists, 136–139
Obsessive-compulsive disorder (OCD)
  biofeedback treatment, 456
  computer-based treatment, 89, 90–91
O'Donnell, Ronald R., 257–275
O'Donohue, William T., xi
  financial dimension, 33–54
  historical developments, 1–16
  quality improvement agenda, 203–222
OEF, see Operation Enduring Freedom (OEF)
Office communications, 75
Office for Minority Health, 360
Olympic athletes, 447
Online Care Anywhere, 412–413
Open culture, 218
OPEN MINDS On-Line news, 409
Operation Desert Storm, 423
Operation Enduring Freedom (OEF)
  extending TriCare eligibility, 430–431
  fundamentals, 418
  managing combat stress importance, 423
  occupational stress differences, 427
  postdeployment health assessment, 420
  suicide, 424
Operation Iraqi Freedom (OIF)
  extending TriCare eligibility, 430–431
  fundamentals, 418
  managing combat stress importance, 423
  occupational stress differences, 427
  postdeployment health assessment, 420
  suicide, 424
Opinions vs. clinical expertise, 183
OptumHealth, 409
Organizations, biofeedback treatment, 457
Originating site, 432
ORS, see Outcome rating scale (ORS)
Oss, Monica E., 395–413

Index   **497**

Outcome data, finance matters, 52
Outcome rating scale (ORS), 271–272
Outcome research, 189
Outcomes *vs.* process, 290–292
Outpatient therapy, hospital emergency room, 25–26
Overarching problem, 204
"Overcoming Depression," 98
Overtime, mandated, 290
Overviews
    e-health and telehealth, 107–110
    practicum program, 269–270

P

Pace, primary care, 242
Panic disorder (PD)
    biofeedback treatment, 455
    choosing a treatment, 187
    computer-based treatment, 88, 89, 91
Papa, Anthony, 83–110
Paper-based office, automating, 75
Paper Kills, 15
Pap smears, 384, 385
Paradigm shifts, diagnostic system innovations, 161, 162
Parkinson's disease, 405
Past lives therapy, 209
Patellofemoral pain, 451
Pathophysiology
    Diagnostic and Statistical Manual of Mental Disorders (DSM), 12
Patient-centered medical/healthcare homes (PCMH/PCHH), *see also* Behavioral health medical homes; Medical homes
    future developments, 252–253
    healthcare overview, 349–350
    primary care, 346–348
"Patient-Centered Primary Care Collaborative," 232
Patient-centric approach, 206, 216, *see also* Consumer-centric approach
Patient characteristics
    difficult, penalized, 287
    evidence-based practice, 183–184
    research focus, 190
Patient contact process, 75
Patient Protection and Affordable Care Act (PPACA)
    access to care, 351–353
    behavioral health practice, expanding, 348
    behavioral health recognition, 1–2
    CHIP/CHIPRA, 351–352
    combined interventions, 136
    community prevention efforts, 353–354
    comparative effectiveness research, 348
    evidence-based practice, 348, 357–358
    fundamentals, 343–344, 351
    healthcare overview, 345–350
    health disparities, 355
    home visiting programs coverage, 354–355
    insurance coverage, 354–355
    integrated care, 349–350
    new opportunities, 344
    patient-centered medical homes, 349–350
    payment issues, 356
    postpartum conditions, 353
    pregnant women, 353
    preventative services, 353–355, 401
    primary care, 346–348
    reforms, children/families, 343
    school-based health centers, 352
    service delivery, 397

technology integration, 350
training opportunities, 356–357
Patient-provider interaction, 75
Patient safety issues, 333
Patient's delusion, joining, 22–23
Pay for performance (P4P) and innovative reimbursement
  behavioral health programs, 285–287
  "Cleveland Clinic" model, 294
  current status, 282–283
  empirically validated psychotherapists, 294–295
  evidence-based treatment, 283–284
  fee scales, 287–288
  free-market healthcare continuation, 293–294
  fundamentals, 279–280, 295
  future developments, 292–295
  historical development, 280–281
  lesser public ownership, healthcare delivery, 293
  lessons learned, 284–285
  present system continuation, 292
  process vs. outcomes, 290–292
  salary models, 288–290
  universal healthcare, 293
Pay market, 400
Payment issues, 14, 356
Payment systems, reforming
  barriers and disincentives, 248–249
  fundamentals, 247–248
  integration support, 249–251
PCMH/PCHH, see Patient-centered medical/healthcare homes (PCMH/PCHH)

PCP, see Primary care physicians (PCP)
PCSAS, see Psychological clinical science accreditation system (PCSAS)
PD, see Panic disorder (PD)
PDHA, see Post-Deployment Health Assessment (PDHA)
PDHRA, see Post-Deployment Health Reassessment (PDHRA)
PEARLS, see Program to Encourage Active, Rewarding Lives for Seniors (PEARLS) intervention
Pediatric behavioral health disorders, 131–132
Pelvic floor training, 445
Perfect Depression Care Initiative, 407–408
Permanente Medical Group, 36, 280
Per-member-per-month payments, 250
Per-member-per-month (pmpm) rate, 250–251
Personal health records (PHRs), 411, see also Electronic health records (EHR)
Personality disorders as mental illnesses, 6
Personality restructuring, 50
Personal responsibility, 228
Perverse incentives, 51–53
Pew Internet and American Life Project, 105–106, 313
Phobic disorders, 29, 88, 91
PHR, see Personal health records (PHRs)
Physical health trends, aging population, 302–303
Physician assistants, 138–139
Physician group practices, 51
Physicians
  adverse drug errors, reducing, 332–333

Index   499

electronic health records
    usage, 59
  evidence against, 331–332
  herd animals, 51
  historical developments,
    34–35
  information, withholding
    from patients, 335–336
  medical centers, 51
  time, leveraging, 44
  unlimited license to practice,
    336–337
pmpm, see Per-member-per-
    month (pmpm) rate
Poisoning, suicide, 425
Political correctness vs. science,
    8–10
Poor health habits, 228
Population-based health
    management course,
    269
Populations, 92, 300, see also
    Aging population
Portability, 84, 93
Postadversity growth, 419
Post-Deployment Health
    Assessment (PDHA),
    421, 422
Post-Deployment Health
    Reassessment (PDHRA),
    421
Postpartum conditions, 353
Posttraumatic amnesia (PTA),
    453
Posttraumatic growth, 419
Posttraumatic stress, 84–85, 419
Posttraumatic stress disorder
    (PTSD)
  biofeedback treatment, 455
  critical incident stress
    debriefing, 173–174
  cultural sensitivity, 375–376
  DESTRESS program, 86–87
  disseminating evidence-
    based care, 101–102
  exposure therapy, 86–87, 88
  Internet delivery, 84, 89
  lack of ESTs use, 209
  military service, 94

  primary care setting, 439
  resiliency, 419
  suicide risk factor, 427
Poverty, 379, see also
    Socioeconomic status
    (SES)
P4P, see Pay for performance
    (P4P) and innovative
    reimbursement
PPACA, see Patient Protection
    and Affordable Care
    Act (PPACA)
Practice-based evidence, 291
Practice/science integration
  basing care on evidence,
    177–179
  fundamentals, 177, 180–182
  historical developments,
    171–172
  scientific mentality, 179–182
Practicum program
  career opportunities, 274–275
  competency assessment,
    271–273
  credentials, 273–274
  overview, 269–270
  sites, 270–271
  supervision, 270
Practitioner-oriented journals,
    191
Prader-Willi syndrome, 159
Preferred practitioners, 283
Pregnant women, 353, 401
Prepaid healthcare, historical
    developments, 35
Prescribing psychologists
  combined interventions,
    133–136
  fundamentals, 129–143
  objections, 136–139
  primary care environment
    preparation, 140–143
  successful treatment, non-
    specialty settings, 133
Prescription medications, see
    also Medications;
    Psychotropic drugs
  behavioral intervention
    replacement, 38

dispensing, nonpsychiatric physicians, 3
historical developments, 2–3
information, lack, 335–336
mental health spending, 1
"syndromes," facilitating, 7
Presentation method, research, 191–192
Present state, 7–8
Present system continuation, 292
Presidential Task Force and Summit on the Future of Psychology Practice, 344
President's New Freedom Commission on Mental Health
evidence-based treatment, 284
mental health informatics, 76
use of technology, 60
Preventative care and services
access issues, 385–386
key provisions, 400–402
reforms, children/family treatment, 353–355
too little emphasis, 207
"Preventing Mental, Emotional, and Behavioral Disorders Among Young People: Progress and Possibilities," 395
Prevention of suicide in primary care elderly: collaborative trial (PROSPECT) model, 311–312
Primary aging, 307
Primary care and primary care settings
environment, preparing psychologists, 140–143
healthcare overview, 346–348
issues, medications as first-line treatment/misuse, 333
pace, 242

preferred site for treatment, 234
vs. primary care physicians, 399
psychology, 349–350
settings, service delivery, 398–399
Primary care physicians (PCP)
cost savings, marketing tool, 44–45
de facto mental health treatment system, 39–40, 233
depressed patients survey, 130
evidence against, 331–332
funding integrated care, 50
integration vs. collaboration, 40
life-history factors, 305
Medicare issues, 301
vs. primary care settings, 399
psychotropic prescriptions, 233
Primary Care Psychology Curriculum Interdivisional Task Force, 238
Primary data, 63
Principle for Accreditation of Programs in Professional Psychology, 274
Principles, lack of clear set, 204
PRISM-E study, 311
Privacy
access from home, 85
e-health and telehealth, 103, 106
smokescreen for accountability, 286
Private funding, financial dimension, 49
Private pay market, 400
Problems, naming, 215
Problem-solving therapy for primary care (PST-PC), 312
Process research, 189

Process *vs.* outcomes, 290–292
ProChange Behavior Systems, 272
Prochaska, James, 272
Productivity measures, 272
Professional education, treatment reforms
   antibusiness, antihealthcare agenda, 260
   blunders, 259–263
   career opportunities, 274–275
   clinical curriculum, 265–266
   clinical training, 261
   competence and competency assessment, 261, 271–273
   controversies, 262–263
   credentials and credentialing, 260–261, 273–274
   doctoral degree, 263–269
   efficiency, 267–268
   emerging reforms, 262–263
   fundamentals, 257–259, 275
   irrelevant course curriculum, 259–260
   licensure, 262
   macrocurriculum, 264–265
   medical cost offset, 267–268
   medical literacy courses, 268
   practicum program, 269–275
   research courses and research project, 269
   sites, 270–271
   supervision, 270
   "unblundering," 263–269
Program to Encourage Active, Rewarding Lives for Seniors (PEARLS) intervention, 310
Project HOPE program, 410
PROSPECT (prevention of suicide in primary care elderly: collaborative trial) model, 311–312
Protocols, adherence, 74
Prozac, 338

PST-PC (problem-solving therapy for primary care), 312
Psychiatric assessment, 90
Psychiatric hospitalization, 25
Psychiatry in crisis, 333
Psychiatry *vs.* psychology, 10–11
Psychoeducational information, insufficiency, 13
Psychological Clinical Science Accreditation System (PCSAS), 189
Psychological clinical science accreditation system (PCSAS), 262
Psychological indicators, statistics, 340
Psychology *vs.* psychiatry, 10–11
Psychoneurosis diagnosis, 5
Psychopathology, end of, 6–7
Psychoreligions, 5, 15, *see also* Religion
"Psychosis risk syndrome," 11
Psychosocial deprivation, 159
Psychosocial indicators, statistics, 347
Psychosprawl, 10
Psychosynthesis, 209
Psychotherapy, combined interventions, 133–136
Psychotropic drugs, 38, 346, *see also* Medications
PTA, *see* Posttraumatic amnesia (PTA)
Public education, 193–194
Public funding, 49
Public healthcare policy issues, 333
Pyramid, healthcare system, 345

Q

QEEG, *see* Quantitative electroenceophalograph (QEEG)
QI, *see* Quality improvement (QI) agenda
Qualitative health data, 63
Quality assurance, 46–48

Quality enhancement research
  initiative (QUERI), 107
Quality improvement (QI)
  agenda
  behavioral healthcare crisis,
    207–211
  consumer-centric approach,
    216–218
  current flawed approach,
    212
  dynamic vs. static approach,
    213
  education and training,
    210–211
  empirically supported
    treatments, 208–210
  fundamentals, 203, 221–222
  healthcare crisis, 204–207
  integrated care, 221
  leadership, 219
  learning organizations,
    213–216
  overarching problem, 204
  reforms, 213–221
  safety, 218
  transparency, 219
  value and costs, 219, 221
Quality of care, payment
  regardless, 288
Quantifiable health data, 61, 63
Quantitative
  electroenceophalograph
  (QEEG), 453, 456

R

Rage vs. love, 21
Range of data, 62–64
Rating scales, 271–272
Raynaud's disease, 443
Readability, intervention
  interfaces, 96
Recommendations
  clarify definition, 195–196
  continuing education,
    194–195
  data integration, 72–73
  diagnostic system
    innovations, 162–163
  dissemination efforts,
    196–197
  education, 192–193, 258–259
  evidence-based treatment,
    192–197
  immigration status, 385
  insurance reimbursement,
    194
  public education, 193–194
  reforms, education, 258–259
  return on investment, 39–72
  small group practices, 74–76
  solo practitioners, 74–76
  texts, biofeedback treatment,
    458
  training, 74, 192–193
  workforce development, 74
Recovered memory techniques,
  174
Reforms
  consumer-centric approach,
    216–218
  dynamic vs. static approach,
    213
  fundamentals, 213
  integrated care, 221
  leadership, 219
  learning organizations,
    213–216
  payment systems, 247–251
  safety, 218
  transparency, 219
  value and costs, 219, 221
Reforms, children/family
  treatment
  access to care, 351–353
  behavioral health practice,
    expanding, 348
  CHIP/CHIPRA, 351–352
  community prevention
    efforts, 353–354
  comparative effectiveness
    research, 348
  evidence-based practice, 348,
    357–358
  fundamentals, 343–344, 351
  healthcare overview,
    345–350
  health disparities, 355

home visiting programs
    coverage, 354–355
insurance coverage, 354–355
integrated care, 349–350
patient-centered medical
    homes, 349–350
payment issues, 356
postpartum conditions, 353
pregnant women, 353
preventative services,
    353–355
primary care, 346–348
school-based health centers,
    352
technology integration, 350
training opportunities,
    356–357
Reforms, ethnic minorities/
    women treatment
access issues, 376–386
barriers, 369–371, 376–377
cost of healthcare, 381
cultural attitudes and
    sensitivity, 368–369,
    374–376, 382
determination of status,
    373–374
e-health access to services,
    376–377
evidence-based treatment,
    368–369
fundamentals, 367, 387–388
health insurance coverage,
    lack, 381
immigration status, 382–385
integrated care, 382, 385–386
Internet access, 377–379
issues, 368–369
language barriers, 381
rural communities, 381
stigma, 382
technology, 376–380
telehealth access to services,
    376–377
treatment delivery, 379–380
two-faced cultural factors,
    372–373
women's preventative care,
    385–386

Reforms, professional education
antibusiness, antihealthcare
    agenda, 260
blunders, 259–263
career opportunities,
    274–275
clinical curriculum, 265–266
clinical training, 261
competence and competency
    assessment, 261,
    271–273
controversies, 262–263
credentials and
    credentialing, 260–261,
    273–274
doctoral degree, 263–269
efficiency, 267–268
emerging reforms, 262–263
fundamentals, 257–259, 275
irrelevant course curriculum,
    259–260
licensure, 262
macrocurriculum, 264–265
medical cost offset, 267–268
medical literacy courses, 268
practicum program, 269–275
research courses and
    research project, 269
sites, 270–271
supervision, 270
"unblundering," 263–269
Reforms, veteran/military
    behavioral health
access to care, 419–424
deployment, 419
eligibility, extending,
    430–431
fitness for duty, 419–424
fundamentals, 417, 437–438
integration into primary care,
    437
military health system,
    417–418
posttraumatic stress, 419
resiliency, 419
stigma, 419–424, 427–430
suicide, 424–427
telemental health network
    development, 431–434

telemental health services, 431
TRICARE Assistance program services, 434–437
TRICARE/TRICARE Behavioral Health Program, 430–437
Reimbursement, *see also* Insurance reimbursement
future developments, 252
issues, 104, 356
Reimbursement, innovation and pay for performance (P4P)
behavioral health programs, 285–287
"Cleveland Clinic" model, 294
current status, 282–283
empirically validated psychotherapists, 294–295
evidence-based treatment, 283–284
fee scales, 287–288
free-market healthcare continuation, 293–294
fundamentals, 279–280, 295
future developments, 292–295
historical development, 280–281
lesser public ownership, healthcare delivery, 293
lessons learned, 284–285
present system continuation, 292
process *vs.* outcomes, 290–292
salary models, 288–290
universal healthcare, 293
Reinhardt, Dave, 327–341
Reintegration programs, 429
Relevance of research, 189–191
Religion, 305, 372, *see also* Clergy; Psychoreligions
Remedicalizing, 2

Replication, treatment criteria, 178
Reporting culture, 218
Research
clinicians, lack of, 185–187
courses and research project reforms, 269
presentation formats, 191–192
"Resilience Training," 430
Resiliency, 419
Resources, biofeedback treatment, 457–459
Respiration, 444
Restoring functioning, 50
Restructuring the personality, 50
Return on investment (ROI)
finance matters, 52
judgment criterion, 251
recommendations, mental health informatics, 39–72
Revenue producers, 288
Reverse seasonal affective disorder (reverse SAD), 10
Risk management, combat stress disorder, 429
Risk sharing arrangements, 250
"Robin Hood medicine," 35
ROI, *see* Return on investment (ROI)
Rorschach inkblot test
irrelevant course curriculum, 259
overdiagnosing psychopathology, 174
problematic practices, 212
Routine immunizations, 402
Rubin, Howard, 327–341
Rummel, Clair, 299–315
Rural communities
access issues, 93–94, 205, 371, 381
depression treatment protocol, 268
older population, 300, 309–310
service delivery, 314

videoconferencing technology, 90
Rust, George, 235–236

S

"Sacred circle," 375
SAD, see Seasonal affective disorder (SAD)
Safety
   healthcare crisis, 205–206
   prescribing psychologists, 138
   psychiatry crisis, 333
   reforms, 218
   unencrypted Internet connections, 106
Safety net funding, service delivery, 398
Salary models, 288–290
SAMHSA, see Substance Abuse and Mental Health Services Administration (SAMHSA)
Sammons, Morgan T., 129–143
SBHC, see School-based health centers (SBHCs)
Schizophrenia
   crisis intervention, 29–30
   Diagnostic and Statistical Manual of Mental Disorders (DSM), 11
   implications for untreated, 384
   improvement through medication, 22
   neuroscience impact, 405
School-based health centers (SBHCs), 352
Science
   biases, 174–176
   clinical *vs.* statistical prediction, 176–177
   heuristics, 174–176
   McFall Manifesto, 177
   vs. political correctness, 8–10
   unchecked clinical expertise, 173–174

Science/practice integration
   basing care on evidence, 177–179
   fundamentals, 177, 180–182
   historical developments, 171–172
   scientific mentality, 179–182
Scientific discoveries, impact on wellness and prevention, 404–406
Scientific mentality, 179–182
Scientist-practitioner model, 172
Scope of practice, 50, 103
Seasonal affective disorder (SAD), 10
Secondary aging, 307
Secondary data, 63
Security, unencrypted Internet connections, 106, *see also* Privacy
Self-correction, 214–215
Self-disclosure, 86
Self-management
   e-health treatment, 85–88, 91
   requirements, 235–236
Selye, Hans, 5
SEMG, see Surface electromyography (SEMG) training
Service delivery
   aging in place, 314–315
   Biodyne model, 267–268
   children, preventative services, 402
   chronic health conditions, 402–403
   comparative effectiveness initiatives, 400
   e-health, 313–314
   evidence-based preventive services, 401–402
   expanded coverage, 400–402
   finance changes, 398–400
   healthcare reform strategic implications, 397–400
   health-plan-based financing, 399–400
   health *vs.* social services, 399–400

home-based services, 310
integrated care, 310–312
primary care settings, 398–399
private pay market, 400
routine immunizations, 402
rural areas, 314
safety net funding, 398
stepped care, 312–313
technology changes, 398–399
traditional model improvement, 309–310
women, preventative services, 402
SES, see Socioeconomic status (SES)
Session rating scale (SRS), 271–272
Sexual initiation, early, 354
SF-36 health survey, 235
SFP 10-14, see Strengthening Families Program for Parents and Youth 10-14 (SFP 10-14)
Short message service (SMS), 84
Silos, 38–39
Sites, practicum program, 270–271
Skin conductance biofeedback treatment, 444, 460
Small group practices, 74–76
Small- vs. large-scale efforts, 70–72
SMS, see Short message service (SMS)
SOC, see Systems of Care (SOC)
Socialized medicine accusations, 36
Social needs, threshold establishment, 163
Social stigma, see Stigma
Social support services, 399–400
Society of Clinical Child and Adolescent Psychology, 194, 357
Society of Clinical Psychology, 178, 194

Socioeconomic status (SES), 370, 380
Software Advice, 76
Solo practitioners, 70–71, 74–76
Somatization, prevalence, 24
South Korea, quality transformation, 213
Spitzer, Rene, 6
Spoke site, 432
SRS, see Session rating scale (SRS)
Staircase treatment, see Stepped care
Standards
  accreditation, 188–189
  cognitive support/comprehension orientation, 74
  homogeneous vs. heterogeneous data formats, 73
  training, 172
Statement of concern, 327–330
Static vs. dynamic approach, 213
Statistical vs. clinical prediction, 176–177
Stepped care
  depressions, 240
  e-health and telehealth, 90–92
  ethnic minorities and women, 378
  service delivery, 312–313
Stigma
  access issues, 382, 384
  active duty service members, 424
  barrier for seeking treatment, 93, 234
  life-history factors, 304
  primary care setting, 439
  removal, wellness and prevention, 396–397
  veteran/military behavioral health reforms, 419–424, 427–430
Strained alliance, 185

Strengthening Families Program for Parents and Youth 10-14 (SFP 10-14), 395
"Stress inoculation," 430
The Stressors of Life, 5
Substance Abuse and Mental Health Services Administration (SAMHSA)
  Annapolis Coalition, 142
  children, evidence-based practice, 357–358
  older adults, 306
Substance use and abuse
  computer-based treatment, 89
  military service, 94
  older adults, 306
  school-based health centers, 354
Successes, identify and build on, 215
Successful treatment, nonspecialty settings, 133
Suffering, reducing, 194
Suicide
  older adults, 306
  posttraumatic stress disorder impact, 422
  prevention training, 428
  PROSPECT model, 311–312
  protective factors, 425–426
  risk factors, 425
  stressors, 427
  veteran/military behavioral health reforms, 424–427
Summative evaluation, 71
Supervision
  model, 261
  practicum program, 270
  videoconferencing, 90
Surface electromyography (SEMG) training, 452
"Syndromes," 6–7
Systems of Care (SOC), 357–358

T

Talk therapy, 2, 38
TAMP, *see* Temporary Assistance to Military Personnel (TAMP)
TAT, *see* Thematic Apperception Test (TAT)
Taxpayers, 329–330
TBI, *see* Traumatic brain injury (TBI)
Technology, *see also* E-health and telehealth; Internet access
  barriers, access to services, 376–380
  changes, service delivery, 398–399
  competitive effectiveness evaluation, 398–399
  costs, 16, 95–97, 103–104
  environment transition, 77
  failure to use, 206
  future improvement costs, 16
  integration, healthcare overview, 350
  reforms, ethnic minorities/ women, 376–380
  treatment delivery, cultural sensitivity, 379–380
  upfront costs, 95–97, 103–104, 109
Telehealth, *see* E-health and telehealth
Telemental health network development, 431–434
Telemental health services, 431–434
Telephone, 13, *see also* E-health and telehealth
Temperature training, 443, 456, 460
Temporary Assistance to Military Personnel (TAMP), 431
Temporomandibular disorder, 442, 450, 452–453
Tension headaches, 442, 449–450, *see also* Chronic headaches; Migraines
Test, Deming's cycle, 214
Text messaging, 84

"The Advanced Medical Home: A Patient-Centered, Physician-Guided Model of Health Care," 231
"The Future of Family Medicine: A Collaborative Project of the Family Medicine Community," 230
Thematic Apperception Test (TAT), 212
The Meaning of Anxiety, 5
Therapeutic drift, 26
Therapeutic shopping spree, 29–30
The Stressors of Life, 5
Thomas, James Lawrence, 441–461
Thorazine, 22
Threshold establishment, 163
Throughput ratio, 98
Tinitus, 94
Tobacco product cessation, 354
TOVA continuous performance test, 455
Traditional therapy costs, 44
Training, *see also* Education
 behavioral healthcare crisis, 210–211
 changes, 262–263
 disseminating evidence-based care, 101–102
 gap, science and practice, 188–189
 mental health informatics, 74
 preparing psychologists, 140–143
 professional education reforms, 261
 recommendations, 74, 192–193, 238
 reforms, children/family treatment, 356–357
 standards, 172
 videoconferencing, 90
Transdisciplinary research, 73
Transition, historical developments, 2–3
Transparency, 219–220
Transportation, lack of as barrier, 95
Traumatic brain injury (TBI)
 biofeedback treatment, 445, 453–454
 returning service members, 422
 suicide risk factor, 427
Traumatic loss, e-health treatment, 84
Treatment
 aged, long-term care, 340–341
 barriers to seeking, 92–93
 compliance, 13
 delivery, 85–86, 379–380
 neuroscience effects, 405–406
 nonspecialty settings, prescribing psychologists, 133
 real doctors, 339
Treatment reforms
 consumer-centric approach, 216–218
 dynamic *vs.* static approach, 213
 fundamentals, 213
 integrated care, 221
 leadership, 219
 learning organizations, 213–216
 payment systems, 247–251
 safety, 218
 transparency, 219
 value and costs, 219, 221
Treatment reforms, children/family
 access to care, 351–353
 behavioral health practice, expanding, 348
 CHIP/CHIPRA, 351–352
 community prevention efforts, 353–354
 comparative effectiveness research, 348
 evidence-based practice, 348, 357–358
 fundamentals, 343–344, 351

Index   509

healthcare overview, 345–350
health disparities, 355
home visiting programs
   coverage, 354–355
insurance coverage, 354–355
integrated care, 349–350
patient-centered medical
   homes, 349–350
payment issues, 356
postpartum conditions, 353
pregnant women, 353
preventative services,
   353–355
primary care, 346–348
school-based health centers,
   352
technology integration, 350
training opportunities,
   356–357
Treatment reforms, ethnic
   minorities/women
access issues, 376–386
barriers, 369–371, 376–377
cost of healthcare, 381
cultural attitudes and
   sensitivity, 368–369,
   374–376, 382
determination of status,
   373–374
e-health access to services,
   376–377
evidence-based treatment,
   368–369
fundamentals, 367, 387–388
health insurance coverage,
   lack, 381
immigration status, 382–385
integrated care, 382, 385–386
Internet access, 377–379
issues, 368–369
language barriers, 381
rural communities, 381
stigma, 382
technology, 376–380
telehealth access to services,
   376–377
treatment delivery, 379–380
two-faced cultural factors,
   372–373

women's preventative care,
   385–386
Treatment reforms, professional
   education
antibusiness, antihealthcare
   agenda, 260
blunders, 259–263
career opportunities, 274–275
clinical curriculum, 265–266
clinical training, 261
competence and competency
   assessment, 261,
   271–273
controversies, 262–263
credentials and
   credentialing, 260–261,
   273–274
doctoral degree, 263–269
efficiency, 267–268
emerging reforms, 262–263
fundamentals, 257–259, 275
irrelevant course curriculum,
   259–260
licensure, 262
macrocurriculum, 264–265
medical cost offset, 267–268
medical literacy courses, 268
practicum program, 269–275
research courses and
   research project, 269
sites, 270–271
supervision, 270
"unblundering," 263–269
Trends, aging America
aging in place, 314–315
behavioral health, 304–309
dementia, 303–304
demographic shift, 299–300
e-health, 313–314
excess disability, 308–309
fundamentals, 299
future directions, 315
healthcare spending,
   300–302
home-based services, 310
integrated care, 310–312
issues, health impact,
   307–308
life-history factors, 304–309

Medicare, 300–302
physical health, 302–303
service delivery, 309–315
stepped care, 312–313
TriCare program services
  eligibility, extending, 430–431
  fundamentals, 430
  funding integrated care, 49
  hallway handoff, 27
  integration *vs.* collaboration, 40
  telemental health network development, 431–434
  telemental health services, 431
  TRICARE Assistance program (TRIAP) services, 434–437
  veteran/military behavioral health reforms, 434–437
  Web-based demo project, 411
TriCare Reserve Select (TRS), 431
Trichotillomania, 84, 94
Tripler Army Medical Center, 437
Trisomy 21, 159
TriWest Healthcare Alliance, 437
TRS, *see* TriCare Reserve Select (TRS)
Tuberous sclerosis, 159
Two-faced cultural factors
  reforms, ethnic minorities/women, 372–373

U

"Unblundering," 263–269
Unchecked clinical expertise, 173–174
Understanding gap, science and practice, 188
Undocumented immigrants, 382, 384–385
Undoing initial information, 175
Unencrypted Internet connections, 106
Unexpected places, 21–22
Uninsured, access issues, 205
Unipolar disorder, 8, 134
UnitedHealth, telehealth, 409–410
United HMO, 47
Unit integrity, 423
Universal healthcare, 293
University of Massachusetts Medical School, 238
Unlimited license to practice, 336–337
Unvalidated interventions, 103
Upfront costs
  federal funding, 109
  technology, 95–97, 103–104
Urinary incontinence, 445
U.S. Department of Health and Human Services (HHS)
  delivery, mental health services, 237
  national health information technology coordinator, 60
  postpartum conditions, 353
  prevention services, 401
  psychological indicators, statistics, 340
U.S. Government Accountability Office (GAO), 106, 137
U.S. Navy, 40
U.S. Preventive Services Task Force (USPSTF), 354, 355, 401–402
U.S. Veterans Administration (VA) system, *see also* TRICARE program services
  e-health and telehealth, 94, 107–108, 110
  electronic health records, 15
  exemplary programs, 68
  failure to ESTs, 209
  funding integrated care, 49
  health data repository, 69
  integration *vs.* collaboration, 40
  stipends/educational funding, 37

videoconferencing, 90, 94
Usability, 65–68, 71, 96
Usage, e-health and telehealth, 103–106
"Use it or lose it" financial dimension, 52

V

VA, *see* U.S. Veterans Administration (VA) system
Validation, categorical diagnosis, 150–151
Valium medication, 5, 7
Value, reforms, 219, 221
Value Options care management organization, 47
Veterans, *see* U.S. Veterans Administration (VA) system
Veterans Health Administration initiative, 196
Veterans Health Information Systems and Technology Architecture (VistA), 68
Videoconferencing
  cost-effectiveness, 90
  cultural sensitivity, 380
  in education, 102
  effectiveness, 94
  vs. e-health interventions, 100
  fundamentals, 84, 90
Video teleconferencing (VTC), 431–433
Vietnam War, 425
VistA, *see* Veterans Health Information Systems and Technology Architecture (VistA)
Vitamin deficiencies, pregnancy, 401
von Recklinghausen's disease, 159
VTC, *see* Video teleconferencing (VTC)
Vulvodynia, 445

W

Wait lists and times, 92, 93, 382
Walker, Elle, 327–341
Waste (muda), 15
Web-based demo project, 411
WebMD example, 188, 191
Web sites
  advantage of e-health sites, 89
  American Health Information Management Association, 76
  American Psychiatric Association, 76
  Annapolis Coalition, 238
  Association for Behavioral and Cognitive Therapies, 194
  British National Heath Service, 217
  BuyerZone, 76
  California HealthCare Foundation, 76
  curriculum, 238
  Department of Family Medicine and Community Health, 238
  DESTRESS program, 86
  Effective Child Therapy, 357, 358
  Google Language Tools, 381
  health performance questionnaire, 273
  Indian Health Care Improvement Act, 367
  Medicare Telehealth Enhancement Act, 104
  National Alliance of Professional Psychology Providers, 327, 341
  National Council for Community Behavioral Healthcare, 76
  National Registry of Evidence-Based Programs and Practices, 358
  Pew Internet and American Life Project, 105–106

psychological treatments, 194
research planning conference, 160–161
Society of Clinical Child and Adolescent Psychology, 194
Software Advice, 76
software regulation, 98
technology transfer grant support, 97
telehealth reimbursement guidelines, 104
U.S. Government Accountability Office, 106
Veterans Health Information Systems and Technology Architecture, 68
Wellness and prevention
　addiction, 412
　Ann-E Smartphone application, 412
　children, preventative services, 402
　chronic health conditions, 402–403
　comparative effectiveness initiatives, 400
　digital coaching programs, 409
　evidence-based preventive services, 401–402
　expanded coverage, 400–402
　finance changes, 398–400
　fundamentals, 395–396
　Google Health, 411–412
　healthcare reform strategic implications, 397–400
　HealthMedia digital coaching programs, 409
　health-plan-based financing, 399–400
　health vs. social services, 399–400
　information technology, impact, 406–413
　integration, fostering, 396–397
　Intel Health Guide, 409–410
　MDLiveCare, 411–412
　Minnesota Blue Cross/Blue Shield, 412–413
　Online Care Anywhere, 412–413
　Perfect Depression Care Initiative, 407–408
　primary care settings, 398–399
　private pay market, 400
　routine immunizations, 402
　safety net funding, 398
　scientific discoveries, impact, 404–406
　service delivery, 397–406
　stigma removal, 396–397
　technology changes, 398–399
　telehealth, 409–410
　TRICARE Web-based demo project, 411
　UnitedHealth, telehealth, 409–410
　Web-based demo project, 411
　women, preventative services, 402
Wellstone-Domenici Mental Health Parity and Addiction Equity Act, 343, 396, 397
WHO, see World Health Organization (WHO)
Whole-person care, 231–232
Widiger, Thomas A., 149–163
Wiggins, Jack G., 327–341
Women, preventative care and services
　access issues, 385–386
　service delivery, 402
Women/ethnic minorities, treatment reforms
　access issues, 376–386
　barriers, 369–371, 376–377
　cost of healthcare, 381
　cultural attitudes and sensitivity, 368–369, 374–376, 382
　determination of status, 373–374

e-health access to services, 376–377
evidence-based treatment, 368–369
fundamentals, 367, 387–388
health insurance coverage, lack, 381
immigration status, 382–385
integrated care, 382, 385–386
Internet access, 377–379
issues, 368–369
language barriers, 381
rural communities, 381
stigma, 382
technology, 376–380
telehealth access to services, 376–377
treatment delivery, 379–380
two-faced cultural factors, 372–373
women's preventative care, 385–386
Work-flow design, 71
Workforce development, 74
World Health Organization (WHO), 154
Wound debridement example, 173

Y

Yoga, 210
Youth, *see* Children